SURGICAL RECALL
2nd edition

SURGICAL RECALL
2nd Edition

RECALL SERIES EDITOR AND SENIOR EDITOR

LORNE H. BLACKBOURNE, M.D.
General Surgeon
Major, Medical Corps
United States Army
Fort Eustis, Virginia

SANS TACHE

Williams & Wilkins
A WAVERLY COMPANY

BALTIMORE • PHILADELPHIA • LONDON • PARIS • BANGKOK
BUENOS AIRES • HONG KONG • MUNICH • SYDNEY • TOKYO • WROCLAW

Editor: Elizabeth A. Nieginski
Manager, Development Editing: Julie Scardiglia
Development Editor: Carol Loyd
Managing Editor: Amy G. Dinkel
Marketing Manager: Rebecca Himmelheber
Production Coordinator: Danielle Hagan
Text/Cover Designer: Karen S. Klinedinst
Typesetter: Port City Press, Inc.
Printer/Binder: Port City Press, Inc.

351 West Camden Street
Baltimore, Maryland 21201-2436 USA

Rose Tree Corporate Center
1400 North Providence Road
Building II, Suite 5025
Media, Pennsylvania 19063-2043 USA

Accurate indications, adverse reactions and dosage schedules for drugs are provided in this book, but it is possible that they may change. The reader is urged to review the package information data of the manufacturers of the medications mentioned.

Printed in the United States of America

First Edition, 1994

Library of Congress Cataloging-in-Publication Data

Surgical recall / senior editor, Lorne H. Blackbourne — 2nd ed.
p. cm. — (Recall series)
Includes index.
ISBN 0-683-30102-0
1. Surgery—Examinations, questions, etc. I. Blackbourne, Lorne H. II. Series.
[DNLM: 1. Surgery, Operative—examination questions. 2. Surgery, Operative—examination questions. WO 18.2 S9618 1997]
RD37.2.S9748 1997
617′.0076—dc21
DNLM/DLC
for Library of Congress 97–25166
CIP

The publishers have made every effort to trace the copyright holders for borrowed material. If they have inadvertently overlooked any, they will be pleased to make the necessary arrangements at the first opportunity.

To purchase additional copies of this book, call our customer service department at **(800) 638-0672** or fax orders to **(800) 447-8438.** For other book services, including chapter reprints and large quantity sales, ask for the Special Sales department.

Canadian customers should call **(800) 665-1148**, or fax **(800) 665-0103.** For all other calls originating outside of the United States, please call **(410) 528-4223** or fax us at **(410) 528-8550.**

Visit Williams & Wilkins on the Internet: **http://www.wwilkins.com** or contact our customer service department at **custserv@wwilkins.com**. Williams & Wilkins customer service representatives are available from 8:30 am to 6:00 pm, EST, Monday through Friday, for telephone access.

97 98 99 00 01
2 3 4 5 6 7 8 9 10

Associate Editors

Jared Antevil, B.A.
Medical Student
University of Virginia Health Sciences Center
Charlottesville, Virginia

Oliver A. R. Binns, M.D.
Resident in General Surgery
Department of Surgery
University of Virginia
Charlottesville, Virginia

Jeffry Claridge, M.D.
Resident
University of Virginia
Charlottesville, Virginia

Eugene Foley, M.D.
Attending General Surgeon
University of Virginia Health Sciences Center
Charlottesville, Virginia

David D. Graham, M.D.
Resident in General Surgery
Department of Surgery
University of Virginia
Charlottesville, Virginia

Charles Hobson, M.D., M.P.H.
Department of Health Services
School of Public Health and Community Medicine
University of Washington
Tacoma, Washington

Christopher Hogan, M.D.
Resident in Orthopedics
University of Virginia
Charlottesville, Virginia

Bradley Kesser, M.D.
Resident in Otolaryngology, Head and Neck Surgery
University of Virginia
Charlottesville, Virginia

John Jane, Jr., M.D.
Resident in Neurosurgery
University of Virginia
Charlottesville, Virginia

Scott E. Langenburg, M.D.
Fellow in Pediatric Surgery
Children's Hospital of Michigan
Detroit, Michigan

John Minasi, M.D.
Assistant Professor
Department of Surgery
Division of General Surgery
University of Virginia
Charlottesville, Virginia

Christopher Moore, B.A.
Medical Student
University of Virginia Health Sciences Center
Charlottesville, Virginia

Paul Mosca, M.D.
Resident in Surgery
Duke University
Durham, North Carolina

Robert Sawyer, M.D.
Attending Transplant Surgeon
University of Virginia
Charlottesville, Virginia

Jonas Sheehan, M.D.
Resident in Neurosurgery
University of Virginia
Charlottesville, Virginia

Paul Shin, M.D.
Resident in Urology
Emory University
Atlanta, Georgia

John Sperling, M.D.
Resident in Surgery
Mayo Clinic
Rochester, Minnesota

Curtis G. Tribble, M.D.
Professor
Department of Surgery
Division of Thoracic-
Cardiovascular Surgery
University of Virginia
Charlottesville, Virginia

Reid Tribble, M.D.
Attending
Division of Cardiothoracic Surgery
Columbia, South Carolina

Albert Weed, B.A.
Medical Student
University of Virginia Health
Sciences Center
Charlottesville, Virginia

Joseph Wells, M.D.
Resident in General Surgery
University of Texas
Dallas, Texas

Jeffrey Young, M.D.
Attending General Surgeon
University of Virginia
Charlottesville, Virginia

Contributors

The following contributed to this book while they were medical students at the University of Virginia Health Sciences Center:

1989 – Lorne H. Blackbourne, M.D.

1990 – Lorne H. Blackbourne, M.D.

1991 – Kirk J. Fleischer, M.D.
Colt Peyton, M.D.

1992 – Oliver A.R. Binns, M.D.
Christopher Bogaev, M.D.
R. Bradford Bowles III, M.D.
James A. Burns, M.D.
David deHoll, M.D.
Hong J. Kim, M.D.
Carolyn Lederman, M.D.
L. Carr McClain, M.D.
Gregory Paine, M.D.
Richard S. Polin, M.D.
Henry M. Prillaman, M.D.
Donald Schmidt, M.D.
Walter Scott, M.D.
Nathan E. Simmons, M.D.
Owen B. Tabor, M.D.
Anne Whitworth, M.D.

1993 – Linda C. Ahn, M.D.
Robert A. Buckmire, M.D.
David C. Cassada, M.D.
John W. Davis, M.D.
Nicolisa DeSouza, M.D.
Barbara M. Fried, M.D.
W. Glover Garner, M.D.
Christopher Hogan, M.D.
Nancy A. Huff, M.D.
Stephen S. Kim, M.D.
Timothy Kwiatkowski, M.D.
J. Pieter Noordzij, M.D.
David M. Powell, M.D.

G. Bino Rucker, M.D.
Julius P. Smith III, M.D.
Mehrdad Soroush, M.D.
John Sperling, M.D.
Sandeep S. Teja, M.D.
Eric E. Walk, M.D.
T. Lisle Whitman, M.D.
William J. Wirostko, M.D.

1996 – David Bentrem, M.D.

1997 – Paul Shin, M.D.
Jennifer Deblasi, M.D.

Dedication

This manual is dedicated to the memory of Leslie E. Rudolf, Professor of Surgery and Vice-Chairman of the Department of Surgery. Dr. Rudolf was born on November 12, 1927 in New Rochelle, New York. He served in the U.S. Army Counter-intelligence Corps in Europe after World War II. He graduated from Union College in 1951 and attended Cornell Medical College, where he graduated in 1955. He then entered his surgical residency at Peter Brigham Hospital in Boston, Massachusetts and completed his residency there serving as Chief Resident Surgeon in 1961.

Dr. Rudolf came to Charlottesville, Virginia as an Assistant Professor of Surgery in 1963. He rapidly rose through the ranks, becoming Professor of Surgery and Vice-Chairman of the Department in 1974 and a Markle Scholar in Academic Medicine from 1966 until 1971. His research interests included organ and tissue transplantation and preservation. Dr. Rudolf was instrumental in initiating the Kidney Transplant Program at the University of Virginia Health Sciences Center. His active involvement in service to the Charlottesville community is particularly exemplified by his early work with the Charlottesville/Albemarle Rescue Squad, and received the Governor's Citation for the Commonwealth of Virginia Emergency Medical Services in 1980.

His colleagues at the University of Virginia Health Sciences Center, including faculty and residents, recognized his keen interests in teaching medical students, evaluating and teaching residents, and helping the young surgical faculty. He took a serious interest in medical student education, and he would have strongly approved of this teaching manual, affectionately known as the "Rudolf" guide, as an extension of ward rounds and textbook reading.

In addition to his distinguished academic accomplishments, Dr. Rudolf was a talented person with many diverse scholarly pursuits and hobbies. His advice and counsel on topics ranging from Chinese cooking to orchid raising were sought by a wide spectrum of friends and admirers.

This manual is a logical extension of Dr. Rudolf's interests in teaching. No one book, operation, or set of rounds can begin to answer all questions of surgical disease processes; however, in a constellation of learning endeavors, this effort would certainly have pleased him.

John B. Hanks, M.D.
Professor of Surgery
University of Virginia
Charlottesville, Virginia

Foreword

Surgical Recall represents the culmination of several years' effort by Lorne Blackbourne and his friends, who began the project when they were third-year medical students. Lorne, who recently completed his residency in General Surgery at the University of Virginia, has involved other surgical residents and medical students to provide annual updates and revisions. This reflects the interest, enthusiasm, and true dedication to learning and teaching that permeates the medical school classes and surgical residencies in our institution. It is an honor, privilege, and a continuing stimulus to work in the midst of this group of dedicated young people. I congratulate all the students and residents involved in this project and also acknowledge the leadership of the surgical faculty. The professor's ultimate satisfaction occurs when all the learners assume ownership of learning and teaching.

This book encompasses the essential information in general surgery and surgical specialties usually imparted to students in our surgical clerkship and reviewed and developed further in electives. Developed from the learner's standpoint, the text includes fundamental information such as a description of the diseases, signs, symptoms, essentials of pathophysiology, treatments, and possible outcomes. The unique format of this study guide exploits the Socratic method by employing a list of questions or problems posed along the left side of the page with answers and responses on the right. In addition, the guide includes numerous practical tips to students and junior residents to facilitate comprehensive and effective management of patients. This material is essential for students in the core course of surgery and for those taking senior electives.

In this second edition, the authors have added several new chapters and have expanded the existing chapters for a fuller and more complete coverage of all subjects, including the new subjects. We hope you find this expanded version of this work stimulating and easy to use.

R. Scott Jones, M.D.
Professor and Chairman
Department of Surgery
University of Virginia
Charlottesville, Virginia

Preface

Surgical Recall began as a source of surgical facts during my Surgery Clerkship when I was a third-year medical student at the University of Virginia. My goal has been to provide concise information that every third-year surgical student should know, placed in a "rapid fire" two-column format.

The format of *Surgical Recall* is conducive to the recall of basic surgical facts because it relies upon repetition and positive feedback. As one repeats the question-and-answer format, one gains success.

We have dedicated our work to the living memory of Professor Leslie Rudolf. It is our hope that those who knew Dr. Rudolf will remember him and those who did not will ask.

Lorne H. Blackbourne, M.D.
General Surgeon
Major, Medical Corps
United States Army
Fort Eustis, Virginia

P.S. We would like to hear from you if you have any corrections, acronyms, classic ward or operating room questions (all contributors will be credited). You can reach me on E-mail in care of Williams & Wilkins at dlong@wwilkins.com.

Contents

Foreword ... xi
Preface ... xiii

SECTION I
OVERVIEW AND BACKGROUND SURGICAL INFORMATION

1 Introduction ... 3
Using the Study Guide ... 3
Surgical Notes ... 8
Common Abbreviations You Should Know ... 11
Glossary of Surgical Terms You Should Know ... 18
Surgery Signs, Triads, etc. You Should Know ... 25
2 Surgical Syndromes ... 31
3 Surgical Most Commons ... 34
4 Surgical Percentages ... 36
5 Surgical History ... 39
6 Surgical Instruments ... 42
7 Sutures and Stitches ... 54
8 Surgical Knot Tying ... 63
9 Incisions ... 69
10 Common Operations ... 75
11 Wounds, Drains, and Tubes ... 84
12 Surgical Anatomy Pearls ... 94
13 Fluids and Electrolytes ... 98
14 Blood and Blood Products ... 111
15 Surgical Hemostasis ... 115
16 Common Surgical Medications ... 117
17 Complications ... 124
18 Common Causes of Ward Emergencies ... 141
19 Surgical Nutrition ... 143
20 Shock ... 147
21 Surgical Infection ... 153
22 Fever ... 163
23 Surgical Prophylaxis ... 165
24 Surgical Radiology ... 167
25 Anesthesia ... 171
26 Surgical Ulcers ... 176

SECTION II
GENERAL SURGERY

27 GI Hormones and Physiology ... 179

28 Acute Abdomen and Referred Pain.....184
29 Hernias.....190
30 Laparoscopy.....201
31 Trauma.....204
32 Burns.....222
33 Upper GI Bleeding.....229
34 The Stomach.....243
35 Bariatric Surgery.....250
36 Ostomies.....252
37 Small Intestine.....255
38 The Appendix.....261
39 Carcinoid Tumors.....267
40 Fistulas.....270
41 Colon and Rectum.....274
42 The Anus.....291
43 Lower GI Bleeding.....298
44 Inflammatory Bowel Disease (IBD): Crohn's Disease and Ulcerative Colitis.....301
45 Liver.....307
46 Portal Hypertension.....318
47 Biliary Tract.....325
48 Pancreas.....341
49 The Breast.....357
50 Endocrine.....373
51 Thyroid Gland.....390
52 Parathyroid.....404
53 Spleen and Splenectomy.....411
54 Surgically Correctable HTN.....416
55 Sarcomas and Lymphomas.....419
56 Skin Lesions.....424
57 Melanoma.....427
58 Surgical Intensive Care.....433
59 Vascular Surgery.....446

SECTION III
SUBSPECIALTY SURGERY

60 Pediatric Surgery.....473
61 Plastic Surgery.....527
62 Otolaryngology: Head and Neck Surgery.....536
63 Thoracic Surgery.....572
64 Cardiovascular Surgery.....599
65 Transplant Surgery.....623
66 Orthopedic Surgery.....639
67 Neurosurgery.....668
68 Urology.....690
69 Ophthalmology.....711
Index.....717

Section I

Overview and Background Surgical Information

1 Introduction

USING THE STUDY GUIDE

This study guide was written to accompany the surgical clerkship. It has evolved over the years through student feedback and continued updating. In this regard, we welcome any feedback (both positive and negative) or suggestions for improvement. The objective of the guide is to provide a rapid overview of common surgical topics, but keep in mind that it **is NOT written as an all-encompassing source (i.e., you will have to consult major textbooks to round out the information in this guide).** The guide is organized in a self-study/quiz format. By covering the information/answers on the right with the bookmark, you can attempt to answer the questions on the left to assess your understanding of the information. Keep the guide with you at all times, and when you have even a few spare minutes (e.g., between cases) hammer out a page or at least a few questions. Many students read this book as a primer before the clerkship even begins!

STUDYING FOR THE SURGERY CLERKSHIP

Your study objectives in surgery should include the following four points:
1. OR question-and-answer periods
2. Ward questioning
3. Oral exam
4. Written exam

The optimal plan of action would include daily reading in a text, such as the Lawrence *Essentials of General Surgery*, anatomy review prior to each OR case, and *Surgical Recall*. But remember, this guide helps you recall basic facts about surgical topics. Reading should be done daily! The average general surgery clerkship is 6 weeks, or 42 days. If you read 10 pages a day, that is 420 pages, or the entire Lawrence text! As you read the text, take notes.

To facilitate the learning of a surgical topic, first break down each topic into the following categories and, in turn, master each category:

1. What is it?
2. Incidence
3. Risk factors
4. Signs and symptoms
5. Lab and radiologic tests
6. Diagnostic criteria
7. Differential diagnoses
8. Medical and surgical treatment
9. Postoperative care

10. Complications
11. Stages and prognosis

Granted, it is hard to read after a full day in the OR. For a change, go to sleep right away and wake up a few hours early the next day and read **before** going to the hospital. It sounds crazy, but it does work.

Appearance

Why is your appearance so important?	The patient sees only the wound dressing, the skin closure, and you. You can wear whatever you want, but **you best look clean.**

What the Perfect Surgical Student Carries in Her/His Coat:

Surgical Recall (of course)
Stethoscope
Penlight
Scissors
Minibook on medications (e.g., trade names, doses)
Tape/4×4s
Sutures to practice tying
Pen/notepad/small notebook to write down pearls
Notebook or clipboard with patient's data (always write down chores with a box next to them so you can check off the box when the chore is completed)
Small calculator
List of commonly used telephone numbers (e.g., radiology)

The Perfect Preparation for Rounds

Interview your patient (e.g., problems, pain, wishes)
Talk with your patient's nurse ("Were there any events during the last shift?")
Examine patient (e.g., cor/pulm/abd/**wound**)
Record vitals (e.g., T_{max})
Record input (e.g., IVF, PO)
Record output (e.g., urine, drains)
Check labs
Check microbiology (e.g., culture reports, Gram stains)
Check x-rays
Check pathology reports
Check allied health updates (e.g., PT, OT)
Read chart
Check medication (don't forget H_2 blocker in the hyperalimentation)
Check nutrition
Always check with the intern for chores, updates, insider information, **before** rounds

Presenting on Rounds

Your presentation on rounds should be like an iceberg. State important points about your patient (the tip of the iceberg visible above the ocean), but know **everything** else about your patient that your chief might ask about (that part of the iceberg under the ocean). Always include:
Name
Postoperative day s/p—procedure
A concise overall assessment of how the patient is doing
Vital signs/temp status/antibiotics day
Change in physical exam
Output—urine/drains
Any complaints (not yours—the patient's)
Plan

Your presentation should be concise, with good eye contact (you should not simply read from a clipboard). The intangible element of confidence cannot be overemphasized; but if you do not know the answer to a question about a patient, the correct response should be "I do not know, but I will find out." Never lie or hedge on an answer because it will only serve to make the remainder of your surgical rotation less than desirable. Furthermore, do your best to be enthusiastic and motivated. **Never, ever whine.** And remember to be a **team player**. Never make your fellow students look bad! Residents pick up on this immediately and will slam you.

The Perfect Surgery Student

Never whines
Never pimps his/her residents or fellow students (or attendings)
Never complains
Is never hungry, thirsty, or tired
Is always enthusiastic
Loves to do scut work and can never get enough
Never makes a fellow student look bad
Is always clean (a patient sees only you and the wound dressing)
Is never late
Smiles a lot and laughs a lot
Makes things happen
Is not a "know it all"
Never corrects anyone **during** rounds unless it will affect patient care
Makes the chief/intern/resident look good at all times, if at all possible
Knows more about her/his patients than anyone else
Loves the OR
Never wants to leave the hospital
Takes correction, direction, and instruction very well
Says "Sir" and "Ma'am" to the scrub nurses (and to the attending, unless corrected)
Never asks questions he can look up for himself

Knows the patient's disease, surgery, indication for surgery, and the anatomy before going to the OR
Is the first one to arrive at clinic and the last one to leave
Always places x-rays up in the OR
Reads from a surgery text **everyday**
Is a team player
Asks for feedback
Never has a chip on his or her shoulder
Loves to suture
Is honest and always admits fault and errors
Knows when her patient is going to the OR (e.g., by calling)
Is confident but **not** cocky
Is **"Can Do"** and can figure out things on his own
Never says **"No"** or **"Maybe"** to involvement in patient care
Treats everyone (e.g., nurses, fellow students) with respect
Follows the chain of command
Never wears scrubs to conference
Praises others when appropriate
Checks with the intern beforehand for information for rounds (test results/ surprises)
RUNS for materials, lab values, test results, etc., during rounds before any house officer
Gives credit where credit is due
Dresses and undresses wounds on rounds
Has a steel bladder, a cast iron stomach, and a heart of gold
Always writes the op note without question
Always checks with the intern after rounds for chores
Always makes sure there is a medical student in **every** case
Always follows the patient to the recovery room
In the OR, always asks permission to ask a question
Always reviews anatomy prior to going to the OR
Does what the intern asks (i.e., the chief will get feedback from the intern)
Is a high speed, low drag, hardcore **HAMMERHEAD**

Define HAMMERHEAD — A hammerhead is an individual who places his/her head to the ground and **hammers** through any and all obstacles to get a job done and then asks for more work. One who gives 110% and never complains. One who **desires** work.

Operating Room

Your job in the OR will be to retract (water-skiing) and answer questions posed by the attending and residents. Retracting is basically idiot-proof. Many students put emphasis on anticipating the surgeon's next move, but stick to following the surgeon's request. Over 75% of the questions asked in the OR deal with anatomy; therefore, read about the anatomy and pathophysiology of the case, which will reduce the "I don't knows."

Never argue with the scrub nurses—they are always right. They are the selfless warriors of the operating suite's sterile field, and arguing with one will only **make matters worse.**

Never touch or take instruments from the Mayo tray (tray with instruments on it over the patient's feet) unless given explicit permission to do so. Everyday when you approach the OR suite door **STOP** and ask yourself if you have on scrubs, shoe covers, a cap, and a mask to avoid the embarrassing situation of being yelled at by the OR staff! When entering the OR, first introduce yourself to the scrub nurse and ask if you can get your gloves or gown. If you have a question in the OR, first **ask** if you can ask a question because it may be a bad time and this way it will not appear as though you are pimping the resident/attending.

Other thoughts on the OR:

When scrubbed, if you need to sneeze, step straight back and do not turn your head. If you feel faint, ask if you can sit down, and try to eat prior to going to the OR. If your feet swell in the OR, try wearing support hose socks. If your back hurts, try taking some ibuprofen (with a meal) **prior** to the case. Also, sit-ups or abdominal crunches help to relieve back pain. At the end of the case, ask the scrub nurse for some leftover ties to practice tying knots with and, if there is time, start writing your OP Note.

Tips For "Driving" the Camera During Laparoscopy

1. Keep the camera **centered** on the action.
2. Watch all trocars as they come into the peritoneal cavity (and the tissues beyond, so they can be avoided!).
3. Watch all instruments as they come through the trocars (unless directed otherwise).
4. Ask if you want to come out and clean or re-FRED the lens.
5. Look outside the body at the trocars and instrument angles to reorient yourself.
6. Keep the camera oriented at all times (i.e., up and down); usually the camera cord is on the bottom of the camera—orient yourself to the camera **before** entering the abdomen.
7. You may clean the camera lens at times by **lightly** touching the lens to the liver or peritoneum.
8. Never let the camera lens come into contact with the bowel because the lens may get very hot and you can burn a hole in the bowel!
9. Put your helmet on (i.e., expect to get yelled at!).
10. Never cop an attitude when the surgeons are a little abrupt (e.g., "Center—center the camera!").
11. Always watch the trocars as they are removed from the abdominal wall for bleeding from the site and view the layers of the abdominal wall looking for bleeding as you pull the camera trocar out at the end of the case.

Surgical Notes

History and Physical Report

The history and physical exam report, better known as the H & P, can make the difference between life and death, and you should take this responsibility very **seriously.** Fatal errors can be made in the H & P, including the incorrect diagnosis, the wrong medications, the wrong allergies, and the wrong PSH. Operative reports of the patient's past surgical procedures are invaluable! The surgical H & P needs to be both accurate and **concise.** To save space, use – for a negative sign/symptom and + for a positive sign/symptom.

Example H & P (very brief—for illustrative purposes only):

Mr. Smith is a 22-year-old white male who was in his normal state of excellent health until he noted the onset of periumbilical pain 1 day prior to admission. This pain was followed approximately 4 hours later by pain in his right lower quadrant that was exacerbated by any movement. + vomiting, anorexia. – fever, urinary tract symptoms, change in bowel habits, constipation, BRBPR, hematemesis, or diarrhea.
Medications: Ibuprofen prn headaches
Allergies: NKDA (no known drug allergies)
PMH: none
PSH: none
SH: ETOH, tobacco
ROS: – resp dz, – cardiac dz, – renal dz
PE:
heent ncat, tms clear
cor nsr, - m,r,g
pulm clear b/l
abd nondistended, + bs, + tender RLQ, + rebound RLQ
rectal guaiac –, nl tone, – mass
ext nt, -c,c,e
neuro wnl
LABS: urinalysis (ua) negative. chem 7, PT/PTT, CBC pending
XRAYS: none
ASSESSMENT: 22 y.o. wm with hx and physical findings of right lower quadrant peritoneal signs consistent with (c/w) appendicitis.
Plan:
Consent
IVF with lactated Ringer's
IV cefoxitin
To OR for appendectomy
Wilson Tyler cc III/

Preop Note

The preop note is written in the progress notes the day before the operation.
Example:
Preop Dx: Colon CA

Labs:	CBC, CHEM 7, PT/PTT
CXR:	- infiltrate
Blood:	T & C × 2 units
ECG:	NSR, wnl
Anesthesia:	Pre-op completed
Consent:	Signed and on front of chart

Orders:
1. Void OCTOR (on call to OR)
2. 1 gm cefoxitin OCTOR
3. Hibiclens scrub this p.m.
4. Bowel prep today
5. NPO P midnight (MN)

Op Note

The op note is written in the OR before the patient is in the PACU (or recovery room) in the progress note section of the chart.

Example:

Preop Dx:	Acute appendicitis
Postop Dx:	Same
Procedure:	Appendectomy
Surgeon:	Halsted
Assistants:	Harvey Cushing, Grayson Stuart cc III
Op findings:	No perforation
Anesthesia:	GET
*I/O:	1000 ml LR/ uo 600 ml
*EBL:	50 ml
Specimen:	Appendix to pathology
Drains:	None
Complications:	None (if there are complications *ask* what you should write)

To PACU in stable condition

cc III = clinical clerk, third year; EBL = estimated blood loss; GET = general endotracheal; I/O = ins and outs; PACU = postanesthesia care unit

*Ask the anesthesiologist for this information.

Postop Note

The postop note is written on the day of the operation in the progress notes.

Example:

Procedure:	Appendectomy
Neuro:	A and O × 3
V/S:	Stable/afebrile
I/O:	1 L LR/ uop 600 ml (urine output)
Labs:	post-op Hct: 36
PE:	cor RRR pulm CTA abd drsg dry & intact
Drains:	JP 30 ml serosanguinous fluid

Assess:	Stable postop

Plan:
1. IV hydration
2. 1 g cefoxitin q 8 hr

Admission Orders

The admission orders are written in the physician orders section of the patient's chart on admission, transfer, or postop.

Example:

Admit to 5E Dr. DeBakey

Dx:	AAA
Condition:	Stable
V/S:	q 4 hr or q shift; if post-op, q 15 min × 2 hr, then q 1 hr × 4, then q 4 hr
Activity:	Bedrest or OOB to chair
Nursing:	Daily wgt; I/O; change drsg q shift; call HO for: Temp > 38.5 UO < 30 ml/hr SBP > 180 < 90 DBP > 100 HR < 60 > 110
Diet:	NPO
IVF:	D5 ½ NS c̄ 20 KCL
Drugs:	ANCEF
Labs:	CBC

HO = House Officer; I/O = ins and outs; OOB = out of bed

Daily Note—Progress Note

Basically an S.O.A.P. note, but it is not necessary to write out S.O.A.P. For many reasons, make your notes very objective and do not mention discharge because this leads to confusion.

Example:

10/1/90 Blue Surgery
POD #4 s/p appendectomy
Day #5 cefoxitin
Pt without c/o
V/S: 120/80 76 12 afebrile (Tmax 38)
I/O: 1000/600
Drains: JP #1 60 last shift (JP = Jackson-Pratt drain)
PE: cor RRR-no m,g,r
  pulm CTA
  abd +BS, +flatus, −rigidity
  ext nt, −cyanosis, −erythema
    (nt = nontender)
ASSESS: Stable POD #4 on IV antibiotics
PLAN:
1. Increase PO intake

2. Increase ambulation
3. Follow cultures

Grayson Stuart, cc III/

** Always sign your notes and leave the room for them to be cosigned!

POD = Postop day (The day after operation is POD 1. The day of operation is the operative day. **But note: antibiotic day #1 is the day the antibiotics were started.)

The acronym for what should be checked on your patient daily before rounding with the surgical team: AVOID WTE

A	Appearance—any subjective complaints
V	Vital signs
O	Output—urine/drains
I	Intake—IV/PO
D	Drains—# of/output/character
W	Wound/dressing/weight
T	Temperature
E	Exam—cor, pulm, abd, etc.

Intensive care note:

The note is by systems:

Neurologic (GCS, MAE)
Pulmonary (vent settings, etc.)
CVS (pressors,swann numbers, etc.)
Heme (CBC)
F.E.N. (Chem 10, nutrition, etc.)
Renal (urine output, bun, cr, etc.)
I.D. (Tmax, WBC, antibiotics, etc.)
Assessment
Plan

(F.E.N. = fluids, electrolytes, nutrition). PE is included in each section. This is also an excellent way to write progress notes for the very complicated floor patient.

Clinic Note

Often the clinic note is a letter to the referring doctor. It should always include:

1. Patient name, history #, date
2. Brief hx, current complaints/symptoms
3. PE, labs, x-rays
4. Assessment
5. Plan

How is a medication prescription written?

Tylenol[R] 500 mg tablet
Disp (dispense): 100 tablets
sig: 1–2 P.O. q 4 hrs PRN pain

Common Abbreviations You Should Know

ā	Before
AAA	Abdominal aortic aneurysm, "triple A"

ABD	Army battle dressing
ABI	Ankle to brachial index
ABG	Arterial blood gas
AKA	Above the knee amputation
A.K.A.	Also known as
AMF YOYO	ADIOS MY FRIEND YOU'RE ON YOUR OWN
APR	Abdominoperineal resection
ARDS	Adult respiratory distress syndrome
ASA	Aspirin
Ao	Aorta
AXR	Abdominal x-ray
B1	Billroth 1 gastroduodenostomy
B2	Billroth 2 gastrojejunostomy
BCP	Birth control pill
BE	Barium enema
BIH	Bilateral inguinal hernia
BKA	Below the knee amputation
BS	Bowel sounds, breath sounds, blood sugar
BRBPR	Bright red blood per rectum
C̄	With
CA	Cancer
CBD	Common bile duct

CVA	Cerebral vascular accident, costovertebral angle
CP	Chest pain
CXR	Chest x-ray
CABG	Coronary artery bypass graft ("CABBAGE")
C/O	Complains of
COPD	Chronic obstructive pulmonary disease
CTA	Clear to auscultation
CVP	Central venous pressure
Dx	Diagnosis
DI	Diabetes insipidus
DDx	Differential diagnosis
DP	Dorsalis pedalis
DT	Delirium tremens
DVT	Deep venous thrombosis
EBL	Estimated blood loss
ECMO	Extracorporeal membrane oxygenation
EGD	Esophagogastroduodenoscopy (UGI scope)
EOMI	Extraocular muscles intact
ERCP	Endoscopic retrograde cholangiopancreatography
ETOH	Alcohol
EUA	Exam under anesthesia
FNA	Fine needle aspiration

FEN	Fluids, electrolytes, nutrition
GCS	Glascow Coma Scale
GET	General endotracheal (anesthesia)
GU	Genitourinary
HEENT	Head, ears, nose, and throat
HO	House officer
IABP	Intra-aortic balloon pump
IBD	Inflammatory bowel disease
ICU	Intensive care unit
I & D	Incision and drainage
I & O	Ins and outs, in and out
IMV	Intermittent mandatory ventilation
IVC	Inferior vena cava
IVF	Intravenous fluids
IVP	Intravenous pyelography
IVPB	Intravenous piggyback
JVD	Jugular venous distention
L	Left
LAP APPY	Laparoscopic appendectomy
LAP CHOLE	Laparoscopic cholecystectomy
LE	Lower extremity
LES	Lower esophageal sphincter
LIH	Left inguinal hernia
LR	Lactated Ringer's

LUQ	Left upper quadrant
LLQ	Left lower quadrant
MAE	Moving all extremities
MAST	Military antishock trousers
MEN	Multiple endocrine neoplasia
MI	Myocardial infarction
MSO_4	Morphine sulfate
NGT	Nasogastric tube
NPO	Nothing per os
NS	Normal saline
OBR	Ortho bowel routine
OOB	Out of bed
OCTOR	On call to OR
ORIF	Open reduction internal fixation
PCWP	Pulmonary capillary wedge pressure
$\bar{P}$	After
PE	Pulmonary embolism
PEEP	Positive end expiration pressure
PEG	Percutaneous endoscopic gastrostomy (via EGD and skin incision)
PERRL	Pupils equal and react to light
PFT	Pulmonary function tests
PICC	Peripherally inserted central catheter

PGV	Proximal gastric vagotomy (i.e., leaves fibers to pylorus intact to preserve emptying)
PID	Pelvic inflammatory disease
PO	Per os (by mouth)
PT	Physical therapy, patient, posterior tibialis
PR	Per rectum
PRN	As needed
PTC	Percutaneous transhepatic cholangiogram (dye injected via a catheter through skin and into dilated intrahepatic bile duct)
PTCA	Percutaneous transluminal coronary angioplasty
PTX	pneumothorax
q̄	Every
QD	Every day
QOD	Every other day
R	Right
RIH	Right inguinal hernia
Rx	Treatment
RTC	Return to clinic
SBO	Small bowel obstruction
SCD	Sequential compression device
SIADH	Syndrome of inappropriate antidiuretic hormone
SICU	Surgical intensive care unit

STSG	Split thickness skin graft
SVC	Superior vena cava
S̄	Without
Sx	Symptoms
TEE	Transesophageal echocardiography
T & C	Type and cross
T & S	Type and screen
TMAX	Maximal temperature
TPN	Total parenteral nutrition
TURP	Transurethral resection of the prostate
UGI	Upper gastrointestinal
UO	Urine output
US	Ultrasound
UE	Upper extremity
UTI	Urinary tract infection
VAD	Ventricular assist device
VOCTOR	Void on call to OR
W→D	Wet-to-dry dressing
XRT	X-ray therapy
ZE	Zollinger-Ellison syndrome
–	No, negative
+	Yes, positive
↑	Increase, more
↓	Decrease, less

<	Less than
>	Greater than

Glossary of Surgical Terms You Should Know

Abscess	Localized collection of pus anywhere in the body, surrounded and walled off by damaged and inflamed tissues
Achlorhydria	Absence of hydrochloric acid in the stomach
Acholic stool	Light-colored stool due to a decreased bile content
Acro-	Prefix denoting extremity or tip
Acronym	Word formed from the initial letter of words
Adeno-	Prefix denoting gland or glands
Adhesion	Union of two normally separate surfaces
Adnexa	Adjoining parts; usually means ovary/ fallopian tube
Adventitia	Outer coat of the wall of a vein or artery (composed of loose connective tissue)
Afferent	Toward
-algia	Suffix denoting pain
Amaurosis fugax	Transient visual loss in one eye
Ampulla	Enlarged or dilated ending of a tube or canal
Analgesic	Drug that prevents pain
Anastomosis	Connection between two tubular organs or parts
Anergy	Lack of response to a specific antigen

Angio-	Prefix denoting blood or lymph vessels
Anomaly	Any deviation from the normal (i.e. congenital or developmental defect)
Apnea	Cessation of breathing
Atelectasis	Collapse of alveoli
Bariatric	Weight reduction; bariatric surgery is performed on the morbidly obese to effect weight loss
Barrett's	Columnar metaplasia of the esophagus
Beta	β-HCG (pregnancy test)
Bifurcation	Point at which division into two branches occurs
Bile salts	Alkaline salts of bile necessary for the emulsification of fats
Bili-	Prefix denoting bile
Boil	Tender inflamed area of the skin containing pus
Bovie	Electrocautery
Cachexia	Condition of abnormally low weight associated with chronic disease
Calculus	Stone
Calor	Heat; one of the classic signs of inflammation
Cannula	Hollow tube designed for insertion into a body cavity or blood vessel
Carbuncle	A collection of boils (furuncle) with multiple drainage channels (**CAR**buncle = car = big)
Caseation	Breakdown of diseased tissue into a cheese-like material

Caudal	Relating to the lower part or tail of the body
Cauterization	Destruction of tissue by direct application of heat
Celiotomy	Surgical incision into the peritoneal cavity (laparotomy = celiotomy)
Cephal-	Prefix denoting the head
Chole-	Prefix denoting bile
Cholecyst-	Prefix denoting gallbladder
Choledocho-	Prefix denoting the common bile duct
Chyme	Semiliquid mass of food that passes from the stomach to the duodenum
Cicatrix	Scar
Cleido-	Prefix denoting the clavicle
Colic	Intermittent abdominal pain usually indicating pathology in a tubular organ (e.g., small bowel)
Colloid	Serum proteins, albumin
Colonoscopy	Endoscopic examination of the colon
Colostomy	Surgical operation in which part of the colon is brought through the abdominal wall
Constipation	Infrequent or difficult passage of stool
Cor pulmonale	Enlargement of the right ventricle caused by lung disease and resultant pulmonary hypertension
Curettage	Scraping of the internal surface of an organ or body cavity by means of a spoon-shaped instrument

Cyst	Abnormal sac or closed cavity lined with epithelium and filled with fluid or semisolid material
Direct bilirubin	Conjugated bilirubin (*in*direct = *un*conjugated)
Dolor	Pain, one of the classic signs of inflammation
-dynia	Suffix denoting pain
Dys-	Prefix: difficult/painful/abnormal
Dysphagia	Difficulty in swallowing
Dyspareunia	Painful sexual intercourse
Ecchymosis	Bruise
-ectomy	Suffix denoting the surgical removal of a part or all of an organ (e.g., gastrectomy)
Efferent	Away from
Endarterectomy	Surgical removal of an atheroma and the inner part of the vessel wall to relieve an obstruction (carotid endarterectomy = CEA)
Enteritis	Inflammation of the small intestine, usually causing diarrhea
Enterolysis	Lysis of peritoneal adhesions; not to be confused with enteroclysis, which is a contrast study of the small bowel
Eschar	Scab produced by the action of heat or a corrosive substance on the skin
Excisional biopsy	Biopsy with removal of entire tumor
Fascia	Sheet of strong connective tissue
Fistula	Abnormal communication between two hollow, epithelialized organs or between a hollow organ and the exterior (skin)

Foley	Bladder catheter
Frequency	Abnormally increased frequency (e.g., urinary frequency)
Furuncle	Boil, small subcutaneous staphylococcal infection of follicle (think *f*uruncle = *f*ollicle < *c*ar = *c*arbuncle)
Gastropexy	Surgical attachment of the stomach to the abdominal wall
Hemangioma	Benign tumor of blood vessels
Hematemesis	Vomiting of blood
Hematoma	Accumulation of blood within the tissues, which clots to form a solid swelling
Hemoptysis	Coughing up blood
Hemothorax	Blood in the pleural cavity
Hepato-	Prefix denoting the liver
Herniorrhaphy	Surgical repair of a hernia
Hesitancy	Difficulty in initiating urination
Hiatus	Opening or aperture
Hidradenitis	Inflammation of the apocrine glands, usually caused by blockage of the glands
Icterus	Jaundice
Ileus	Abnormal intestinal motility (usually paralytic)
Ileostomy	Surgical connection between the lumen of the ileum and the skin of the abdominal wall
Incisional biopsy	Biopsy with only a “slice” of tumor removed

Induration	Abnormal hardening of a tissue or organ
Intussusception	Telescoping of one part of the bowel into another
-itis	Suffix denoting inflammation of an organ, tissue, etc. (e.g., gastritis)
Laparotomy	Surgical incision into the abdominal cavity (laparotomy = celiotomy)
Laparoscopy	Visualization of the peritoneal cavity via a laparoscope
Lap appy	Appendectomy via laparoscopy
Lap chole	Cholecystectomy via laparoscopy
Leiomyoma	Benign tumor of smooth muscle
Leiomyosarcoma	Malignant tumor of smooth muscle
Melena	Black tarry feces due to the presence of partly digested blood; occurs when more than 100 ml (approximately) of blood has entered the gut (Melenic, not melanotic stools)
Necrotic	Dead
Obstipation	Failure to pass flatus or stool
Odynophagia	Painful swallowing
-orraphy	Surgical repair (e.g., herniorrhaphy)
-ostomy	General term referring to any operation in which an artificial opening is created between two hollow organs or between one viscera and the abdominal wall for drainage purposes (e.g., colostomy) or for feeding (e.g., gastrostomy)
-otomy	Suffix denoting surgical incision into an organ
Percutaneous	Performed through the skin

-pexy	Suffix denoting fixation
Phleb-	Prefix denoting vein or relating to veins
Phlebolith	Concretion in a vein
Phlegmon	Solid, swollen, inflamed mass of pancreatic tissue
Plica	Fold or ridge
Plicae semilunares	Folds (semicircular) into lumen of the large intestine
Plicae circulares	Circular (complete circles) folds in the lumen of the small intestine (A.K.A. valvulae conniventes)
Pneumaturia	Passage of urine containing air
Pneumothorax	Collapse of lung with **air** in pleural space
Pseudocyst	Dilated cavity resembling a true cyst, but **not** lined with epithelium
Pus	Liquid product of inflammation, consisting of dying leukocytes and other fluids from the inflammatory response
Rubor	Redness, classic sign of inflammation
Steatorrhea	Fatty stools due to decreased fat absorption
Stenosis	Abnormal narrowing of a passage or opening
Sterile field	Area covered by sterile drapes or prepped in sterile fashion using antiseptics (e.g., Betadine)
Succus	Fluid (e.g., succus entericus is fluid from the bowel lumen)
Tenesmus	Urge to defecate with ineffectual (and often painful) straining

Thoracotomy — Surgical opening of the chest cavity

Transect — To divide transversely (to cut in half)

Trendelenburg — Patient posture with pelvis higher than the head, inclined about 45° (A.K.A. "Headdownenburg")

Urgency — Sudden strong urge to urinate; often seen with a UTI

Wet-to-dry dressing — Damp gauze dressing placed on wound and removed after the dressing dries to the wound, providing microdebridement

Surgery Signs, Triads, Etc. You Should Know

What are the A,B,C,Ds of melanoma?

Signs of melanoma:
- A-Asymmetric
- B-Border irregularities
- C-Color variation
- D-Diameter > 0.6 cm **and** dark black color

What is Allen's test?

Test for patency of ulnar artery prior to placing a radial arterial line or performing an ABG. Simply stated, occlude both ulnar and radial arteries with the examiner's fingers with the patient's hand in a fist; open fist and release ulnar artery occlusion and assess blood flow to hand

Define the following terms:

Ballance's sign — Tender mass in the left upper quadrant due to a spleen hematoma (e.g., after spleen trauma); think: Ball in LUQ = **BALL**ANCE'S

Battle's sign — Ecchymoses over the mastoid process in patients with basilar skull fractures

Beck's triad — Seen in patients with cardiac tamponade:
1. JVD
2. Decreased or muffled heart sounds
3. Decreased blood pressure

Bergman's triad Seen with fat emboli syndrome:
1. Mental status changes
2. Petechiae (often in the axilla/thorax)
3. Dyspnea

Blumer's shelf Metastatic disease to the rectouterine (pouch of Douglas) or rectovesical pouch creating a "shelf" that is palpable on rectal exam

Boas's sign Right subcapular pain due to cholelithiasis

Carcinoid triad Seen with carcinoid syndrome:
1. Flushing
2. Diarrhea
3. Right-sided heart failure (FDR)

Charcot's triad Seen with cholangitis:
1. Fever (chills)
2. Jaundice
3. Right upper quadrant pain

(Pronounced "char-cows")

Chovstek's sign Twitching of facial muscles upon tapping the facial nerve in patients with hypocalcemia

Courvoisier's law An enlarged nontender gallbladder seen with obstruction of the common bile duct, most commonly with pancreatic cancer

Note: not seen with acute cholecystitis because the gallbladder is scarred secondary to chronic cholelithiasis (pronounced "core-va-see-a").

Cullen's sign Bluish discoloration of the periumbilical area due to retroperitoneal hemorrhage tracking around to the anterior abdominal wall through fascial planes (e.g., acute hemorrhagic pancreatitis)

Cushing's triad Signs of increased intracranial pressure:
1. Hypertension
2. Bradycardia
3. Irregular respirations

Dance's sign	Empty right lower quadrant in children with ileocecal intussusception
Fothergill's sign	Used to differentiate an intraabdominal mass from one in the abdominal wall; if mass is felt while there is tension on the musculature, then it is in the wall (i.e., sitting halfway upright)
Fox's sign	Ecchymosis of inguinal ligament seen with retroperitoneal bleeding
Goodsall's rule	Anal fistulae course in a straight path anteriorly and take a curved path posteriorly (think of a dog with a straight anterior nose and a curved posterior tail)
Grey Turner's sign	Ecchymosis or discoloration of the flank in patients with retroperitoneal hemorrhage due to dissecting blood from the retroperitoneum (think: turn side-to-side = flank)
Hamman's sign/crunch	Crunching sound on auscultation of the heart due to emphysematous mediastinum, seen with Boerhaave's syndrome, pneumomediastinum, etc.
Homans' sign	Calf pain on forced dorsiflexion of the foot in patients with DVT
Howship-Romberg sign	Pain along the inner aspect of the thigh; seen with an obturator hernia due to nerve compression
Kehr's sign	Severe left shoulder in patients with splenic rupture (due to referred pain from diaphragmatic irritation)
Krukenburg tumor	Metastatic tumor to the ovary (classically from gastric cancer)
Kelly's sign	Visible peristalsis of the ureter in response to squeezing or retraction; used to identify the ureter during surgery

Laplace's law	Wall tension = pressure × radius (thus, the colon perforates preferentially at the cecum because of the increased radius and resultant increased wall tension)
McBurney's point	One-third the distance from the anterior iliac spine to the umbilicus on a line connecting the two
McBurney's sign	Tenderness at McBurney's point in patients with appendicitis
Meckel's diverticulum rule of 2s	Two percent of the population have a Meckel's diverticulum, 2% of those are symptomatic, and they occur within approximately 2 feet from the ileocecal valve
Mittelschmerz	Lower quadrant pain due to ovulation
Murphy's sign	Pain in the right upper quadrant during inspiration, while palpating under the right costal margin; the patient cannot continue to inspire deeply because it brings an inflamed gallbladder under pressure (seen in acute cholecystitis)
Obturator sign	Pain upon internal rotation of the leg with the hip and knee flexed; seen in patients with appendicitis/pelvic abscess
Psoas sign	Pain elicited by extending the hip with the knee in full extension, seen with appendicitis and psoas inflammation
Pheochromocytoma SYMPTOMS triad	Think of the first three letters in the word pheochromocytoma—P-H-E: 1. **P**alpitations 2. **H**eadache 3. **E**pisodic diaphoresis
Pheochromocytoma rule of 10s	10% bilateral, 10% malignant, 10% in children, 10% extraadrenal, 10% have multiple tumors
Raccoon eyes	Bilateral black eyes due to basilar skull fracture

Reynold's pentad	1. Fever 2. Jaundice 3. Right upper quadrant pain 4. Mental status changes 5. Shock/sepsis Thus, Charcot's triad plus # 4 and # 5; seen in patients with suppurative cholangitis
Rovsing's sign	Palpation of the left lower quadrant resulting in pain in the right lower quadrant; seen in appendicitis; (helps differentiate abdominal source of pain from thoracic)
Saint's triad	1. Cholelithiasis 2. Hiatal hernia 3. Diverticular disease
Silk glove sign	Indirect hernia sac in the pediatric patient; the sac feels like a finger of a silk glove when rolled under the examining finger
Sister Mary Joseph's sign (A.K.A. Sister Mary Joseph's node)	Metastatic tumor to umbilical lymph node(s)
Virchow's node	Metastatic tumor to left supraclavicular node (classically due to gastric cancer)
Virchow's triad	Risk factors for thrombosis: 1. Stasis 2. Abnormal endothelium 3. Hypercoagulability
Trousseau's sign	Carpal spasm after occlusion of blood to the forearm with a BP cuff in patients with hypocalcemia
Westermark's sign	Decreased pulmonary vascular markings on CXR in a patient with pulmonary embolus

Whipple's triad

Evidence for insulinoma:

1. Hypoglycemia (< 50)
2. CNS and vasomotor symptoms (e.g., syncope, diaphoresis)
3. Relief of symptoms with administration of glucose

2

Surgical Syndromes

What is Leriche's syndrome?

Claudication of buttocks
Impotence
Atrophy of buttocks (seen with iliac occlusive disease)
(Think: **CIA**)

What is RED reaction syndrome?

Syndrome of rapid vancomycin infusion, resulting in skin erythema

What is Ogilvie's syndrome?

Massive **nonobstructive** colonic dilatation

What is Gardner's syndrome?

GI polyps and associated findings of **s**ebaceous cysts, **o**steomas, and **d**esmoid tumors **(SOD)**; polyps have high malignancy potential (think: a Gardner plants **SOD**)

What is Peutz-Jeghers syndrome?

Benign GI polyps and buccal pigmentation (think: **P**eutz = **P**igmentation)

What is Fitz-Hugh and Curtis syndrome?

Perihepatic gonorrhea infection

What is SIADH?

Syndrome of inappropriate antidiuretic hormone (think: **I**nappropriately **I**ncreased ADH)

What is toxic shock syndrome?

Staphylococcus aureus sepsis, marked by fever, sepsis, and **rash**

What is Tietze's syndrome?

Costochondritis of rib cartilage; aseptic (treat with NSAIDs)

What is Plummer-Vinson syndrome?

Syndrome of:
1. Esophageal web
2. Fe-deficiency anemia
3. Dysphagia
4. Spoon-shaped nails
5. Atrophic oral and tongue mucosa

Usually occurs in elderly women; 10% develop squamous cell carcinoma

What is carcinoid syndrome?	Syndrome of **B FDR:** **B**ronchospasm **F**lushing **D**iarrhea **R**ight-sided heart failure (caused by factors released by carcinoid tumor)
What does ARDS stand for?	Adult respiratory distress syndrome (poor oxygenation caused by leaky capillaries)
What is dumping syndrome?	Delivery of a large amount of hyperosmolar chyme into the small bowel, usually after vagotomy and a gastric drainage procedure (pyloroplasty/gastrojejunostomy); results in autonomic instability, abdominal pain, and diarrhea
What is afferent loop syndrome?	Obstruction of the afferent loop of a Billroth II gastrojejunostomy
What is short-gut syndrome?	Malnutrition resulting from less than 100 cm of viable small bowel
What is blind loop syndrome?	Bacterial overgrowth of intestine caused by stasis
What is Cushing's syndrome?	Excessive cortisol production
What is Rendu-Osler-Weber (ROW) syndrome?	Syndrome of GI-tract telangiectasia
What is Boerhaave's syndrome?	Esophageal perforation
What is thoracic outlet syndrome?	Compression of the structures exiting from the thoracic outlet
What is Munchausen syndrome?	Self-induced illness
What is superior vena cava (SVC) syndrome?	Obstruction of the SVC (e.g., by tumor, thrombosis)
What is another name for Sipple's syndrome?	MEN II

What is another name for Werner's syndrome?	MEN I
What is Trousseau's syndrome?	Syndrome of deep venous thrombosis (DVT) associated with carcinoma
What is Mirrizi's syndrome?	Extrinsic obstruction of the common bile duct from a cystic duct gallstone
What is refeeding syndrome?	Hypokalemia, hypomagnesemia, and hypophosphoremia after refeeding a starved patient
What is compartment syndrome?	Compartmental hypertension due to edema, resulting in muscle necrosis of the lower extremity, seen in the calf; patient may have a distal pulse
What is heparin-induced thrombocytopenic thrombosis (Hitt) syndrome?	Heparin-induced platelet antibodies cause platelets to thrombose vessels, often resulting in loss of limb or life.
What is Budd-Chiari syndrome?	Thrombosis of hepatic veins
What is Mendelson's syndrome?	Chemical pneumonitis after aspiration of gastric contents
What is Zollinger-Ellison's syndrome?	Gastrinoma and PUD

3

Surgical Most Commons

What is the most common: **Indication for surgery with Crohn's disease?**	Small bowel obstruction (SBO)
Type of melanoma?	Superficial spreading
Type of breast cancer?	Infiltrating ductal
Site of breast cancer?	Upper outer quadrant
Vessel involved with a bleeding duodenal ulcer?	Gastroduodenal artery
Cause of common bile duct obstruction?	Choledocholithiasis
Cause of cholangitis?	Bile duct obstruction due to choledocholithiasis
Cause of pancreatitis?	ETOH
Bacteria in stool?	*Bacillus fragilis*
Cause of SBO in adults in the United States?	Adhesions
Cause of SBO in children?	Hernias
Cause of emergency abdominal surgery in the United States?	Acute appendicitis
Site of GI carcinoids?	Appendix

Abdominal x-ray (AXR) finding with SBO?	Air-fluid levels
Cause of large bowel obstruction?	Colon cancer
Type of colonic volvulus?	Sigmoid volvulus
Cause of fever < 48 postoperative hours?	Atelectasis
Bacterial cause of urinary tract infection (UTI)?	*Escherichia coli*
Chest x-ray (CXR) finding with traumatic thoracic aortic injury?	Widened mediastinum
Abdominal organ injured in blunt abdominal trauma?	Spleen
Abdominal organ injured in penetrating abdominal trauma?	Small bowel
Benign tumor of the liver?	Hemangioma
Malignancy of the liver	Mets
Pneumonia in the ICU?	Gram-negative bacteria
Cause of epidural hematoma?	Middle meningeal artery injury

4 Surgical Percentages

What percentage of people in the United States will develop acute appendicitis?

Approximately 7%

What is the acceptable percentage of normal appendices removed with the preoperative diagnosis of appendicitis?

Up to 20%; it is better to remove some normal appendices than to miss a case of acute appendicitis, which could result in a ruptured appendix

In what percentage of cases can ultrasound diagnose cholelithiasis?

98%

In what percentage of cases does a thoracic aortogram to rule out a torn thoracic aorta after blunt trauma yield a positive study?

Approximately 10%

In what percentage of cases does abdominal CT diagnose liver metastasis?

Approximately 90%

In what percentage of cases does a lower GI bleed stop spontaneously?

Approximately 90%

In what percentage of cases does a UGI bleed stop spontaneously?

Approximately 80%

What is the 5-year survival rate after liver resection with clean margins for colon cancer liver metastasis?

Approximately 25%

What is the 5-year survival rate after diagnosis of unresectable colon cancer liver metastasis?	0%
What percentage of patients undergoing laparotomy develop a postoperative small bowel obstruction sometime in their lives?	Approximately 5%
What percentage of American women develop breast cancer sometime in their lives?	10%
What percentage of patients with acute appendicitis will have a radiopaque fecalith on abdominal x-ray (AXR)?	Only about 5%
What percentage of patients with gallstones will have radiopaque gallstones on AXR?	Approximately 10%
What percentage of kidney stones are radiopaque on AXR?	Approximately 90%
At 6 weeks, wounds have achieved what percentage of their total tensile strength?	Approximately 90%
What percentage of patients with ARDS will die?	Approximately 50%
What percentage of the population has a Meckel's diverticulum?	2%

What is the risk of appendiceal rupture 24 hours after the onset of symptoms?

Approximately 25%

What percentage of colonic villous adenomas contain cancer?

Approximately 40% (**think: VILLous** = **VILL**ian)

5

Surgical History

Identify the following people:

Halsted

William Halsted (1852–1922)—**Father of the American surgical residency system** of progressive responsibility at Johns Hopkins
Developed the radical mastectomy and inguinal hernia repair
Advocated surgical gloves
Developed metallic clips

Lister

Joseph Lister (1827–1912)—Father of antiseptic surgery
(used carbolic acid in surgery)

Billroth

Theodor Billroth (1829–1894)—
Performed the first gastric resection (1881)

McBurney

Charles McBurney (1845–1913)—
Developed surgery for appendicitis

Bassini

Edoardo Bassini (1844–1924)—
Developed surgical "radical cure" for inguinal hernias (1887, same time as Halsted)

Kocher

Theodor Kocher (1841–1917)—Nobel prize winner for **thyroid surgery** (1908)
Designed the Kocher clamp for clamping thyroid arteries during thyroidectomy
Right subcostal incision for gallbladder surgery bears his name

Cushing

Harvey Cushing (1869–1939)—**Father of American neurosurgery**
Developed anesthesia records for vital signs (ether notes)
Won the Pulitzer Prize for his biography on Osler

Bovie	Developed electrocautery for surgery with Cushing (1928)
Sister Mary Joseph	Nun and OR scrub nurse Worked with the Mayo Brothers Described periumbilical lymph node metastases from gastric cancer
Gibbon	John Gibbon (1903–1973)—Developed cardiopulmonary bypass
Debakey	Michael Debakey (1908–)—Pioneer in cardiovascular surgery; performed the first carotid endarterectomy (CEA) in 1953 Developed prosthetic grafts for abdominal aortic aneurysm (AAA) Widely-used atraumatic forceps bear his name
Sabiston	David Sabiston Jr.—Pioneer in cardiovascular surgery and academic surgery; performed the first coronary artery bypass grafting (CABG)

Identify the year the following procedures were first performed and the physician who performed them:

Renal transplant	1954; Murray
CABG?	1962; Sabiston
CEA	1953; Debakey
Heart transplant	1967; Barnard
Artificial heart valve	1960; Starr
Liver transplant	1963; Starzl
Total parenteral nutrition (TPN)	1968; Rhoades
Vascular anastomosis	1902; Carrel

Lung transplant	1964; Hardy
Pancreatic transplant	1966; Najarian
Heart–lung transplant	1982; Reitz
AAA rx	1951; Dubost

Who was the first surgeon to advocate wearing surgical gloves?

Halsted

Who was the only surgeon to win the Pulitzer Prize?

Cushing

Which surgeons have won the Nobel Prize?

Kocher (thyroid surgery)
Murray (kidney transplant)
Banting (insulin)
Hess (brain physiology)
Forssman (cardiac catheterization)
Huggins (oncology)
Barany (inner ear disease)
Carrel (transplantation)

6

Surgical Instruments

How should a pair of scissors/needle-driver/ clamp be held?

With the thumb and **fourth** finger, using the index finger to steady

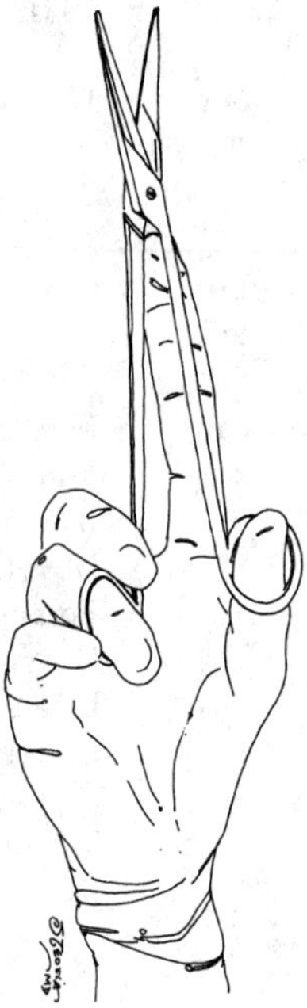

What helps steady the scissor- or bovie-hand?

Resting it on the opposite hand

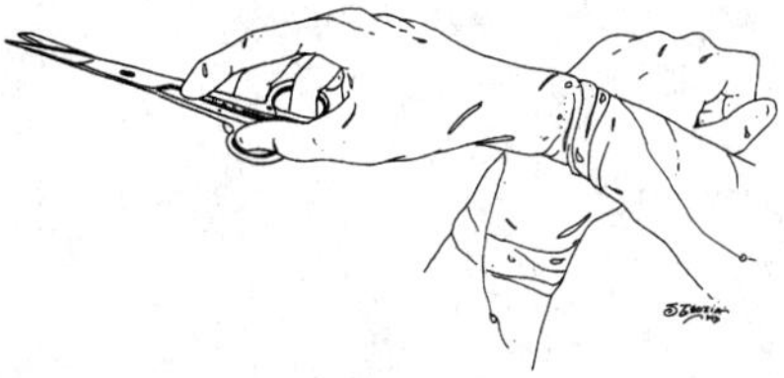

How should a pair of forceps be held?

Like a pencil

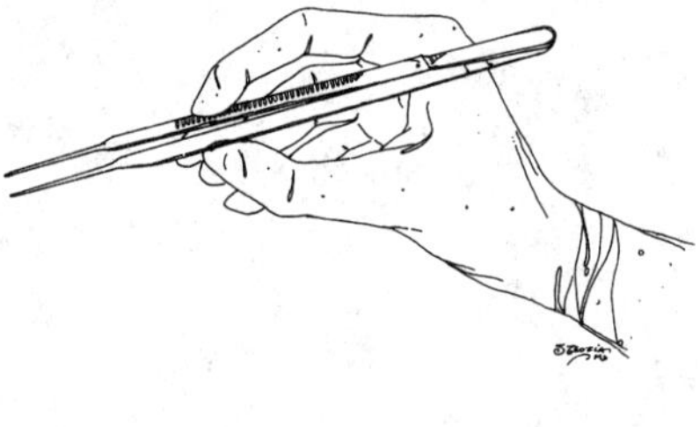

Identify the following instruments:

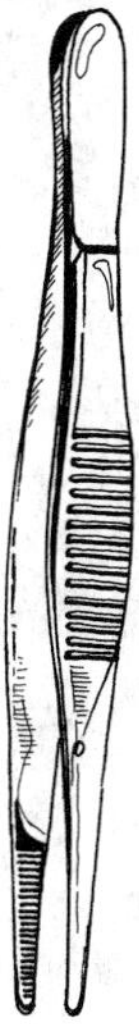

Forcep

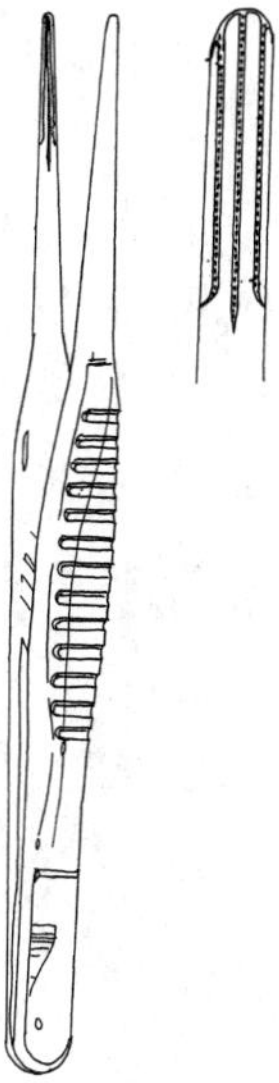

Debakey pickup

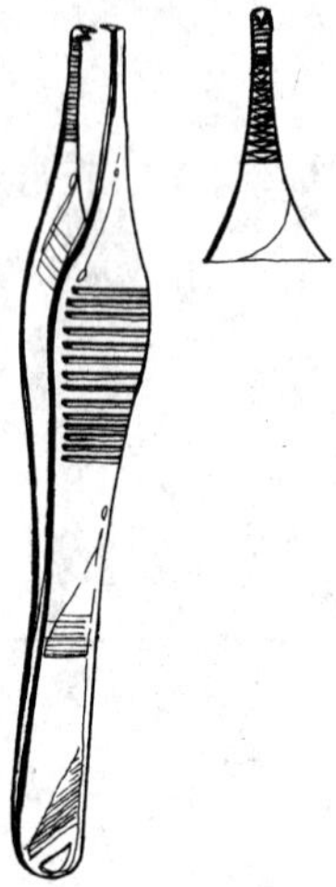

Adson pickup

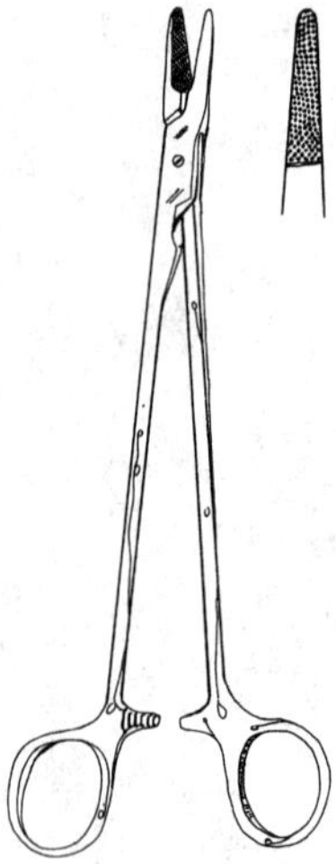

Needle-driver

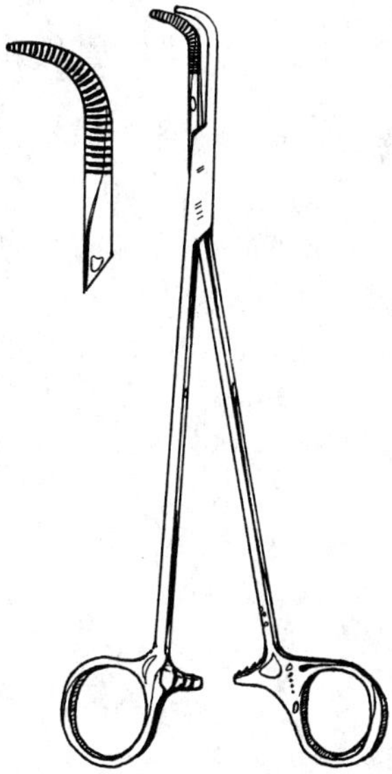

Right-angle clamp

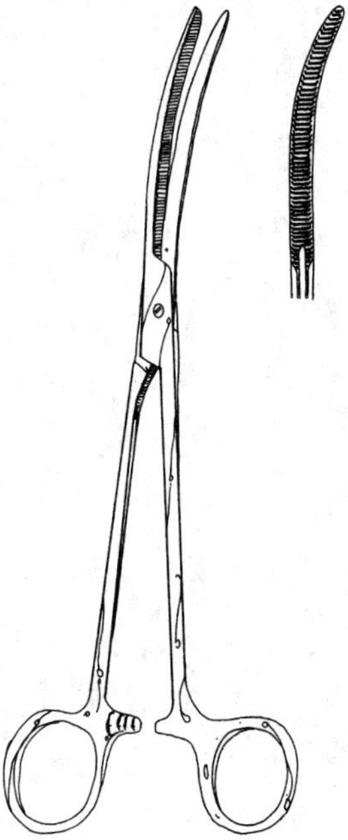

Kelly clamp

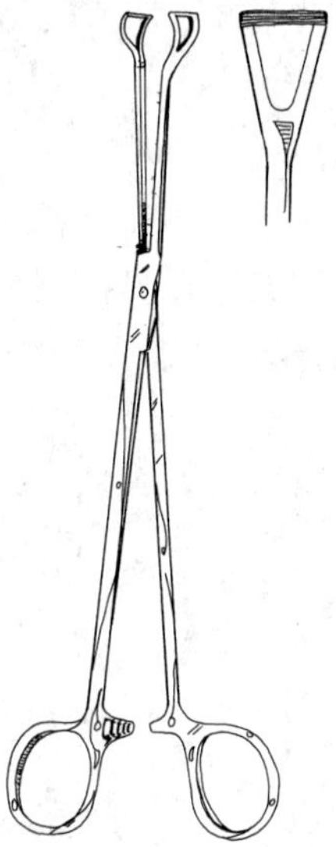

Babcock clamp

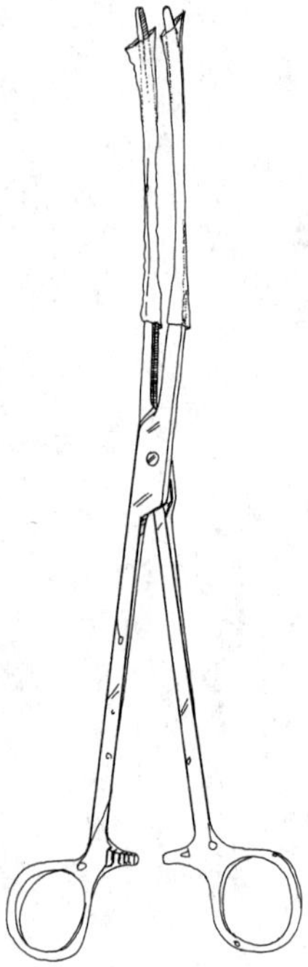

Atraumatic bowel clamp

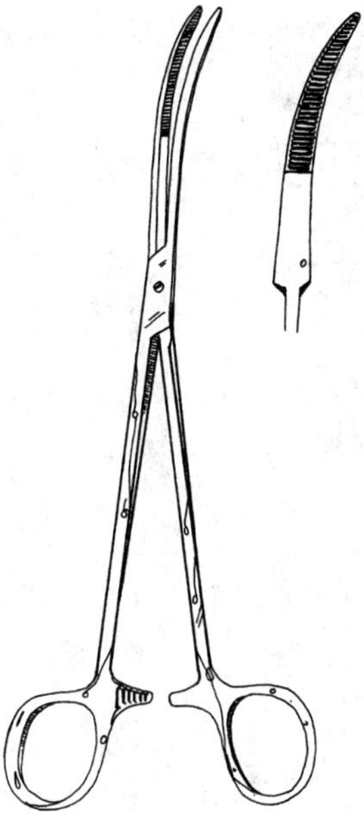

Tonsil clamp

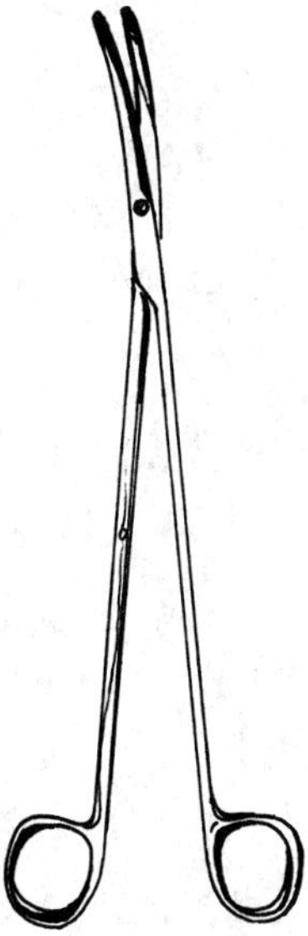

Metzenbaum scissors

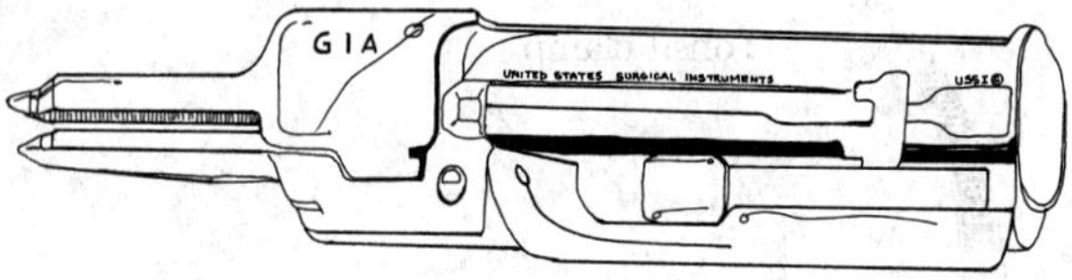

GIA stapler

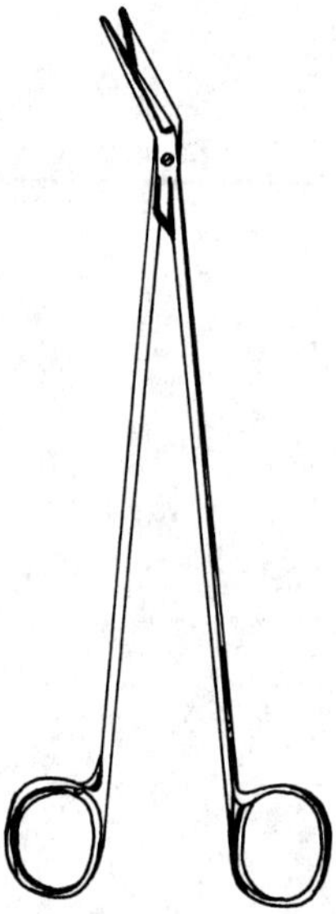

Pott's scissors

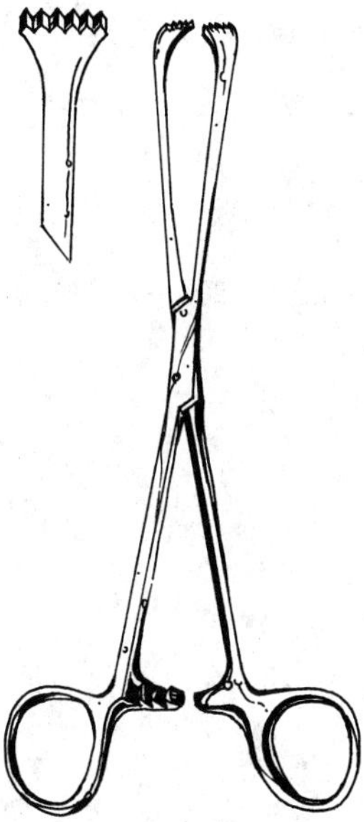

Allis clamp

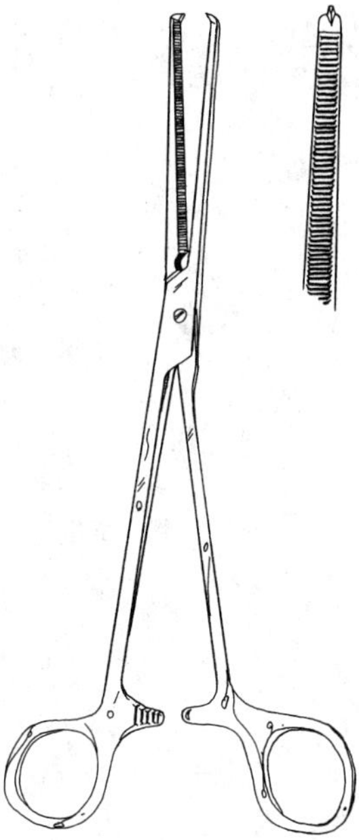

Kocher clamp, for very thick tissue (e.g., fascia)

Tip:

Define the following scalpel blades:

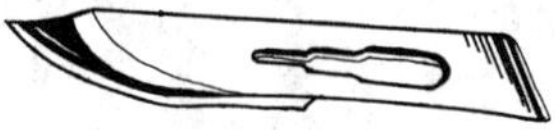

Number 10 or number 20

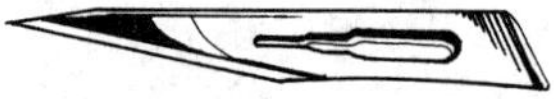

Number 11

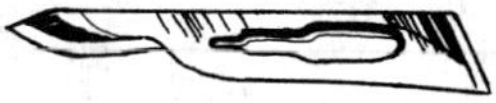

Number 15

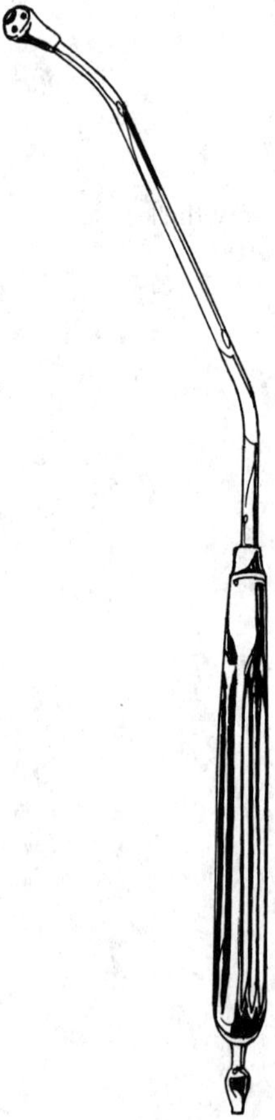

Yankuer suction (sucker)

RETRACTORS (YOU WILL GET TO KNOW THEM WELL!)

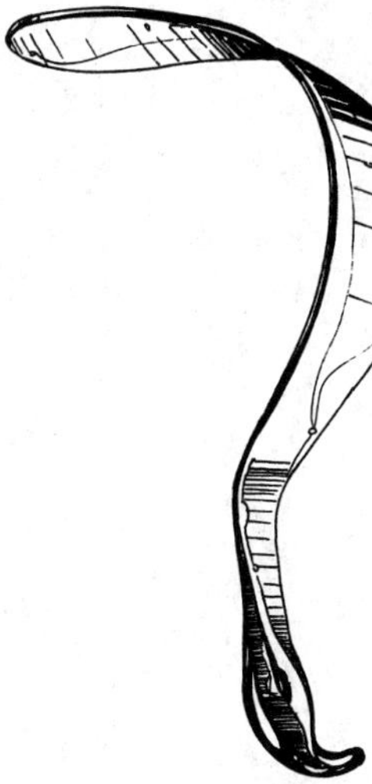

Deaver retractor

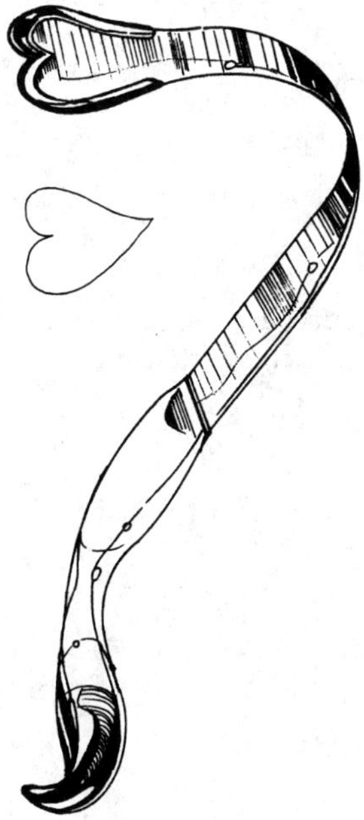

Sweetheart retractor (Harrington)

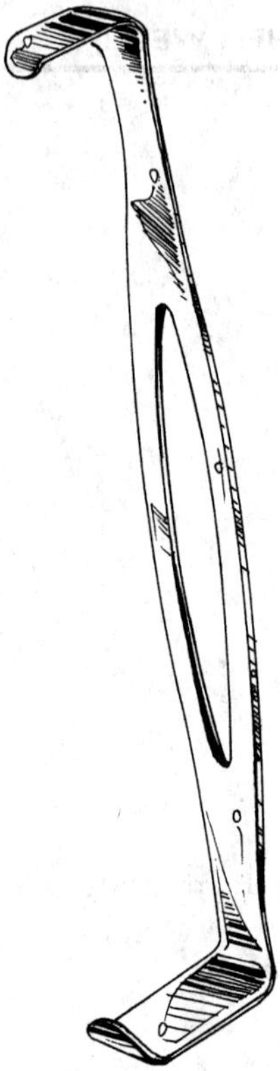

Army–Navy retractor

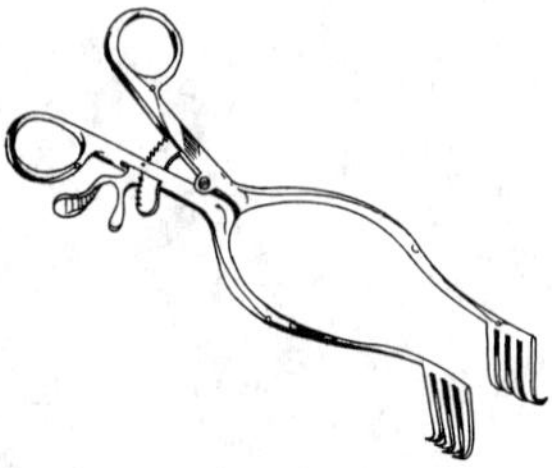

Weitlander retractor (self-retaining retractor; sorry, operates without a student!)

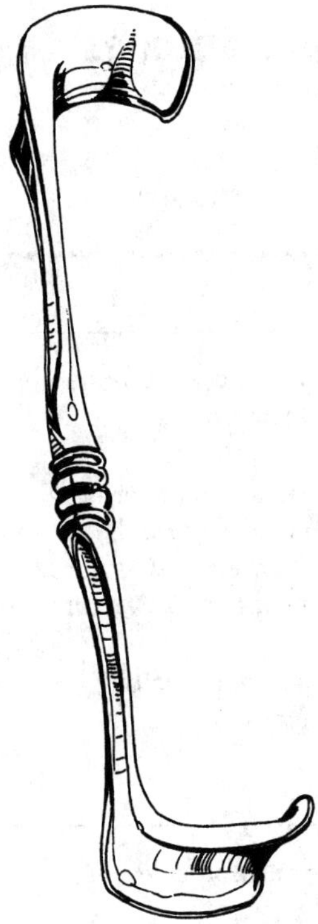

Richardson retractor

7 Sutures and Stitches

SUTURE MATERIALS

GENERAL INFORMATION

What is a suture?
Any strand of material used to ligate blood vessels or to approximate tissues

How are sutures sized?
By diameter; stated as a number of O's: the higher the number of O's, the smaller the diameter (e.g., 2-O suture has a larger diameter than 5-O suture)

Which is thicker, 1-O suture or 3-O suture?
1-O suture (pronounced "one oh")

CLASSIFICATION

What are the two most basic suture types?
Absorbable and nonabsorbable

What do these terms mean?
Absorbable—broken down and eventually dissolved by the body
Nonabsorbable—not broken down

SUTURES

Catgut

What are "catgut" sutures made of?
Purified collagen fibers from the intestines of healthy cows or sheep (no cats)

What are the two types of gut sutures?
Regular and chromic

What is the difference between the two types?
Chromic gut is soaked in chromium salts, which cause it to resist breakdown and to be less irritating to tissues than regular gut

Vicryl® Suture

What is it? Absorbable, braided, multifilamentous copolymer of lactide and glycolide

How long does it retain its strength? 60% at 2 weeks, 8% at 4 weeks

PDS®

What is it? Absorbable, monofilament polymer of polydioxanone (absorbable fishing line)

How long does it maintain its tensile strength? 70% to 74% at 2 weeks, 50% to 58% at 4 weeks, 25% to 41% at 6 weeks

How long does it take to complete absorption? 180 days (6 months)

What is silk? Braided protein filaments spun by the silkworm larva; known as a nonabsorbable suture

What is prolene? Nonabsorbable suture used for vascular anastomoses

What is nylon? Nonabsorbable "fishing line"

WOUND CLOSURE

GENERAL INFORMATION

What is the purpose of a suture closure? To approximate divided tissues to enhance wound healing

What are the three types of wound healing?

1. Primary intention
2. Secondary intention
3. Tertiary intention (delayed primary intention)

What is primary intention? When the edges of a (relatively) clean wound are closed in some manner (e.g., suture, Steri-Strips®, staples)

What is secondary intention? When a wound is allowed to remain open and heal by granulation

What is tertiary intention?

When a wound is allowed to remain open for a time and then closed, allowing for debridement and other wound care to reduce bacterial counts prior to closure (i.e., delayed primary closure)

What rule is constantly told to medical students about wound closure?

"Approximate, don't strangulate!"

What does it mean?

If a suture is tied too tightly, the wound edges may become ischemic and either fail to heal, or even become necrotic.

SUTURE TECHNIQUES

What is a taper-point needle?

Round body, leaves a round hole in tissue

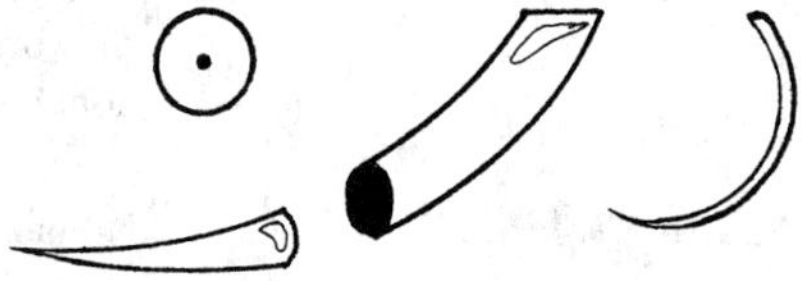

What is it used for?

Suturing of soft tissues other than skin (e.g., GI tract, muscle, nerve, peritoneum, fascia)

What is a conventional cutting needle?

Triangular body with the sharp edge toward the inner circumference; leaves a triangular hole in tissue

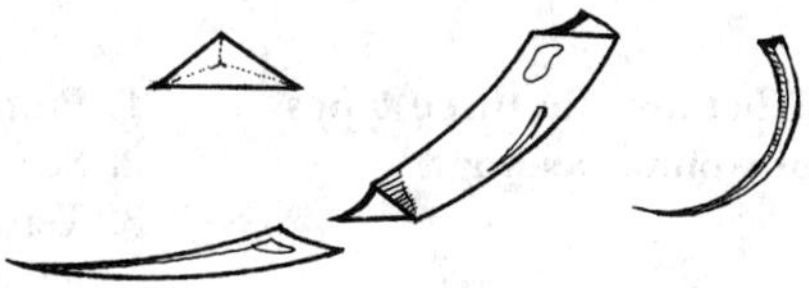

What are its uses?

Suturing of **skin**

What is a simple interrupted stitch?

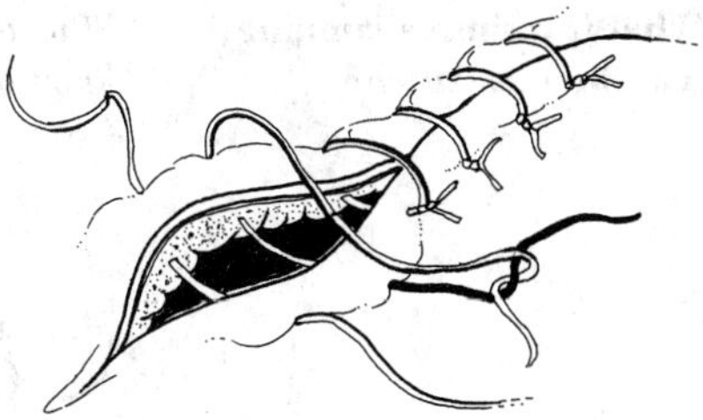

What is a vertical mattress stitch?

A simple stitch is made, the needle reversed, and a small bite taken from each wound edge; the knot ends up on one side of the wound.

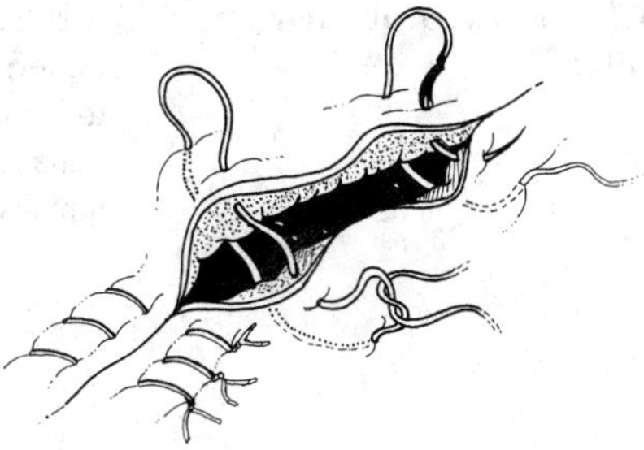

What is it also known as?

Far-far, near-near stitch

What is it used for?

Difficult-to-approximate skin edges; everts tissue well

What is a horizontal mattress stitch?

A simple stitch is made, the needle reversed, and the same size bite taken again.

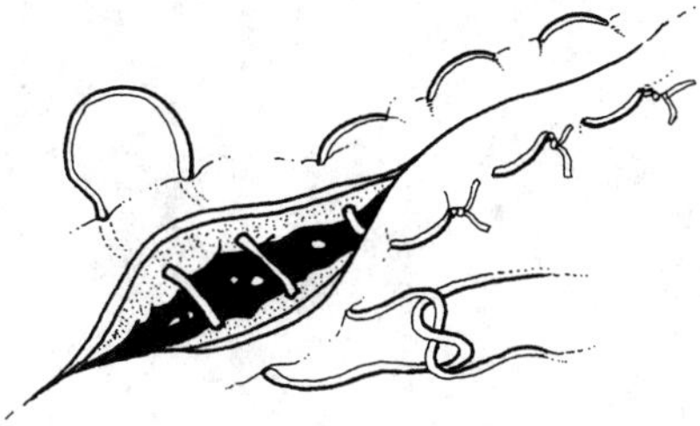

What is a simple running (continuous) stitch?

Stitches made in succession without knotting each stitch

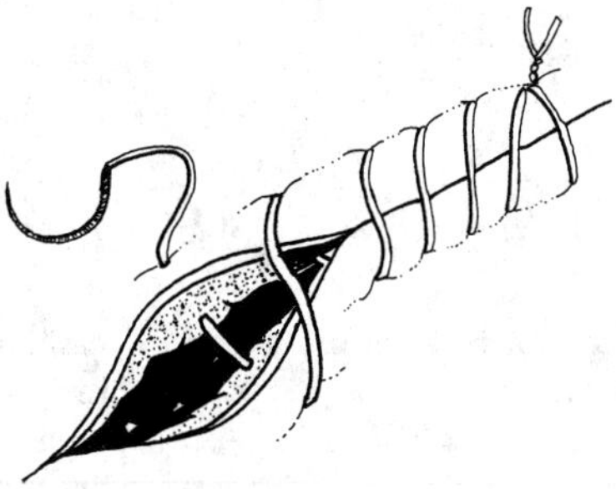

What is a subcuticular stitch?

A stitch, usually running, placed just underneath the epidermis; allows suture to remain in longer without leaving scars; can be either absorbable or nonabsorbable (e.g., pull-out stitch)

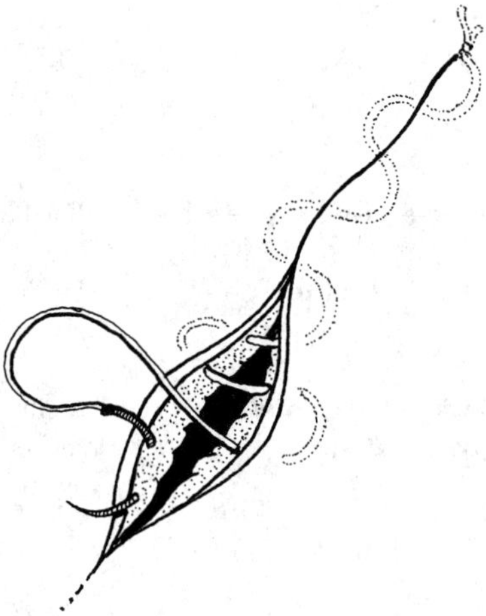

What is a pursestring suture?

A stitch that encircles a tube perforating a hollow viscus (e.g., gastrostomy tube), allowing the hole to be drawn tight and thus preventing leakage

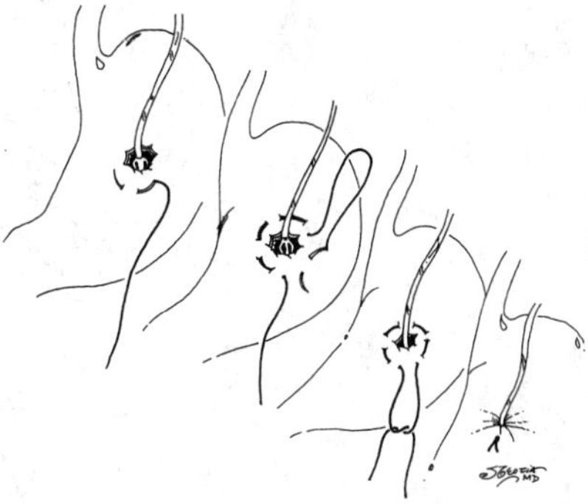

What are metallic skin staples?

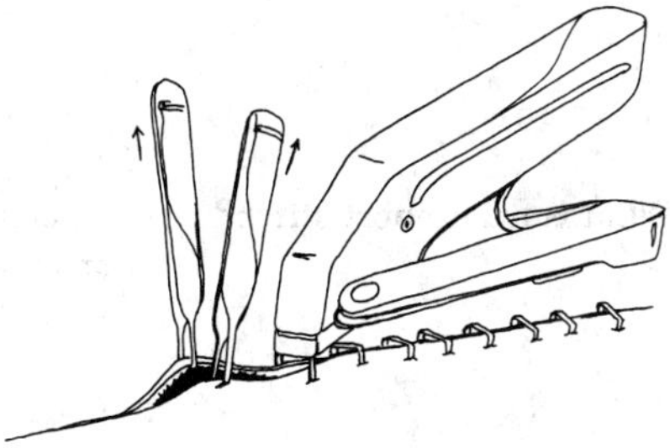

What is a staple removal device?

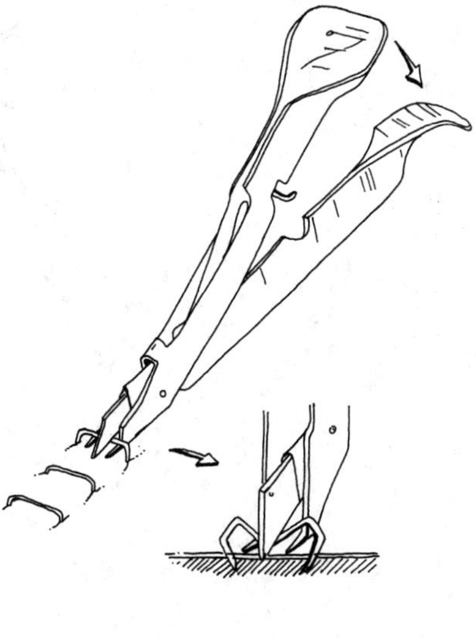

What is a gastrointestinal anastomosis (GIA) device?

A stapling device that lays two rows of small staples in a hemostatic row and **automatically cuts** in between them

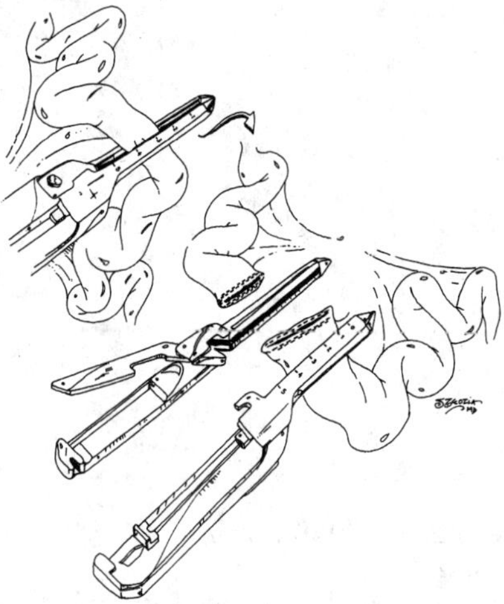

What is a Lembert stitch?

A reinforcing vertical stitch placed over an existing suture line, inverting the suture line; used in GI cases

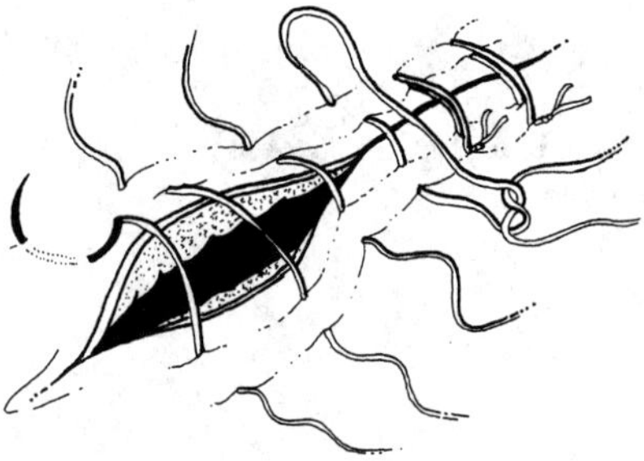

What is a stick tie?

The suture is anchored by passing it through the vessel **on a needle** before wrapping it around and occluding the vessel; prevents slippage of knot

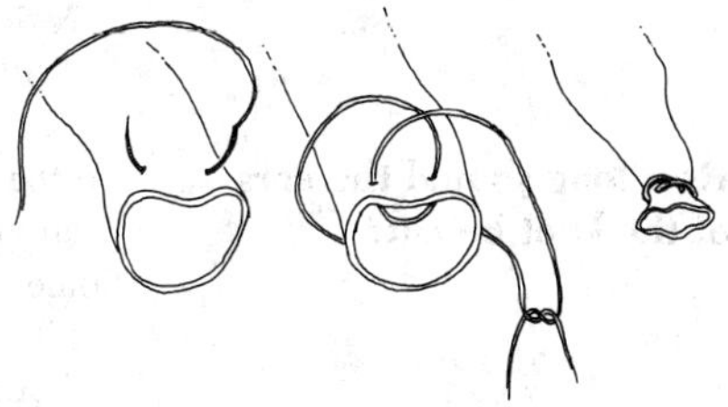

What is a pop-off suture?

A suture that is not permanently swaged to the needle, allowing the surgeon to "pop" off the needle from the suture without cutting the suture

KNOTS AND EARS

What is the basic surgical knot?

The square knot (note that the ear and the loop exit the knot on the same side)

What is a surgeon's knot?

A square knot with two twists in the first throw

How many (correct) throws are necessary to insure that your knots do not slip?

As many as the attending surgeon wants

What are the guidelines for the number of throws needed?	Depends on the suture material **Silk**—3 **Gut**—4 **Vicryl®, Dexon®, other braided synthetics**—4 **Nylon, polyester, polypropylene, PDS, Maxon**—6
How long should the ears of the knot be cut?	To the length requested by the attending surgeon Some guidelines are: **Silk vessel ties**—1 to 2 mm **Abdominal fascia closure**—5 mm **Skin sutures, drain sutures**—5 to 10 mm (makes them easier to find and remove)
How should the suture be cut?	Use the tips of the scissors to avoid cutting other tissues Try to remove the cut ends (less foreign material decreases risk of infection) Rest the scissor-hand on the nonscissor-hand to steady
When should skin sutures be removed?	As soon as the wound has healed enough to withstand expected mechanical trauma Any stitch left in more than approximately 10 days will leave a scar (railroad tracks) Some guidelines are: **Face**—3 to 5 days **Extremities**—7 days **Joints**—7 to 10 days **Back**—2 weeks **Abdomen**—7 days
How can strength be added to an incision during and after suture removal?	With Steri-Strips®
In general, which group of patients should skin sutures be left in longer than normal?	Patients on steroids

8

Surgical Knot Tying

What is the first knot that should be mastered?	Instrument knot
How is an instrument knot tied?	Always start with a double wrap, known as a "surgeon's knot," and then use a single wrap, pulling the suture in the opposite directions after every "throw."

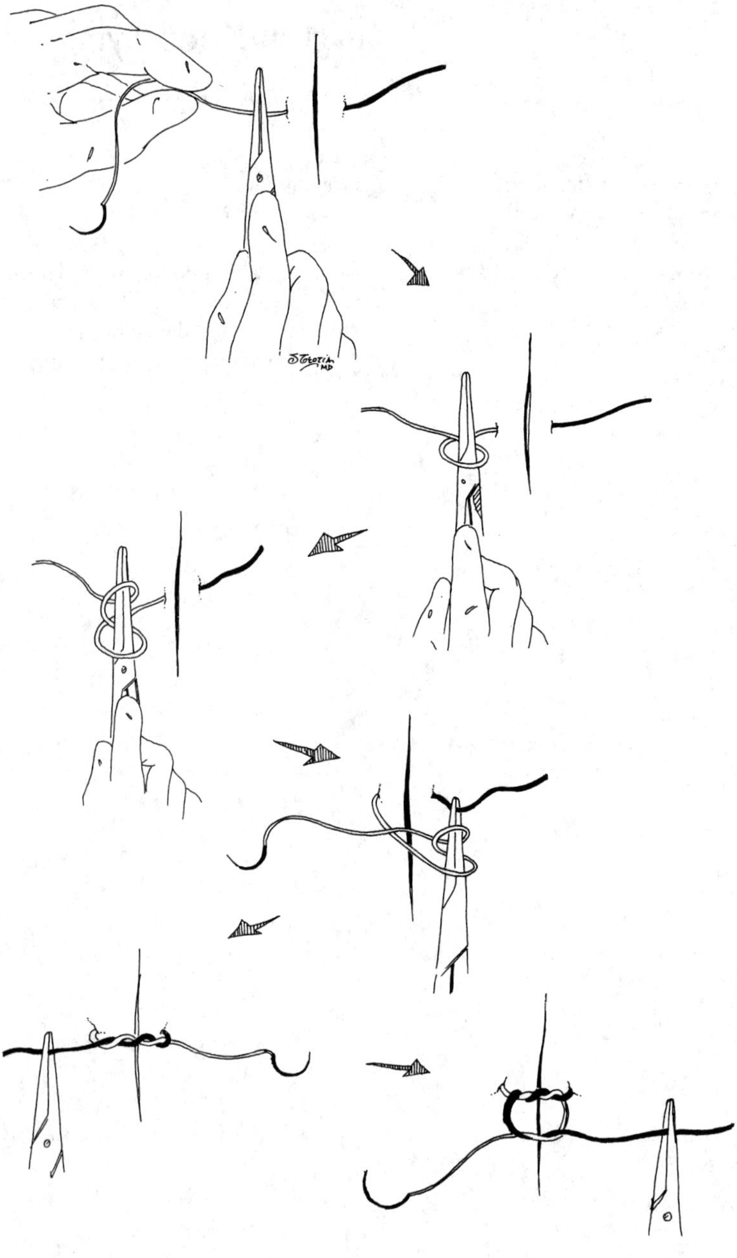

Does a student need to know a one-hand tie?

No! Master the two-hand tie and the instrument tie.

TWO-HAND TIE

What is the basic position for the two-hand tie?

The "C" position, formed by the thumb and index finger; the suture will **alternate** over the thumb and then the index finger for each throw

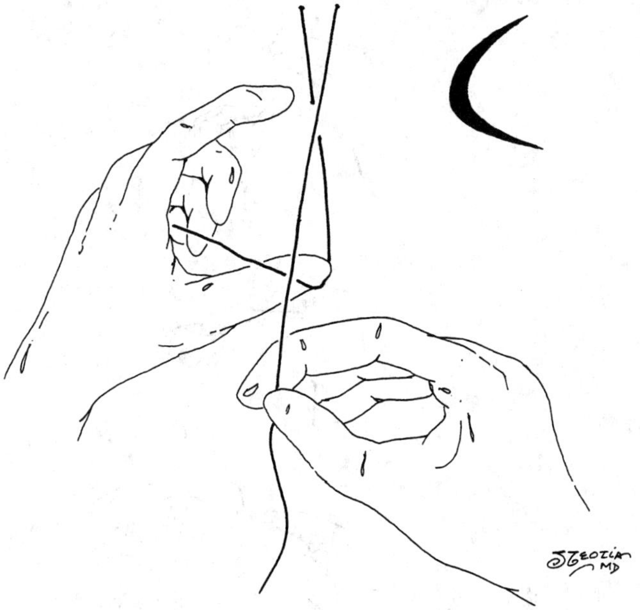

How is a two-hand knot tied?

First, use the index to lead
Then, use the thumb to lead

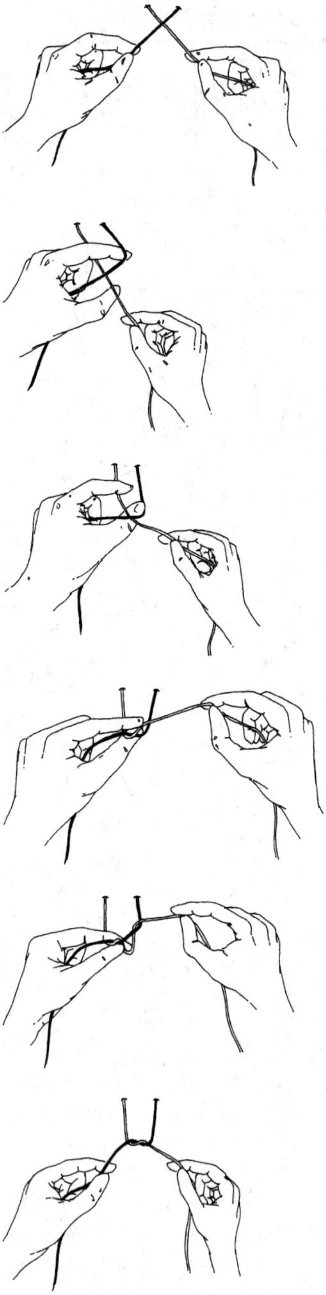

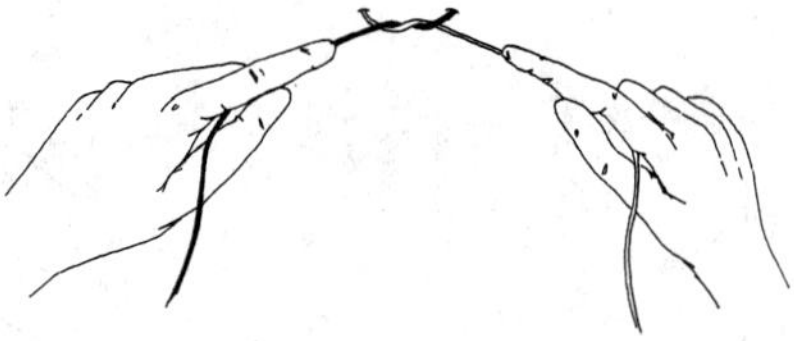

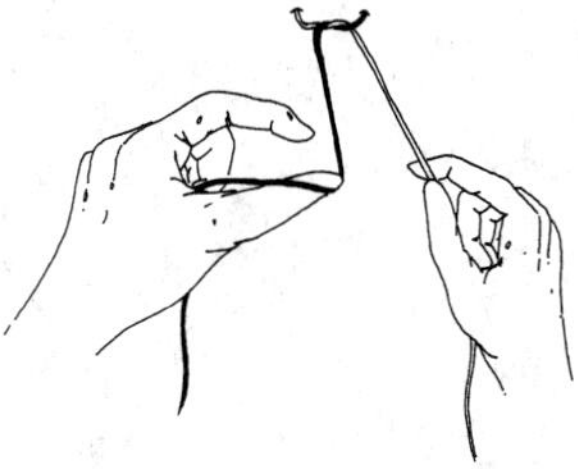

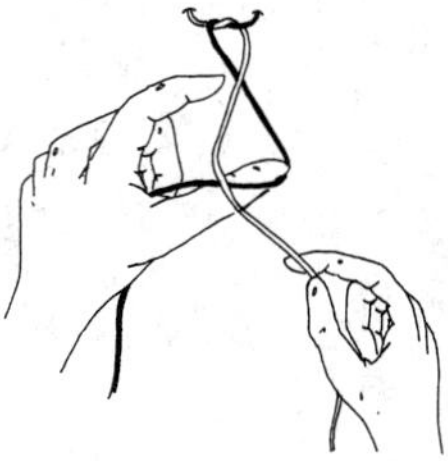

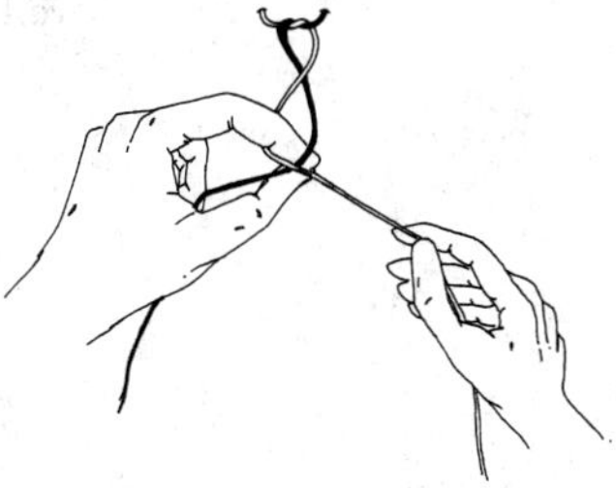

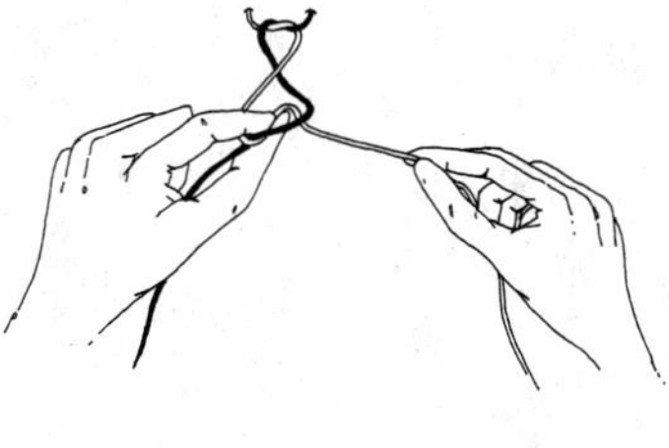

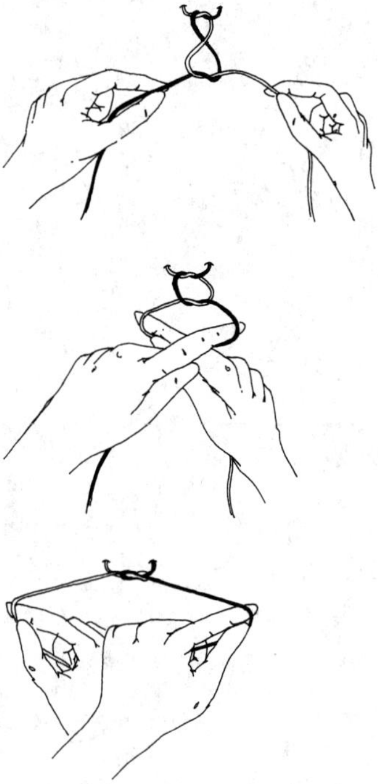

Ask a resident to help you after you have tried for awhile.

9 Incisions

If a patient has an old incision, is it best to make a subsequent incision next to or through the old incision?

Through the old incision, or excise the old incision, because it has scar tissue that limits the amount of collaterals that would be needed to heal an incision placed next to it

What is used to incise the epidermis?

Scalpel blade

What is used to incise the dermis?

Scalpel or electrocautery

Describe the following incisions:

Kocher's

Right subcostal incision for open cholecystectomy

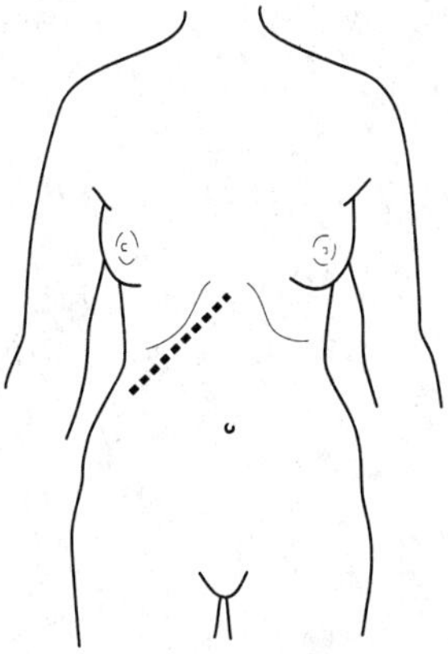

Midline laparotomy Incision down the abdomen along and through the linea alba

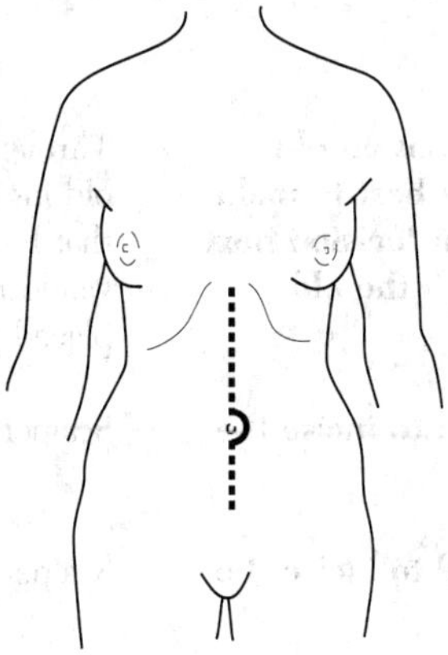

McBurney's Small right lower quadrant incision for an appendectomy through McBurney's point (one-third from the anterior superior iliac spine to the umbilicus)

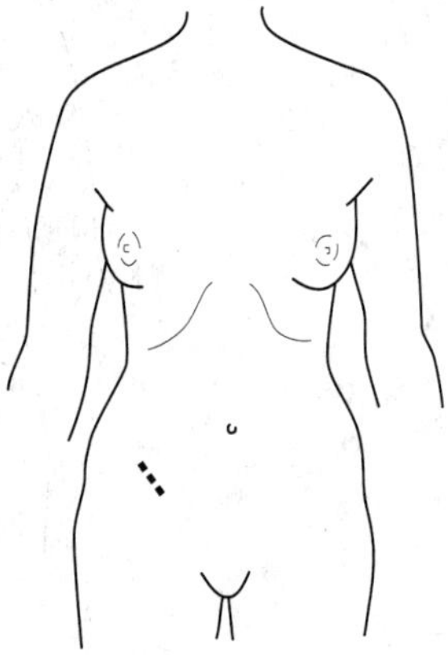

Paramedian

Incision that is longitudinal, but lateral to the linea alba (rarely used)

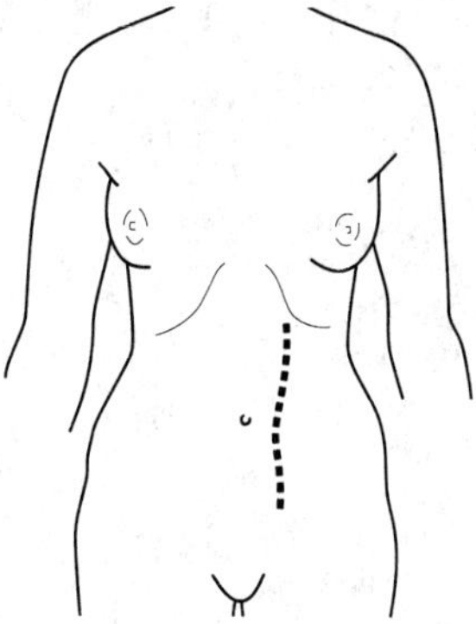

Pfannenstiel's

Low transverse abdominal incision with retraction of the rectus muscles laterally; most often used for gynecologic procedures

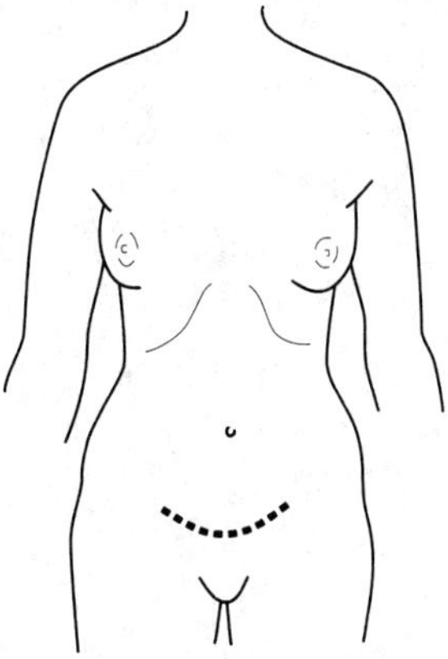

Kidney transplant Lower quadrant; kidney placed extraperitoneally

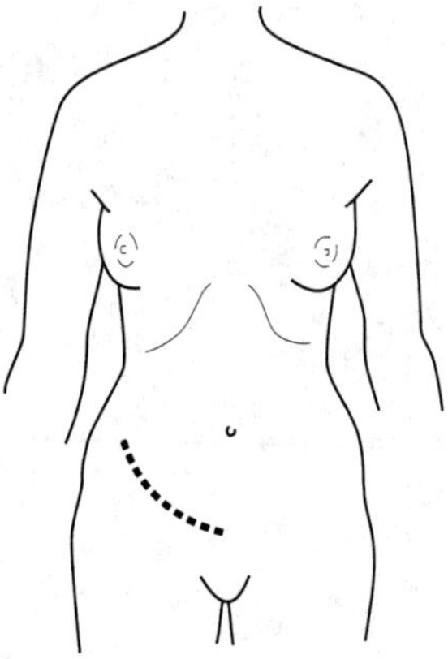

Liver transplant Chevron or Mercedes-Benz® incision in the upper abdomen

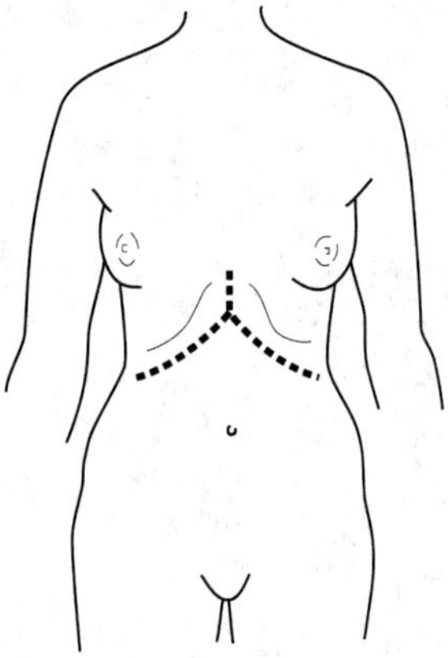

Transverse abdominal

Used mainly in infants and children or for splenectomy/hemicolectomy

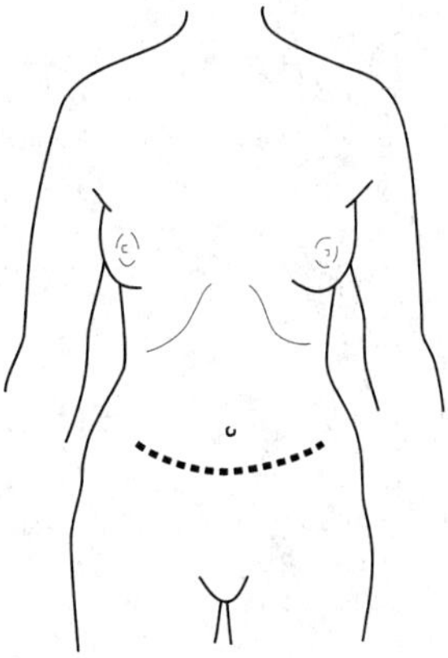

Sternotomy

Midline sternotomy incision for heart procedures; less painful than a lateral thoracotomy

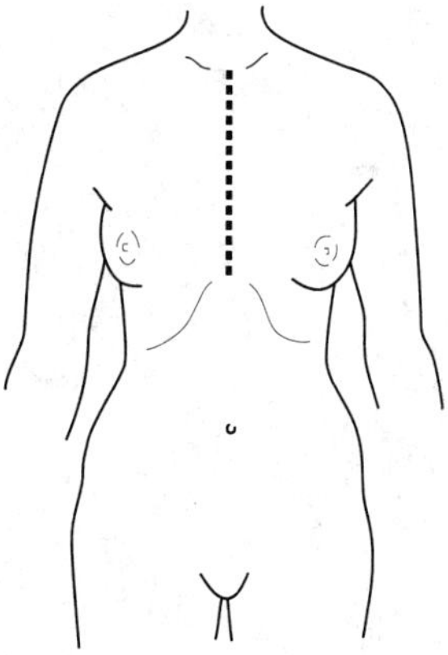

Thoracotomy

Usually through the fourth or fifth intercostal space; may be anterior or posterior lateral incisions
Very painful, but many are performed with muscle sparing (muscle retraction and not muscle transection)

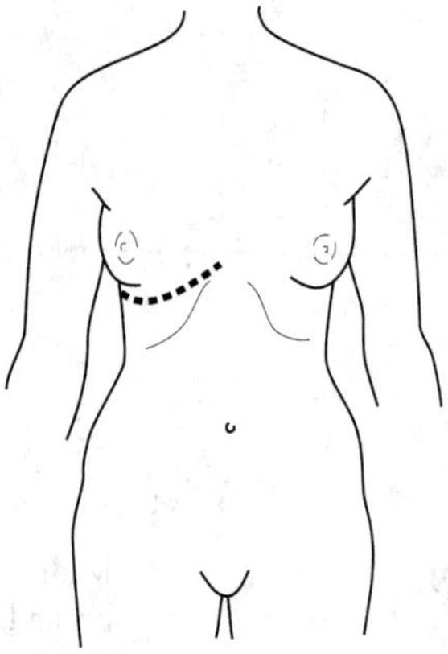

10

Common Operations

Define the following procedures:

Billroth I

Antrectomy with gastroduodenostomy

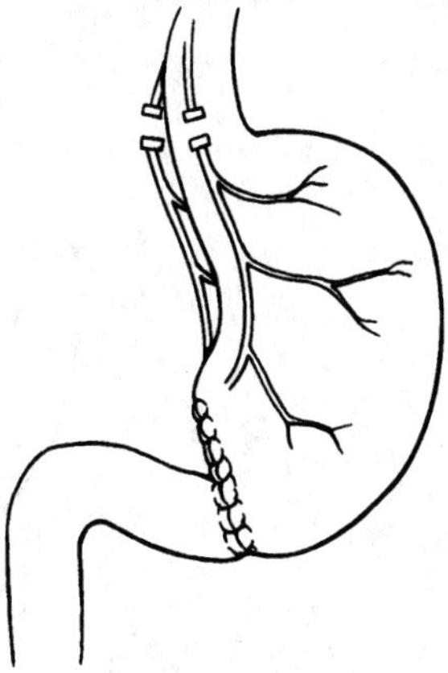

Billroth II

Antrectomy with gastrojejunostomy

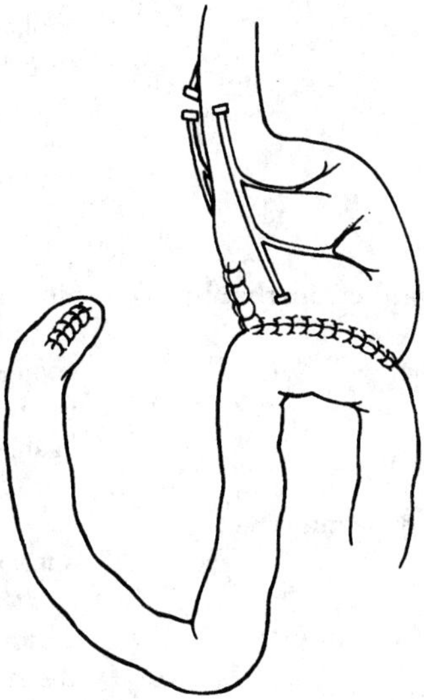

Roux-en-Y limb

Jejunojejunostomy forming a Y-shaped figure of small bowel; the free end can then be anastomosed to a second hollow structure (e.g., gastrojejunostomy)

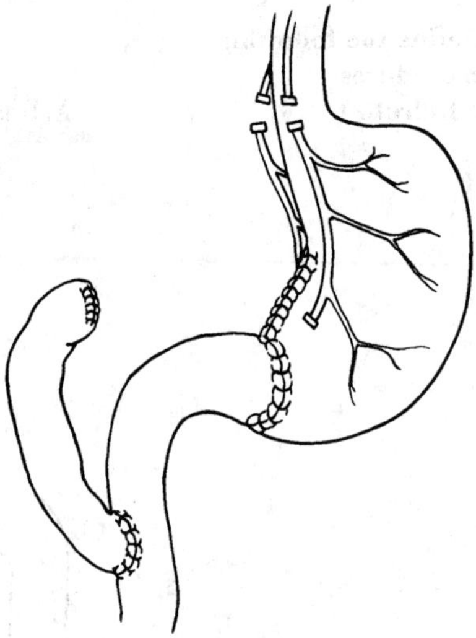

Brooke ileostomy

Standard ileostomy that is **folded on itself** to protrude from the abdomen approximately 2 cm to allow easy appliance placement and collection of succus

CEA

Carotid **E**nd**a**rterectomy; removal of atherosclerotic plaque from a carotid artery

Bassini herniorrhaphy

Repair of inguinal hernia by approximating transversus abdominis aponeurosis and the conjoint tendon to the reflection of **Poupart's** (inguinal) ligament

McVay herniorrhaphy

Repair of inguinal hernia by approximating the transversus abdominis aponeurosis and the conjoint tendon to **Cooper's** ligament (which is basically the superior pubic bone periosteum)

Lichtenstein herniorrhaphy

"Tension-free" inguinal hernia repair using **synthetic** graft material

Shouldice herniorrhaphy

Repair of inguinal hernia by **imbrication** of the transversalis fascia, transversus abdominis aponeurosis, and the conjoint tendon and approximation of the transversus abdominis aponeurosis and the conjoint tendon to the inguinal ligament

APR

Abdomino**p**erineal **R**esection; removal of the rectum and sigmoid colon through abdominal and perineal incisions (patient is left with a colostomy); used for low rectal cancers less than 8 cm from the anal verge

LAR

Low **A**nterior **R**esection; **resection** of **low** rectal tumors (> 8 cm from the anal verge) through an **anterior** abdominal incision

Hartman's procedure

1. Proximal colostomy
2. Distal stapled off colon or rectum that is left in peritoneal cavity

Mucus fistula

Distal end of the colon is brought to the abdominal skin as a stoma (proximal end is brought up to skin as an end colostomy)

Kocher maneuver

Dissection of the duodenum from the right-sided peritoneal attachment to allow mobilization and visualization of the back of the duodenum/pancreas

Seldinger technique

Placement of a central line by first placing a wire in the vein, followed by placing the catheter over the wire

Peustow procedure Side-to-side anastomosis of the pancreas and jejunum (pancreatic duct is filleted open)

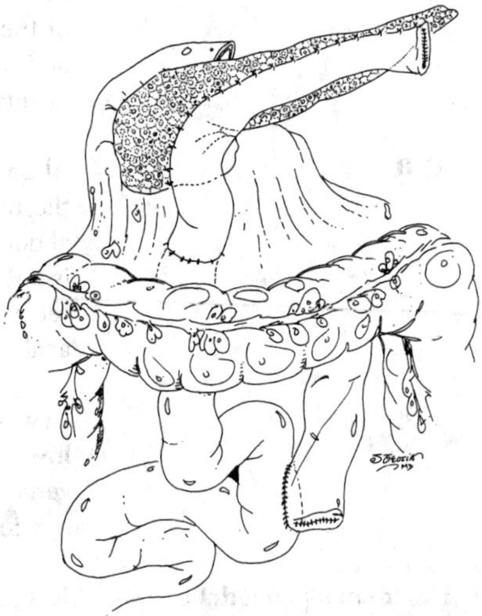

Stamm gastrostomy Gastrostomy placed by open surgical incision and tacked to the abdominal wall

Highly selective vagotomy Transection of vagal fibers to the body of the stomach without interruption of fibers to the pylorus (does not need pyloroplasty or other drainage procedure because the pylorus should still function)

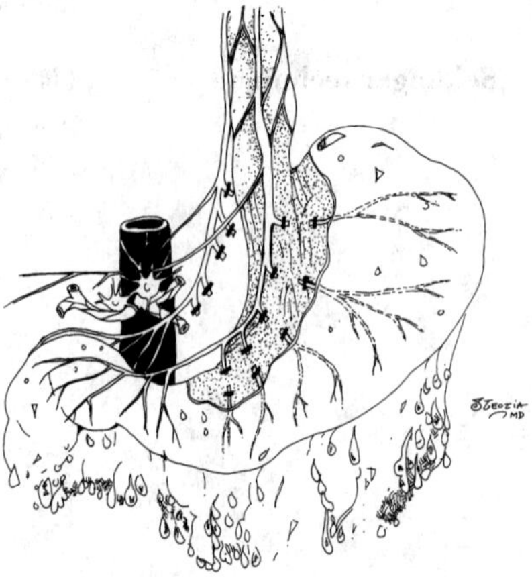

Enterolysis	Lysis of peritoneal adhesions
Appendectomy	Removal of the appendix
Lap appy	Laparoscopic removal of the appendix
Cholecystectomy	Removal of the gallbladder
Lap chole	Laparoscopic removal of the gallbladder
Nissen	Nissen fundoplication; 360° wrap of the stomach by the fundus of the stomach around the distal esophagus to prevent reflux

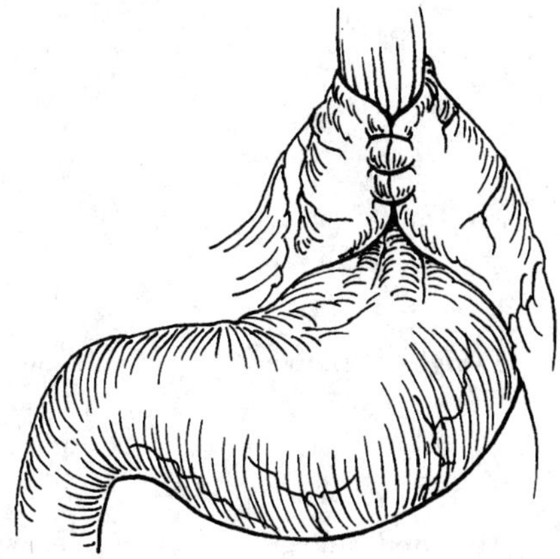

Simple mastectomy	Removal of breast and nipple without removal of nodes
Choledochojejunostomy	Anastomosis of the common bile duct to the jejunum (end to side)
Graham patch	Placement of omentum with stitches over a gastric or duodenal perforation (i.e., omentum is used to plug the hole)

Heineke-Mukulicz pyloroplasty

Longitudinal incision through all layers of the pylorus, sewing closed in a transverse direction to make the pylorus nonfunctional (used after truncal vagotomy)

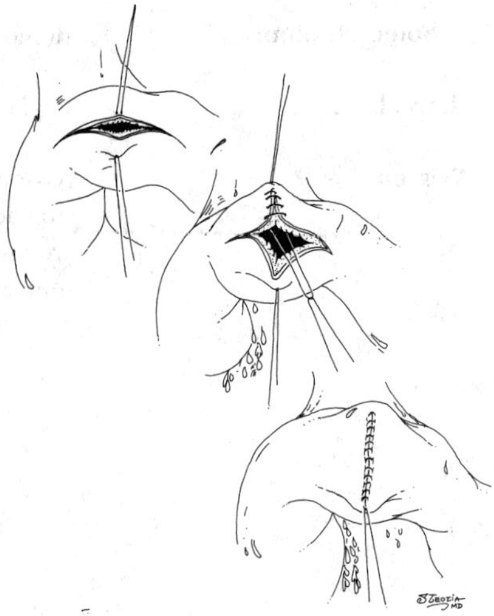

Pringle maneuver

Temporary occlusion of the porta hepatis (for temporary control of liver blood flow when liver parenchyma is actively bleeding)

Modified radical mastectomy

Removal of the breast, nipple, **and axillary lymph nodes** (no muscle is removed)

Lumpectomy and radiation

Removal of breast mass and axillary lymph nodes; normal surrounding breast tissue is spared; patient then undergoes postoperative radiation treatments

I and D

Incision and **D**rainage of pus; the wound is then packed open

PEG

Percutaneous **E**ndoscopic **G**astrostomy; the endoscope is placed in the stomach, which is then inflated with air. A needle is passed into the stomach percutaneously, string is passed through the needle traversing the abdominal wall, and gastrostomy is then placed by using the Seldinger technique over the wire.

Exploratory laparotomy Laparotomy to explore the peritoneal cavity looking for the cause of pain/peritoneal signs/obstruction/hemorrhage/etc.

TURP **T**ran**su**rethral **R**esection of the **P**rostate; removal of obstructing prostatic tissue via scope in the urethral lumen

Fem pop bypass **Fem**oral artery to **pop**liteal artery bypass using synthetic graft or saphenous vein; used to bypass blockage in the femoral artery

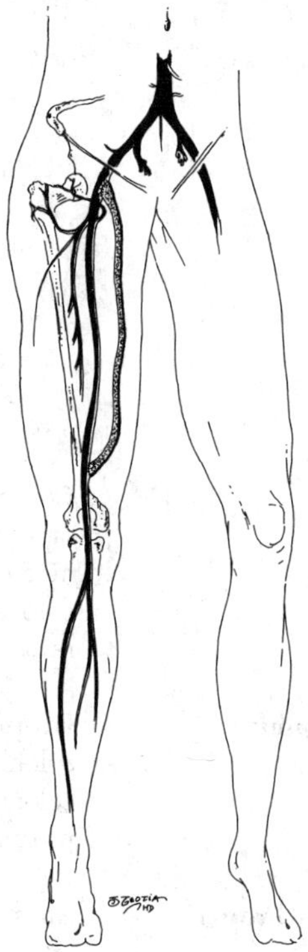

AX FEM — Long prosthetic graft tunneled under the skin placed from the **ax**illary artery to the **fem**oral artery

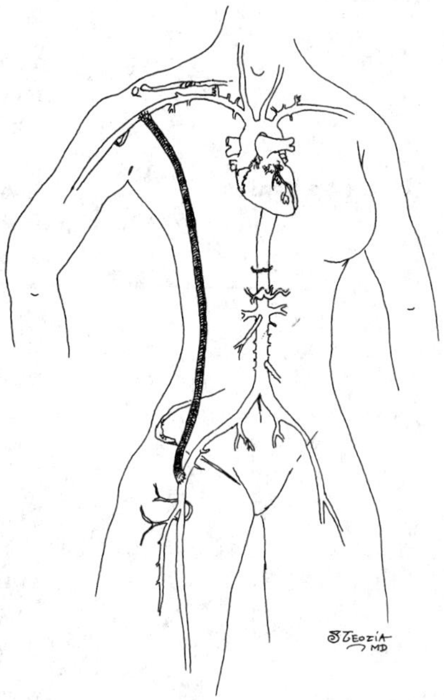

CABG — **C**oronary **A**rtery **B**ypass **G**rafting; via saphenous vein graft or internal mammary artery bypass grafts to coronary arteries from aorta (cardiac revascularization)

Hartmann's pouch — Oversewing of a rectal stump (or distal colonic stump) after resection of a colonic segment; patient is left with a proximal colostomy

Ileoanal pull-through — Anastomosis of the ileum to the anus after total proctocolectomy

Hemicolectomy — Removal of a colonic segment (i.e., partial colectomy)

Truncal vagotomy — Transection of the vagus nerve trunks; must provide drainage procedure to stomach (e.g., gastrojejunostomy or pyloroplasty) because after truncal vagotomy, the **pylorus does not relax**

Antrectomy Removal of stomach antrum

Whipple procedure Pancreaticoduodenectomy:
- Cholecystectomy
- Truncal vagotomy
- Antrectomy
- Pancreaticoduodenectomy—removal of the head of the pancreas and duodenum
- Choledochojejunostomy (anastomosis of common bile duct to jejunum)
- Pancreaticojejunostomy (anastomosis of distal pancreas remnant to the jejunum)
- Gastrojejunostomy (anastomosis of stomach to jejunum)

11 Wounds, Drains, and Tubes

Define the following terms:

Primary wound closure — Immediate suture wound closure

Delayed primary closure — Suture wound closure usually 3 to 5 days after incision

Secondary wound closure — Wound closure over time **without sutures;** heals by contraction and epithelialization (leaves a large scar)

How long until a sutured wound epithelializes?

~ 48 hours

After a primary closure, when should the dressing be removed?

Postoperative day 2

When can a patient take a shower after a primary closure?

Anytime after postoperative day 2

What is a wet-to-dry dressing?

A damp (not wet) gauze dressing placed over a granulating wound and then allowed to dry to the wound; removal allows for debridement of the wound

What inhibits wound healing?

Malnutrition, anemia, hypoxia, steroids, cancer, radiation

What reverses the deleterious effects of steroids on wound healing?

Vitamin A

What is Dakin solution?

Dilute sodium hypochlorite (**bleach**) used in contaminated wounds

PigTail Drain.

What is the purpose of drains?

1. Withdrawal of fluids
2. Apposition of tissues to remove a potential space by suction

What is a Jackson-Pratt (JP) drain?

A closed drainage system attached to a suction bulb ("grenade")
(Always remember to detach the suction before pulling!)

What are the "three S's" of Jackson-Pratt drain removal?

1. **S**titch removal
2. **S**uction discontinuation
3. **S**low, steady pull

What is a Penrose drain?

An open drainage system composed of a thin rubber hose; associated with increased infection rate in clean wounds

Define the following terms:

G-tube

Gastrostomy tube; used for drainage or feeding

D-tube

Duodenostomy tube; used for drainage, usually after duodenal trauma (rare)

J-tube

Jejunostomy tube; used for feeding; may be a small-needle catheter (remember to flush after use or it will clog) or a large, red rubber catheter

Cholecystostomy tube
C

Tube placed surgically or percutaneously with ultrasound guidance to drain the gallbladder

T-tube

A tube placed in the common bile duct with an ascending and descending limb that forms a "T"
Drains percutaneously
Usually placed after common bile duct exploration

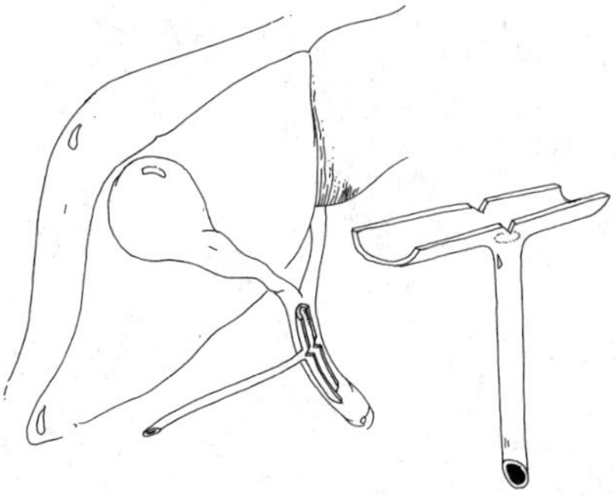

When can a T-tube be removed?

Usually after 3 weeks; may be removed if bilirubin level does not increase and there are no signs/symptoms of cholangitis after clamping, and after normal T-tube cholangiogram

Why doesn't the bile duct leak bile after removal of a T-tube?

A fibrous tract forms around the T-tube prior to removal; the fibrous tract then scleroses down after removal of the T-tube, resulting in a patent and closed bile duct.

Define the following terms:

Chest tube

Thoracostomy tube
Drains the pleural cavity
Attached to suction to appose the parietal and visceral pleura
Used to drain blood, pus, fluid, chyle, and air

Cecostomy tube

Tube placed into the cecum after colonic distention to decompress the colon (rare)

Malicot Drain: Common Bile duct drain.

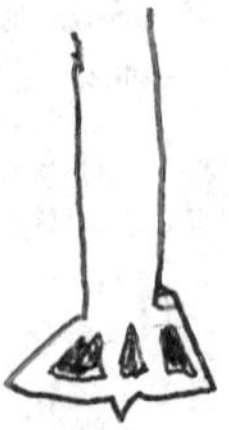

CHEST TUBES

How is a chest tube inserted?

1. Administer local anesthetic
2. Incise skin in the fourth intercostal space between the mid- and anterior-axillary lines
3. Perform blunt Kelly-clamp dissection **over** the rib into the pleural space
4. Perform finger exploration to confirm intrapleural placement
5. Place tube posteriorly and superiorly

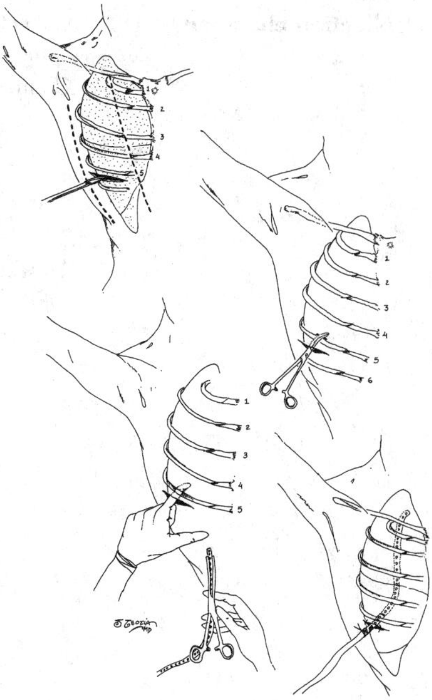

What are the goals of chest tube insertion?

Drain
Appose parietal and visceral pleura to seal any visceral pleural holes

In most cases, where should the chest tube be positioned?

Posteriorly into the apex

How can you tell on CXR if the last hole on the chest tube is in the pleural cavity?

The last hole is cut through the radiopaque line in the chest tube and is seen on CXR as a break in the line, which should be within the pleural cavity.

What is the chest tube connected to?

A Pleurovac® (three-chambered box)

What are the three chambers of the Pleurovac®?

1. Collection chamber
2. Water seal
3. Suction control

Describe how each chamber of the Pleurovac® box works as the old three-bottle system:

Collection chamber

Collects fluid, pus, blood, or chyle and measures the amount

Connects to the water seal bottle and to the chest tube

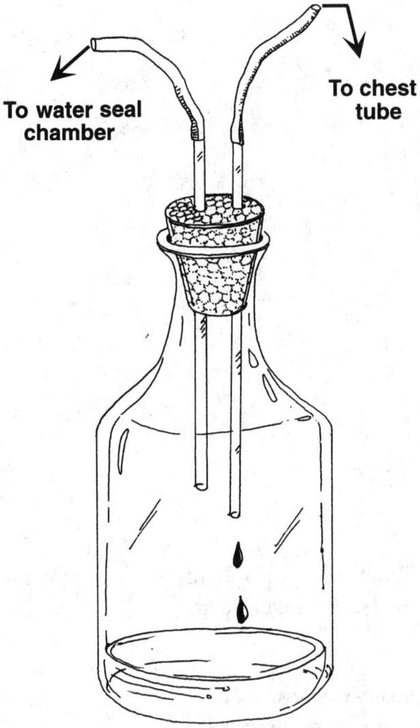

Water-seal chamber

One-way valve—allows air to be removed from the pleural space; does not allow air to enter pleural cavity; connects to the suction control bottle and to the collection chamber

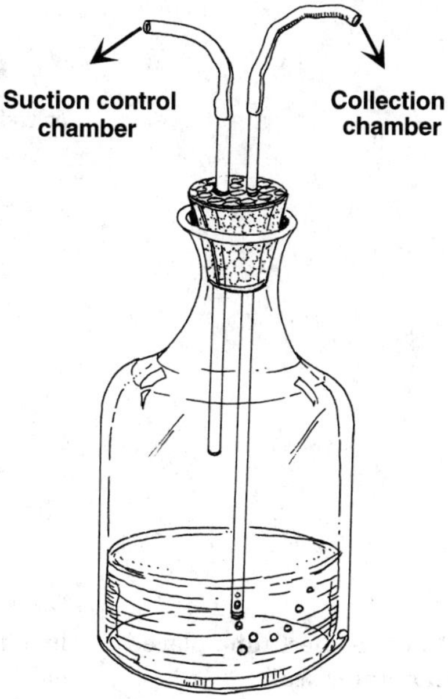

Suction-control chamber

Controls the amount of suction by the height of the water column
Excessive suction is released by sucking in room air
Connects to wall suction and to the water seal bottle

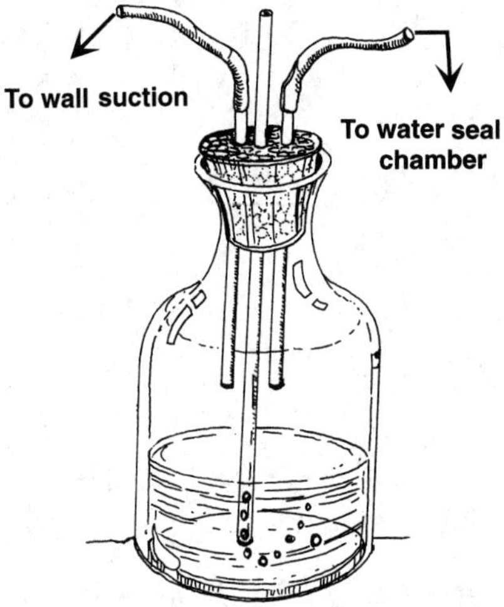

How is a chest tube placed on a water seal?

By removing the suction; a tension pneumothorax (PTX) cannot form because the one-way valve allows release of air buildup

Should a chest tube ever be clamped off?

No, except to "run the system" **momentarily**

What does it mean "to run the system" of a chest tube?

To see if the air leak is from a leak in the pleural cavity (i.e., visceral hole) or from a leak in the tubing
Momentarily occlude the chest tube and if the air leak is still present, it is from the tubing or tubing connection, not from the chest.

How can an air leak be checked for?

Look at the water seal chamber on suction; if bubbles pass through the water seal fluid, a large air leak (i.e., air leaking into chest tube) is present. If no air leak is evident on suction, remove suction and ask the patient to cough. If air bubbles through the water seal, a small air leak is present.

What is the usual course for removing a chest tube placed for a PTX?

1. Suction until the PTX resolves and the air leak is gone
2. Water seal for 24 hours
3. Remove the chest tube if no PTX or air leak is present after 24 hours of water seal

How fast is a small, stable PTX absorbed?

Approximately 1% daily; therefore, a 10% PTX by volume will absorb in 10 days

How should a chest tube be removed?

1. Cut the stitch
2. Ask the patient to expire (breathe out, not die!)
3. Rapidly remove the tube (split second) as the patient forcefully expires; at same time, place petroleum jelly gauze covered by 4 x 4, tape
4. Obtain a CXR

NASOGASTRIC TUBES (NGT)

How should an NGT be placed?

1. Use lubrication and have suction up on the bed.
2. Slightly numb nose.
3. Place head in flexion.
4. Ask patient to drink a small amount of H_2O when the tube is in the back of the throat and to swallow the tube; if the patient can talk without difficulty and succus returns, the tube should be in the stomach (get an x-ray if there is any question).

What test should be performed before feeding via any tube?

Low chest x-ray to confirm placement into the GI tract

How does an NGT work?

Sump pump, dual lumen tube—the large clear tube is hooked to suction and the small blue tube allows for air sump (i.e., circuit sump pump with air in the blue tube and air and succus sucked out through the large clear lumen)

Should an NGT be placed on continuous or intermittent suction?

Continuous low suction—side holes disengage if they are against mucosa because of the sump mechanism and multiple holes

What happens if the NGT is clogged?

The tube will not decompress the stomach and keeps the low esophageal sphincter (LES) open (i.e., a setup for aspiration)

How should an NGT be unclogged?

Saline-flush the clear port, reconnect to suction, and flush air down the blue sump port

What is a common cause of excessive NGT drainage?

The tip of the NGT is inadvertently placed in the duodenum and drains the pancreatic fluid and bile; an x-ray should be taken and the tube repositioned into the stomach.

FOLEY CATHETER

What is a Foley catheter?

Catheter into the bladder, allowing accurate urine output determination

What is a coudé catheter?

A Foley catheter with a small, curved tip to help maneuver around a large prostate

If a Foley catheter cannot be inserted, what are the next steps?

1. Anesthetize the urethra with a sterile local anesthetic (e.g., lidocaine jelly)
2. Try a **larger** Foley catheter

CENTRAL LINES

What are they?

Catheters placed into the major veins (central veins) via subclavian-, internal–jugular-, or femoral-vein approaches

What major complications result from placement?

PTX (always obtain postplacement CXR), bleeding, malposition (e.g., into the neck from subclavian approach)

In long-term central lines, what does the "cuff" do?

Allows ingrowth of fibrous tissue, which:
- Holds the line in place
- Forms a barrier to the advance of bacteria

What is a Hickman® or Hickman-type catheter?	External central line tunneled under the skin with a "cuff"
What is a Portacath®?	Central line that has a port buried under the skin that must be accessed through the skin (percutaneously)

MISCELLANEOUS

How can diameter in mm be determined from a French measurement?	Divide the French size by pi or 3.14 (e.g., a 15 French tube has a diameter of 5 mm)
How can needle-gauge size be determined?	A 14-gauge needle is 1/14 of an inch (and thus a 14-gauge needle is larger than a 21-gauge needle)
What is a Tenckhoff catheter?	Catheter placed into the peritoneal cavity for peritoneal dialysis

12

Surgical Anatomy Pearls

What is the drainage of the left testicular vein?	Left renal vein
What is the drainage of the right testicular vein?	IVC
What is Gerota's fascia?	Fascia surrounding the kidney
What are the prominent collateral circulations seen in portal hypertension?	Esophageal varices, hemorrhoids (inferior hemorrhoidal vein to internal iliac vein), patent umbilical vein (caput medusa), and retroperitoneal vein via lumbar tributaries
What parts of the GI tract are retroperitoneal?	Most of the duodenum, the ascending colon, the descending colon, and the pancreas
What is the gubernaculum?	Embryologic structure that adheres the testes to the scrotal sac; used to help manipulate the testes during indirect hernia repair
Which artery bleeds in bleeding duodenal ulcers?	Gastroduodenal artery
What is the name of the lymph nodes between the pectoralis minor and major muscles?	Rotter's lymph nodes
Is the left vagus nerve anterior or posterior?	Anterior; remember the esophagus rotates during development
What is Morrison's pouch?	The hepatorenal recess; the most posterior cavity in the peritoneal cavity

Give the locations of the following structures:

Foregut — Mouth to ampulla of Vater

Midgut — Ampulla of Vater to distal third of transverse colon

Hindgut — Distal third of transverse colon to the anus

Where are the blood vessels on a rib?

The vein, artery, and nerve (VAN) are underneath the rib (thus, place chest tubes and thoracentesis needles above the rib!)

What is the order of the femoral vessels?

The femoral vein is medial to the femoral artery (think: **NAVEL** for the order of the right femoral vessels—**n**erve, **a**rtery, **v**ein, **e**xtralymphatic tissue, **l**ymphatics).

What is Hesselbach's triangle?

The area bordered by:
1. Inguinal canal
2. Epigastric vessels
3. Lateral border of the rectus sheath

What nerve is located on top of the spermatic cord?

Ilioinguinal nerve

What is Calot's triangle?

The area bordered by:
1. Cystic duct
2. Common hepatic duct
3. Lower edge of the liver

What is Calot's (Lund's) node?

Lymph node found in Calot's triangle

What separates the right and left lobes of the liver?

Cantlie's line—a line drawn from the IVC to just left of the gallbladder fossa

What is the gastrinoma triangle?

A triangle where more than 90% of extrapancreatic gastrinomas are located, bordered by:
1. Third portion of the duodenum
2. Cystic duct
3. Pancreatic neck

Which artery is responsible for anterior spinal syndrome?	Artery of Adamkiewicz
Where is McBurney's point?	One-third the distance from the anterior superior spine to the umbilicus (estimate of the position of the appendix)
How can you find the appendix after you find the cecum?	Trace the taenia back as they converge on the origin of the appendix.
Where is the space of Retzius?	The preperitoneal space anterior to the bladder
What are the white lines of Toldt?	The lateral peritoneal reflections of the ascending and descending colon
What is the strongest layer of the small bowel?	Submucosa (not the serosa)
Which parts of the GI tract do not have a serosa?	Esophagus Middle and distal rectum
What is the vein that overlies the pylorus?	Vein of Mayo
What is the pouch of Douglas?	Pouch between the rectum and bladder or uterus
What does the thoracic duct empty into?	Left subclavian vein; left internal jugular vein junction
What is the coronary vein?	Left gastric vein
What is the hypogastric artery?	Internal iliac artery
What is longer, the left or right renal vein?	The left
What are the layers of the abdominal wall?	1. Skin, then fat 2. Scarpa's fascia, then more fat 3. External oblique 4. Internal oblique 5. Transversus abdominis 6. Transversalis fascia 7. Preperitoneal fat 8. Peritoneum

What are the plicae circulares?

Plicae = folds, circulares = circular; thus, the circular folds of mucosa (valvulae conniventes) of the small bowel

What are the major structural differences between the jejunum and ileum?

Jejunum—long vasa rectae; large plicae circulares; thicker wall
Ileum—shorter vasa rectae; smaller plicae circulares; thinner wall (think: **I**leum = **I**nferior vasa rectae, **I**nferior plicae circulares, and **I**nferior wall)

What are the major anatomic differences between the colon and the small bowel?

The colon has taenia coli, haustra, and appendices epiploicae (fat appendages), whereas the small intestine is smooth.

How far up does the diaphragm extend?

To the nipples in men (fourth intercostal space)

13 Fluids and Electrolytes

What are the two major body fluid compartments?

1. Intracellular
2. Extracellular

What are the two subcompartments of extracellular fluid?

1. Interstitial fluid (in between cells)
2. Intravascular fluid (plasma)

What percentage of body weight is in fluid?

60%

What percentage of body fluid is intracellular?

66%

What percentage of body fluid is extracellular?

33%

What percentage of extracellular fluid is in plasma?

25%

What percentage of extracellular fluid is interstitial?

75%

Body fluid composition?

Fluids = 60% total body weight
- Intracellular—40%
- Extracellular—20% (think: 60,40,20)
  - Interstitial—15%
  - Plasma—5% (think: 20,15,5)

On average, what percentage of body weight does blood account for in adults?

≈ 7%

How many liters of blood are in a 70-kg man?

$0.07 \times 70 = 5$ liters

What are the fluid requirements every 24 hours for each of the following substances:

Water? ≈ 30 to 35 ml/kg

Sodium and potassium? ≈ 1 mEq/kg

Chloride? ≈ 1.5 mEq/kg

What are the levels and sources of normal daily water loss?

Urine—1200 to 1500 ml (25–30 ml/kg)
Sweat—200 to 400 ml
Respiratory losses—500 to 700 ml
Feces—100 to 200 ml

What are the levels and sources of normal daily electrolyte loss?

Sodium and potassium = 100 mEq
Chloride = 150 mEq
(40 mEq/l sodium and chloride lost as sweat)

What is the physiologic response to hypovolemia?

Sodium/H_2O retention via renin → aldosterone, water retention via ADH, vasoconstriction via angiotensin II and sympathetics, low urine output and tachycardia (early), hypotension (late)

THIRD SPACING

What is it?

Fluid accumulation in the interstitium of tissues, as in edema, e.g., loss of fluid into the interstitium and lumen of a paralytic bowel following surgery (think of the intravascular and intracellular spaces as the first two spaces)

Note: third-spaced fluid tends to mobilize back into the intravascular space around the third postoperative day; beware of overhydration once the fluid begins to return to the intravascular space

What are the signs of third spacing?

Tachycardia
Decreased urine output

What is the treatment?

IV hydration with isotonic fluids

What are the surgical causes of the following conditions:

Metabolic acidosis?
Diarrhea, ileus, fistula, high-output ileostomy, renal tubular acidosis, carbonic anhydrase inhibitors (due to loss of bicarbonate), lactic acidosis, ketoacidosis, dehydration, renal failure, TPN, low flow, ischemia, necrotic tissue

Hypochloremic alkalosis?
NGT suction, loss of gastric HCl through vomiting/NGT

Metabolic alkalosis?
Vomiting, NG suction, diuretics, alkali ingestion, mineralocorticoid excess

Respiratory acidosis?
Hypoventilation (e.g., CNS depression), drugs (e.g., morphine), PTX, pleural effusion, parenchymal lung disease, acute airway obstruction

Respiratory alkalosis?
Hyperventilation (e.g., anxiety, pain, fever, wrong ventilator settings)

What is paradoxic alkalotic aciduria?
Occurs with hypokalemic or hypovolemic alkalosis (e.g., gastric fluid loss); H^+ is lost in the urine in exchange for Na^+ in an attempt to restore volume
H^+ is exchanged preferentially instead of K^+ because of the low concentration of K^+

With volume derangements (hypovolemia/hypervolemia), what changes are evident on physical exam?
Weight changes, skin turgor, jugular venous distention (JVD), mucosal membranes, rales (crackles)

With hypovolemia, what changes occur in vital signs?
Tachycardia, tachypnea, initial rise in diastolic blood pressure because of clamping down (peripheral vasoconstriction) with subsequent decrease in both systolic and diastolic blood pressure

What are the insensible fluid losses?

Feces—100 to 200 ml/24 hours
Breathing—500 to 700 ml/24 hours (**Note:** increases with fever and tachypnea)
Skin—approximately 300 ml/24 hours, increased with fever; thus, insensible fluid loss is not directly measured

What are the quantities of daily secretions?

Bile—approximately 1000 ml/24 hours
Gastric—approximately 2000 ml/24 hours
Pancreatic—approximately 600 ml/24 hours
Small intestine—approximately 3000 ml/day
Saliva—approximately 1500 ml/24 hours
Note: almost all secretions are reabsorbed

How can the estimated levels of daily secretions from bile, gastric, and small-bowel sources be remembered?

Alphabetically and numerically: B,G,S and 1,2,3; or B1, G2, S3 as bile, gastric, and small bowel produce roughly 1 L, 2 L, and 3 L, respectively!

What are the principles of fluid and electrolyte replacement?

1. Replace deficits
2. Fulfill daily maintenance requirements
3. Replace ongoing losses

COMMON IV REPLACEMENT FLUIDS (ALL VALUES ARE PER LITER)

What comprises normal saline (NS)?

154 mEq of Cl^-
154 mEq of Na^+

What comprises ½ NS?

77 mEq of Cl^-
77 mEq of Na^+

What comprises 1/4 NS?

39 mEq of Cl^-
39 mEq of Na^+

What comprises lactated Ringer's (LR)?

130 mEq Na^+
110 mEq Cl^-
28 mEq lactate
4 mEq K^+
3 mEq Ca^+

D5W?	5% dextrose (50 g) in H_2O
What accounts for tonicity?	Mainly electrolytes; thus, NS and LR are both isotonic, whereas ½ NS is hypotonic to serum
What happens to the lactate in LR in the body?	Converted into bicarbonate; thus, LR cannot be used as a maintenance fluid because patients would become alkalotic

CALCULATION OF MAINTENANCE FLUIDS

What is the 100/50/20 rule?	Maintenance IV fluids for a 24-hour period 100 ml/kg for the first 10 kg 50 ml/kg for the next 10 kg 20 ml/kg for every kg over 20 (divide by 24 for hourly rate)
What is the 4/2/1 rule?	Maintenance IV fluids—hourly rate 4 ml/kg for the first 10 kg 2 ml/kg for the next 10 kg 1 ml/kg for every kg over 20
What is the maintenance for a 70-kg man?	Using 100/50/20: 100 × 10 kg = 1000 50 × 10 kg = 500 20 × 50 kg = 1000 Total = 2500 Divided by 24 hours: 104 ml/hr maintenance rate Using 4/2/1: 4 × 10 kg = 40 2 × 10 kg = 20 1 × 50 kg = 50 Total = 110 ml/hr maintenance rate
What is the common adult maintenance fluid?	D5 ½ NS with 20 mEq KCl/L
What is the common pediatric maintenance fluid?	D5 1/4 NS with 20 mEq KCl/L (use 1/4 NS because of decreased ability of children to concentrate urine)
Why should sugar be added to maintenance fluid?	To inhibit muscle breakdown

What is the best way to assess fluid status?	Urine output (unless the patient has cardiac or renal dysfunction, in which case central venous pressure or wedge pressure is often used)
What is the minimal urine output for an adult on maintenance IV?	30 ml/hr
What is the minimal urine output for an adult trauma patient?	50 ml/hr
How many ml are in 12 oz?	356
How many ml are in 1 oz?	30
How many ml are in 1 tsp?	5
What are common isotonic fluids?	NS, LR
What is a bolus?	A volume of fluid given IV in a rapid manner (e.g., 1 L over 1 hour); used for increasing intravascular volume and isotonic fluids should be used (i.e., NS or LR)
Why not combine bolus fluids with dextrose?	Hyperglycemia may result
What is the possible consequence of hyperglycemia in the hypovolemic patient?	Osmotic diuresis
Why not combine bolus fluids with a significant amount of potassium?	Hyperkalemia may result (the potassium in LR is very low: 4 mEg/L)
Why should isotonic fluids be given for resuscitation (i.e., to restore intravascular volume)?	If hypotonic fluid is given, the tonicity of the intravascular space will be decreased and H_2O will freely diffuse into the interstitial and intracellular spaces. Thus, use isotonic fluids to expand the intravascular space.

What portion of 1 L NS will stay in the intravascular space after a laparotomy?	In 5 hours, only approximately 200 cc will remain in the intravascular space!
What is the most common trauma resuscitation fluid?	LR
What is the most common postoperative IV fluid after a laparotomy?	D5LR for 24 to 36 hours, followed by maintenance fluid
After a laparotomy, when should a patient's fluid be "mobilized"?	Classically, postoperative day 3; the patient begins to mobilize the "third-space fluid" back into the intravascular space

ELECTROLYTE IMBALANCES

What is a common cause of electrolyte abnormalities?	Lab error!

HYPERKALEMIA

What are the surgical causes?	Iatrogenic overdose, blood transfusion, renal failure, diuretics, acidosis, tissue destruction (injury/hemolysis)
What are the signs/ symptoms?	Decreased deep tendon reflex (DTR) or areflexia, weakness, paraesthesia, paralysis, respiratory failure
What are the EKG findings?	**Peaked T waves,** depressed ST segment, prolonged PR, wide QRS, bradycardia, ventricular fibrillation
What are the critical values?	$K^+ > 6.5$
What is the urgent treatment?	IV calcium, EKG monitoring, IV (cardioprotective) Sodium bicarbonate IV (alkalosis drives K^+ intracellularly) Glucose and insulin Albuterol Sodium polystyrene sulfonate (Kayexalate) and **furosemide** (Lasix) Dialysis

What is the nonacute treatment?	Furosemide (Lasix), sodium polystyrene sulfonate (Kayexalate)

HYPOKALEMIA

What are the surgical causes?	Diuretics, certain antibiotics, steroids, alkalosis, diarrhea, intestinal fistulae, NG aspiration, vomiting, insulin, insufficient supplementation, amphotericin
What are the signs/ symptoms?	Weakness, tetany, nausea, vomiting, **ileus,** paraesthesia
What are the EKG findings?	**Flattening of T waves, U waves,** ST segment depression, PAC, PVC, atrial fibrillation
What is the rapid treatment?	KCl IV
What is the chronic treatment?	KCl PO
What is the most common electrolyte-mediated ileus in the surgical patient?	Hypokalemia
What electrolyte condition exacerbates digitalis toxicity?	Hypokalemia

HYPERNATREMIA

What are the surgical causes?	Inadequate hydration, diabetes insipidus, diuresis, vomiting, diarrhea, diaphoresis, tachypnea, iatrogenic (e.g., TPN)
What are the signs/ symptoms?	Seizures, confusion, stupor, pulmonary or peripheral edema, tremors, respiratory paralysis
What is the treatment supplementation slowly over days?	D5W or ½ NS

HYPONATREMIA

What are the surgical causes of the following types:

Hypovolemic? Diuretic excess, hypoaldosteronism, vomiting, NG suction, burns, pancreatitis, diaphoresis

Euvolemic? SIADH, CNS abnormalities, drugs

Hypervolemic? Renal failure, CHF, liver failure (cirrhosis), iatrogenic fluid overload (dilutional)

What are the signs/ symptoms? Seizures, coma, nausea, vomiting, ileus, lethargy, confusion, weakness

What is the treatment of the following types:

Hypovolemic? NS IV, correct underlying cause

Euvolemic? SIADH: furosemide and NS acutely, fluid restriction

Hypervolemic? Dilutional: fluid restriction and diuretics

"PSEUDOHYPONATREMIA"

What is it? Spurious lab value of hyponatremia due to hyperglycemia, hyperlipidemia, or hyperproteinemia

HYPERCALCEMIA

What are the causes? "C.H.I.M.P.A.N.Z.E.E.S.":

Calcium supplementation IV
Hyperparathyroidism (1°/3°) hyperthyroidism
Immobility/iatrogenic (thiazide diuretics)
Mets/Milk alkali syndrome
Paget's disease (bone)
Addison's disease/acromegaly
Neoplasm (colon, lung, breast, prostate, multiple myeloma)
Zollinger-Ellison syndrome (as part of MEN I)
Excessive vitamin D
Excessive vitamin A
Sarcoid

What are the signs/ symptoms?	Hypercalcemia—"Stones, bones, abdominal groans, and psychiatric overtones"
What are the EKG findings?	Short QT interval, prolonged PR interval
What is the acute treatment?	Volume expansion with NS, diuresis with furosemide (not thiazides), steroids, calcitonin, phosphate, dialysis
What is the chronic treatment?	Restrict calcium intake, steroids, phosphate

HYPOCALCEMIA

What are the surgical causes?	Short bowel syndrome, intestinal bypass, vitamin D deficiency, sepsis, acute pancreatitis, osteoblastic metastasis, aminoglycosides, diuretics, renal failure, hypomagnesemia, rhabdomyolysis
What is Chvostek's sign?	Facial muscle spasm with tapping of facial nerve
What is Trousseau's sign?	Carpal spasm after occluding blood flow in forearm with blood pressure cuff
What are the signs/ symptoms?	Chvostek's and Trousseau's signs, paraesthesia (early), increased deep tendon reflexes (late), confusion, abdominal cramps, laryngospasm, stridor, seizures, tetany, psychiatric abnormalities (e.g., paranoia, depression, hallucinations)
What are the EKG findings?	Prolonged QT and ST interval (peaked T-waves are also possible, as in hyperkalemia)
What is the acute treatment?	Calcium gluconate IV
What is the chronic treatment?	Calcium PO, vitamin D

What is the possible complication of infused calcium if the IV infiltrates?	**Tissue necrosis;** never administer peripherally unless absolutely necessary (calcium gluconate is less toxic than calcium chloride during an infiltration)

HYPERMAGNESEMIA

What is the surgical cause?	TPN, renal failure, IV over supplementation
What are the signs/ symptoms?	Respiratory failure, CNS depression, decreased deep tendon reflexes (Remember on Obstetrics–Gynecology)
What is the treatment?	Calcium gluconate IV, insulin plus glucose, dialysis (similar to treatment of hyperkalemia), furosemide (Lasix)

HYPOMAGNESEMIA

What are the surgical causes?	TPN, hypocalcemia, gastric suctioning, aminoglycosides, renal failure, diarrhea, vomiting
What are the signs/ symptoms?	Increased deep tendon reflexes, tetany, asterixis, tremor, Chvostek's sign, ventricular ectopy, vertigo, tachycardia, arrhythmias
What is the acute treatment?	$MgSO_4$ IV
What is the chronic treatment?	Magnesium oxide PO (side effect: diarrhea)

HYPERGLYCEMIA

What are the surgical causes?	Diabetes (poor control), infection, stress, TPN, drugs, lab error (drawing over IV site)
What are the signs/ symptoms?	Polyuria, hypovolemia, confusion/coma, polydipsia, ileus, DKA (Kussmaul breathing), abdominal pain, hyporeflexia
What is the treatment?	IVF, insulin, monitoring of glucose and electrolytes

HYPOGLYCEMIA

What are the surgical causes?
Excess insulin, decreased caloric intake, insulinoma, drugs, liver failure, adrenal insufficiency, gastrojejunostomy

What are the signs/ symptoms?
Sympathetic response (diaphoresis, tachycardia, palpitations), confusion, coma, headache, diplopia, neurologic deficits, seizures

What is the treatment?
Glucose (IV or PO)

How is Ca^{++} level corrected in hypoalbuminemia?
(4 – measured albumin level) × 0.8, added to the measured Ca_2^+ level

MISCELLANEOUS

This EKG pattern is consistent with which electrolyte abnormality?
Hyperkalemia: Peaked T-waves

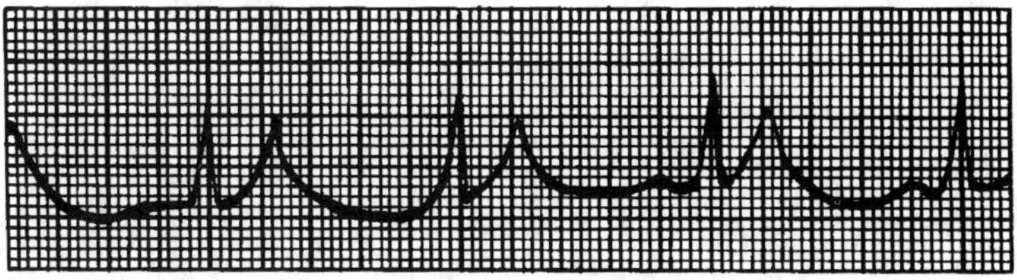

If hyperkalemia is left untreated, what can occur?
Ventricular tachycardia/fibrillation → death

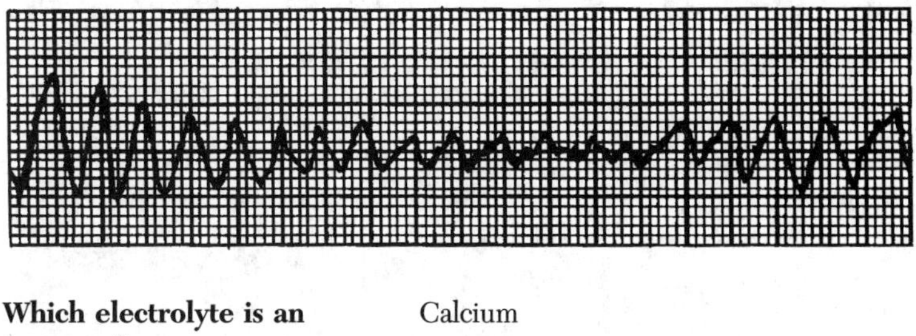

Which electrolyte is an inotrope?
Calcium

What are the major cardiac electrolytes?
Potassium (arrhythmias), magnesium (arrhythmias), calcium (arrhythmias/ inotrope)

Which electrolyte must be monitored closely in patients on digitalis?	Potassium
What is the most common cause of electrolyte-mediated ileus?	Potassium
What is a colloid fluid?	Protein-containing fluid (albumin)
What is the rationale for using an albumin-furosemide "sandwich"?	The albumin will pull interstitial fluid into the intravascular space and the furosemide will then help excrete the fluid as urine.

14

Blood and Blood Products

Define the following terms:	
Whole blood	One unit = 450 ml (±50 ml); deficient in platelets and clotting factors V, VIII, and XI; **rarely used**
Packed red blood cells (PRBCs)	One unit ≈ 300 ml (±50 ml); no platelets or clotting factors; can be mixed with NS to infuse faster
Platelets	Replace platelets; 1 (random donor) unit ≈ 50 ml; usually 6 to 8 units or one single donor unit (250–300 ml) are infused
Fresh frozen plasma (FFP)?	Replaces **clotting factors;** no RBCs/WBCs/platelets
Cryoprecipitate (cryo)?	Replaces fibrinogen and some clotting factors
Which electrolyte is most likely to fall with the infusion of stored blood? Why?	Ionized calcium; the citrate preservative used for the storage of blood binds serum calcium
What changes occur in the storage of whole blood?	↓ $Ca2^{+}$, ↑ K^{+}, ↓ 2,3-DPG, ↑ H^{+} (↓ pH), ↓ clotting factors (V, VII, & XI), ↓ PMNs
What is the rough formula for converting Hgb to Hct?	Hbg × 3 ≈ Hct
One unit PRBC ↑ Hct by how much?	≈ 3% to 4%
Which blood type is the universal donor?	O negative

What is a type and screen?
Blood clot in blood bank; patient's blood type is determined and the blood is screened for antibodies; a type and cross from that sample can then be ordered if needed later

What is a type and cross?
Patient's blood is sent to the blood bank and cross-matched for **specific units for possible blood transfusion.**

Define thrombocytopenia.
Low platelet count

What are the common causes of thrombocytopenia in the surgical patient?
Sepsis, H_2 blockers, heparin, massive transfusion, DIC, antibiotics, spurious lab value, Swann-Ganz catheter

What can be given to help correct uremic platelet dysfunction?
DDAVP

What common medication causes platelets to irreversibly malfunction?
Aspirin (inhibits cyclooxygenase)

What platelet count is associated with spontaneous bleeding?
Less than 20,000

What should the platelet count be before a surgical procedure?
Greater than 50,000

What is microcytic anemia "until proven otherwise" in a man or postmenopausal woman?
Colon cancer

Why not infuse PRBCs with lactated Ringer's?
The calcium will result in coagulation within the IV line

What is the most common cause of transfusion hemolysis?
ABO incompatibility due to **clerical error**

What is widely stated to be the optimal Hct?
Approximately 30%

What is the optimal Hct in a patient with a history of heart disease or strokes?	Approximately 30%
When should aspirin administration be discontinued preoperatively?	At 1 week because platelets live 7 to 10 days
What can move the oxyhemoglobin dissociation curve to the right?	Acidosis, 2,3-DPG, fever, elevated PCO_2 (to the right means greater ability to release the O_2)
What is the normal life of RBCs?	120 days
What is the normal life of platelets?	From 7 to 10 days
What factor is deficient in hemophilia A?	Factor VIII
How do you remember the clotting factor for hemophilia A?	Think: **Eight** sounds like **A**
What is the preoperative treatment of hemophilia A?	Factor VIII infusion to ≥ 100% normal preoperative levels
What coagulation study is elevated with hemophila A?	PTT
How do you remember which coagulation study is affected by the hemophilias?	There are two major hemophilias and two t's in PTT
What factor is deficient in hemophilia B?	Factor IX
How do you remember which factors are deficient with hemophilia A and hemophilia B?	Alphabetically and chronologically: A before B and VIII before IX; thus, hemophilia A is factor VIII and hemophilia B is factor IX
What is Christmas disease?	Hemophilia B

How are Hemophilias A and B inherited?

Sex-linked recessive

What is von Willebrand's disease?

Deficiency of von Willebrand factor (vWF) and factor VIII:C

What coagulation is abnormal with the following disorders:

Hemophilia A?

PTT (elevated)

Hemophilia B?

PTT (elevated)

Von Willebrand's disease?

Bleeding time

What is the effect on the coagulation system if the patient has a deficiency in protein C, protein S, or antithrombin III?

A hypercoagulable state

What is a "left shift" on a CBC?

Juvenile polymorphonuclear leukocytes (bands),and most now include neutrophils greater than 80%

15 Surgical Hemostasis

What motto is associated with surgical hemostasis?

"All bleeding stops."

What is the most immediate method of obtaining hemostasis?

Pressure (finger)

What is the "Bovie"?

Electrocautery (designed by Bovie with Cushing for neurosurgery in the 1920s)

What is the CUT mode on the Bovie?

Continuous electrical current (20,000 Hz); cuts well with a decreased ability to coagulate

What is the COAG mode on the Bovie?

Intermittent electrical current (20,000 Hz); results in excellent vessel coagulation with decreased ability to cut

Where should a Bovie be applied to a clamp or pick-up to coagulate a vessel?

Anywhere on the clamp/pick-up

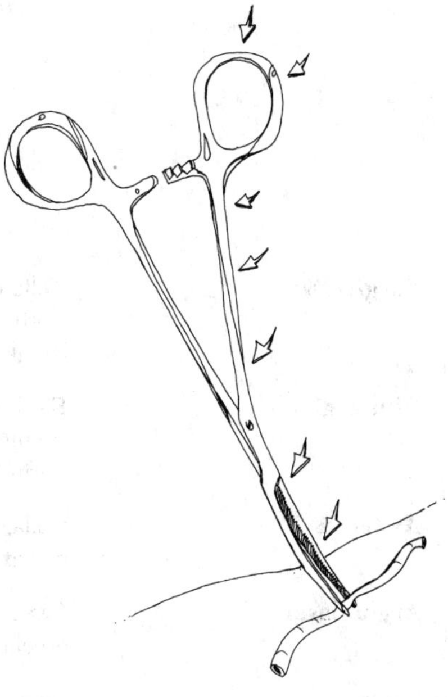

Define the following terms:

Figure of eight suture — Suture ligature placed **twice** in the tissue prior to being tied

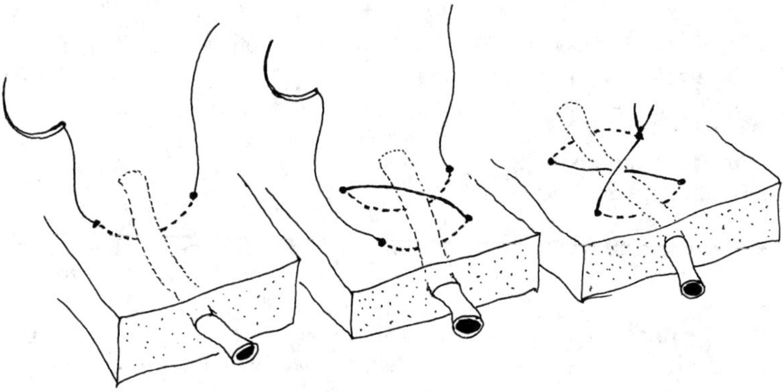

Vessel "tied in continuity" — Tie, tie, cut in between

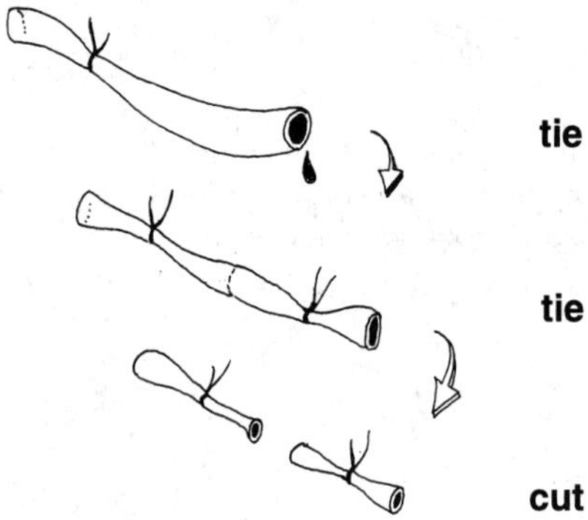

Surgicel® — Cellulose sheets—act as framework for clotting factors/platelets to adhere to (think: Surgi**cel** = **cel**lulose)

Fibrin glue — Fibrinogen and thrombin sprayed simultaneously and mixed to produce a fibrin "glue"

Avitene® — Collagen powder or sheets; act as a matrix for clotting factors/platelets

Argon laser — Laser for topical hemostasis by heat; excellent for liver oozing

Clips — Metallic clips for clipping vessels

16

Common Surgical Medications

ANTIBIOTICS

What do first-, second-, and third-generation cephalosporin refer to in regard to spectrum?	Gram-negative activity (third-generation has the most)
Which antibiotics are commonly used for anaerobic infections?	Metronidazole, clindamycin, cefoxitin, cefotetan, imipenem, ticarcillin-clavulanic acid, ampicillin-sulbactam
Which antibiotics are commonly used for gram-negative infections?	Gentamicin and other aminoglycosides, ciprofloxacin, aztreonam, third-generation cephalosporins, sulfamethoxazole-trimethoprim
How do the following agents work:	
Penicillins?	β-lactam (inhibits cell-wall synthesis)
Cephalosporins?	β-lactam
Ciprofloxin (Cipro)?	Binds DNA helicase
Gentamycin?	Inhibits bacterial ribosomes
Vancomycin?	Inhibits cell wall by inhibiting peptidoglycan polymers
Imipenem (Primaxin)?	β-lactam
Clindamycin?	Binds bacterial ribosomes
Which antibiotic, if taken with alcohol, will give a disulfiram-like reaction?	Metronidazole (Flagyl); disulfiram is Antabuse

What is the drug of choice for treating amoebic infections?

Metronidazole (Flagyl)

Which antibiotic is associated with cholestasis?

Ceftriaxone (Rocephin)

Which antibiotic cannot be given to children?

Ciprofloxacin (interferes with the growth plate)

With which medications must serum levels be determined?

Aminoglycosides (most commonly gentamicin peak and "trough"; some experts also believe in determining serum levels with vancomycin

Is rash (only) in response to penicillins a contraindication to cephalosporins?

No, but breathing problems, urticaria, and edema in response to penicillins are contraindications to the cephalosporins

Describe the following medications:

Cefazolin (Ancef)

First-generation cephalosporin; surgical prophylaxis for **skin flora**

Cefoxitin (Mefoxin)

Second-generation cephalosporin; used for mixed aerobic/anaerobic infections; effective against *Bacteroides fragilis*; effective against **anaerobic bacteria**

Ceftazidime (Ceftaz)

Third-generation cephalosporin; strong activity against Pseudomonas

Clindamycin

Strong activity against gram-negative **anaerobes,** such as *B. fragilis,* adequate gram-positive activity

Gentamicin

Aminoglycoside used to treat **gram-negative** bacteria; nephrotoxic, ototoxic; blood peak/trough levels should be monitored

Imipenem and cilastatin (Primaxin)

Often used as a last resort against serious, multiresistant organisms

Usually combined with cilastin, which inhibits the renal excretion of imipenem

Has a very wide spectrum

Metronidazole (Flagyl)	Used for serious **anaerobic** infections (e.g., diverticulitis); also used to treat amebiasis; patient must abstain from alcohol use during therapy
Mezlocillin (Mezlo)	An antipseudomonal penicillin with good activity against Enterobacteriaceae; commonly used for cholangitis because it covers the common biliary tract organisms
What is mezlocillin's (Mezlo's) claim to fame?	The concentration in bile is much greater than that of serum.
Nafcillin (Nafcil)	Antistaphylococcal penicillin commonly used for cellulitis
Vancomycin	Used to treat methicillin-resistant Staphylococcus aureus (MRSA); used orally to treat *C. difficile* pseudomembranous colitis (poorly absorbed from the gut); with IV administration, peak/trough levels should be monitored
Meperidine (Demerol)	Injectable narcotic; used commonly with acute pancreatitis/biliary pathology because morphine may cause sphincter of Oddi spasm/constriction
Percocet	PO narcotic pain reliever with acetominphen and oxycodone
Ciprofloxicin (Cipro)	Quinoline antibiotic with broad-spectrum activity, especially against gram-negative bacteria, including *Pseudomonas*
Aztreonam (Azactam)	Monobactam with gram-negative spectrum
Amphotericin	IV antifungal antibiotic associated with renal toxicity
Dantrolene (Dantrium)	Medication used to treat malignant hyperthermia

Fluconazole (Diflucan)	Antifungal agent (IV or PO) **not** associated with renal toxicity
Nystatin	PO and topical antifungal

STEROIDS

What are the side effects?	Adrenal suppression, immunosuppression, weight gain with central obesity, cushingoid facies, acne, hirsutism, purple striae, hyperglycemia, sodium retention/hypokalemia, hypertension, osteopenia, myopathy, ischemic bone necrosis (avascular necrosis of the hip), gastrointestinal perforations
What are its uses?	Immunosuppression (transplant), autoimmune diseases, hormone replacement (Addison's disease), spinal cord trauma **Steroids should never be stopped acutely; always taper.**
Which patients need stress-dose steroids before surgery?	Those who are on steroids, have suspected hypoadrenalism, or are about to undergo adrenalectomy
What is the "stress dose" for steroids?	**100** mg of hydrocortisone IV Q 8 hours and then taper
Which vitamin helps counteract the deleterious effects of steroids on wound healing?	Vitamin A

HEPARIN

Describe the action.	Binds with and **activates antithrombin III; PTT** level should be monitored and maintained at about **one-and-a-half** to two times the normal rate
What are its uses?	Prophylaxis/treatment—DVT, pulmonary embolism, stroke, atrial fibrillation, acute occlusion of an artery, cardiopulmonary bypass

What are the side effects? Bleeding complications; can cause thrombocytopenia

What reverses the effects? **Protamine** IV (**1**:**100**, **1** mg of protamine to every **100** units of heparin)

Who is at risk for a protamine anaphylactic reaction? Patients with IDDM

What is the half-life of heparin? Approximately 90 minutes

How long before surgery should it be discontinued? From 4 to 6 hours preoperatively

Does heparin dissolve clots? No; it stops the progression of clot formation and allows the body's own fibrinolytic systems to dissolve the clot

WARFARIN (COUMADIN)

Describe its action. **Inhibits vitamin K–dependent clotting factors II, VII, IX, X,** (i.e., 2, 7, 9, **10**) produced in the liver; monitor PT levels, maintain at **one-and-a-half to two** times the normal level

What are its uses? Long-term anticoagulation (PO)

What risk is it associated with? Bleeding complications, teratogenic in pregnancy

What is the half-life of effect? **48 hours;** thus, it takes 2 days to observe a change in the PT

What reverses the action? **Cessation,** vitamin K, fresh-frozen plasma (in emergencies)

How long before surgery should it be discontinued? From 3 to 5 days preoperatively and IV heparin should be begun; heparin should be discontinued from 4 to 6 hours preoperatively, and can be restarted postoperatively; coumadin can be restarted in a few days

Describe the following drugs:	
Sucralfate (Carafate)	Treats peptic ulcers by forming an acid-resistant barrier; binds to ulcer craters; needs acid to activate and thus should not be used with H_2 blockers
Cimetidine (Tagamet)	H_2 blocker (ulcers/gastritis)
Ranitidine (Zantac)	H_2 blocker (ulcers/gastritis)
Omeprazole (Prilosec)	Gastric acid–secretion inhibitor; works by inhibiting the **K^+/H^+-ATPase** (Note: causes carcinoid tumors in rats)
Promethazine (Phenergan)	Acute antinausea agent; used postoperatively
Metoclopramide (Reglan)	Increases gastric emptying with increase in LES pressure; **dopamine antagonist;** used in diabetic gastroparesis and to help move feeding tubes past the pylorus
Albumin	5% albumin—expands plasma volume 25% albumin—draws extravascular fluid into intravascular space by oncotic pressure
Famotidine (Pepcid)	H_2 blocker
Aspirin	Irreversibly inhibits platelets by irreversibly inhibiting cyclooxygenase
Furosemide (Lasix)	Loop diuretic (watch for hypokalemia)
If the patient does not respond to a dose of furosemide, should the dose be repeated? Increased? Decreased?	The dose should be doubled if there is no response to the initial dose.
What medication is used to treat promethazine-induced dystonia?	Diphenhydramine hydrochloride (Benadryl)

How does cisapride (Propulsid) work?	Increases ACH release from myenteric nerve cells (Auerbach's plexus) and increases enteric smooth-muscle contraction
What are the effects of cisapride (Propulsid)?	Increase esophageal peristalsis Increases LES tone Increases gastric emptying
What are the indications for cisapride (Propulsid)?	GE reflux (heartburn), gastroparesis
Which medication is classically associated with mesenteric ischemia?	Digitalis
What type of antihypertensive medication is contraindicated in patients with renal artery stenosis?	Ace inhibitors
Does acetaminophen (Tylenol) inhibit platelets?	No
What medications are used to stop seizures?	Bezodiazepines (e.g., lorazepam [Ativan]); phenytoin (Dilantin)

17 Complications

ATELECTASIS

What is it?
Collapse of the alveoli

What is the etiology?
Inadequate alveolar expansion (i.e., poor ventilation of lungs during surgery, inability to fully inspire secondary to pain, excessive sputum retarding air flow)

What are the signs?
Fever, decreased breath sounds with rales present, tachypnea, tachycardia, and increased density on CXR

What are the risk factors?
Chronic obstructive pulmonary disease (COPD), smoking, abdominal or thoracic surgery, oversedation, poor pain control **(patient unable to breathe in deeply secondary to pain on inspiration)**

What is its claim to fame?
Most common cause of postoperative fever during POD 1 to 2

What prophylactic measures can be taken?
Preoperative cessation of smoking, incentive spirometry, good pain control

What is the treatment?
Postoperative deep breathing, coughing, postural drainage, suctioning, chest PT, and incentive spirometry

POSTOPERATIVE RESPIRATORY FAILURE

What is it?
RR > 25
pH < 7.20
$P_{CO_2} > 50$
$PO_2 < 60$
Note: these values are approximations and must be compared with baseline values and clinical picture

What is the differential diagnosis?

Hypovolemia, pulmonary embolism, impaired respiratory drive with administration of O_2 to a patient with chronic CO_2 retention (i.e., COPD), atelectasis, pneumonia, increased intraabdominal pressure, pneumothorax, chylothorax, hemothorax, narcotic overdose, mucus plug

What is the treatment?

O_2 and intubation/ventilation if necessary; chest PT; suctioning

What are the possible causes of postoperative pleural effusion?

Diaphragmatic inflammation with possible subphrenic abscess formation, fluid overload, pneumonia

What is the treatment of postoperative wheezing?

Albuterol nebulizer

PULMONARY EMBOLISM

What is it?

Blood clot from the venous system (usually lower extremity or pelvic veins are site of origin) that embolizes to the pulmonary arterial system

What are the risk factors?

Postoperative status, immobility, CHF, obesity, use of oral contraceptives, neoplastic disease, advanced age, polycythemia, MI, hypercoagulable state (protein C/protein S deficiency)

What are the signs/ symptoms?

Shortness of breath, tachypnea, hypotension, CP, occasionally fever, tender LE, loud pulmonic component of S_2, hemoptysis with pulmonary infarct

What is Homan's sign?

Calf pain with dorsiflexion of the foot seen classically with DVT, but actually found in fewer than one-third of patients with DVT

What are the associated lab findings?

Arterial blood gas (ABG)—decreased PO_2 and Pco_2 (from hyperventilation)

Which diagnostic tests are indicated?

V-Q scan (ventilation–perfusion scan), **pulmonary A-gram is the gold standard**

What are the associated CXR findings?	Westermark's sign (wedge-shaped area of decreased pulmonary vasculature) or, rarely, a wedge-shaped area of infarction.
What are the associated EKG findings?	More than 50% are abnormal; classic finding is cor pulmonale (S1Q3T3 RBBB, and right-axis deviation); EKG most commonly shows flipped T waves or ST depression
What is a "saddle" embolus?	Pulmonary embolism (PE) that "straddles" the pulmonary artery and is in the lumen of both the right and left pulmonary arteries
What is the treatment if the patient is stable?	Anticoagulation (heparin bolus followed by infusion) Greenfield filter, if anticoagulation is contraindicated or if patient has further PE on adequate anticoagulation PA gram with local infusion of thrombolytics via PA catheter is now an option Long-term warfarin (Coumadin) anticoagulation
What is the treatment if the patient is unstable?	Consult thoracic surgeon for possible thoracotomy and operative embolectomy; consider thrombolytic therapy; consider catheter suction embolectomy
What prophylactic measures can be taken for DVT/PE?	Sub-Q heparin (5,000 units sub-Q every 8–12 hrs; must be started preoperatively), sequential compression device BOOTS beginning in OR (often used with sub-Q heparin), compression hose, early ambulation

What is a Greenfield filter?

Metallic filter placed into IVC via femoral or subclavian vein to catch emboli prior to lodging in the pulmonary artery

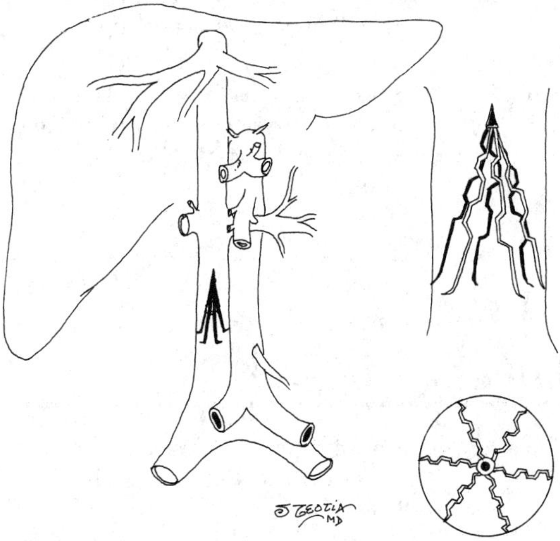

ASPIRATION PNEUMONIA

What is it?

Pneumonia following aspiration of vomitus

What are the risk factors?

Intubation/extubation, impaired consciousness, (i.e., drug or ETOH overdose), dysphagia (esophageal disease), nonfunctioning NGT, Trendelenburg position, OR emergent intubation with full stomach

What are the signs/ symptoms?

Respiratory failure, CP, increased sputum production, fever, cough, mental status changes, tachycardia, cyanosis, infiltrate on CXR

What are the associated CXR findings?

Early—fluffy infiltrate or normal CXR
Late—pneumonia, ARDS

Which lobes are commonly involved?

Supine—RUL
Sitting/semirecumbent—RLL

Which organisms are commonly involved?
Community acquired—gram-positive/mixed
Hospital/ICU—gram-negative rods

Which diagnostic tests are indicated?
CXR, sputum, Gram stain, sputum culture, bronchoalveolar lavage

What is the treatment?
Bronchoscopy, antibiotics if pneumonia develops, intubation if respiratory failure occurs, ventilation with PEEP if ARDS develops

What is Mendelson's syndrome?
Chemical pneumonitis secondary to aspiration of the stomach contents (i.e., gastric acid)

GASTROINTESTINAL COMPLICATIONS

What are the possible NGT complications?
Aspiration-pneumonia/atelectasis (especially if NGT is clogged)
Sinusitis
Minor UGI bleeding
Epistaxisis
Pharyngeal irritation

GASTRIC DILATATION

What are the risk factors?
Abdominal surgery, gastric outlet obstruction, splenectomy

What are the signs/symptoms?
Abdominal distension, hiccups, electrolyte abnormalities, and nausea

What is the treatment?
NGT decompression

POSTOPERATIVE PANCREATITIS

What is it?
Pancreatitis due to manipulation of the pancreas during surgery or low blood flow during the procedure (i.e., cardiopulmonary bypass)

What is the treatment?
Same as that of the other causes of pancreatitis (e.g., NPO, ± NGT, fluid resuscitation)

CONSTIPATION

What is the treatment?	OBR
What is OBR?	**O**rtho **B**owel **R**outine: docusate sodium (daily), dicacodyl suppository if no bowel movement occurs, Fleet® enema if suppository is ineffective

SHORT BOWEL SYNDROME

What is it?	Malabsorption and diarrhea resulting from extensive bowel resection (approximately ≤ 100 cm of small bowel remaining)
What is the initial treatment?	TPN early, followed by many small meals chronically

POSTOPERATIVE SBO/ILEUS

What causes are related to small bowel obstruction?	**Adhesions** (most of which resolve spontaneously), incarcerated hernia (internal or fascial/dehiscence), intussusception
What causes are related to ileus?	Adynamic ileus (normal after laparotomy), ileus due to hypokalemia, ileus due to narcotics, intraperitoneal infection
What are the signs of resolving ileus/small bowel obstruction?	Flatus PR, stool PR
What is the order of recovery of bowel function after abdominal surgery?	**First**—small intestine **Second**—stomach **Third**—colon
When can a postoperative patient be fed through a J tube?	From 12 to 24 postoperative hours because the small intestine recovers function first in that period

What are the causes of the following types of postoperative jaundice:

Prehepatic?

Hemolysis (prosthetic valve), resolving hematoma, transfusion reaction, postcardiopulmonary bypass, blood transfusions (decreased RBC compliance leading to cell rupture)

Hepatic?

Drugs, hypotension, hypoxia, sepsis, hepatitis, "sympathetic" hepatic inflammation from adjacent right lower lobe infarction of the lung or pneumonia, preexisting cirrhosis, right-sided heart failure, hepatic abscess, pylephlebitis (thrombosis of portal vein), Gilbert syndrome, Crigler-Najjar syndrome, Dubin-Johnson syndrome, fatty infiltrate from TPN

Posthepatic?

Obstruction (stone), cholangitis, cholecystitis, biliary-duct injury, pancreatitis, sclerosing cholangitis, tumors (e.g., cholangiocarcinoma, pancreatic cancer, gallbladder cancer, metastases), biliary stasis (e.g., ceftriaxone [Rocephin])

What blood tests would support the assumption that hemolysis was causing jaundice in a patient?

Decreased—Haptoglobin, Hct
Increased—LDH, reticulocytes
Also, fragmented RBCs on a peripheral smear

BLIND LOOP SYNDROME

What is it?

Bacterial overgrowth in the small intestine.
The organisms that tend to overgrow are not the normal flora of the small bowel (such as gram-positive, aerobic organisms resembling oropharyngeal flora). Rather, they are more representative of colonic flora (e.g., gram-negative bacteria like *Escherichia coli*, *Clostridium* and *Bacteroides* species)

What are the causes?

Anything that disrupts the normal flow of intestinal contents (i.e., causes stasis), stricture of the intestine, Crohn's disease, postvagotomy syndromes, scleroderma, small bowel diverticula, decreased gastric acid secretion, incompetent ileocecal valve

What are the signs/ symptoms?

Diarrhea, steatorrhea, malnutrition, abdominal pain, hypocalcemia, megaloblastic anemia (due to B_{12} deficiency)

What is the pathogenesis of B_{12} deficiency?

Two hypotheses:

1. Bacterial utilization of B_{12}
2. Bacterial toxins inhibit the absorption of B_{12} across the small bowel mucosa

Which diagnostic tests are indicated?

Schilling test: demonstrating an intrinsic factor–resistant B_{12} malabsorption

Hydrogen breath test: lactose is swallowed and expiration of H_2 is monitored. With bacterial overgrowth there is increased H_2 production earlier than normal.

What is the treatment?

Surgical correction of the underlying disorder causing the stasis, if feasible; otherwise, antibiotics to inhibit bacterial overgrowth

What are the other causes of B_{12} deficiency?

Gastrectomy (decreased secretion of intrinsic factor) and excision of the terminal ileum (site of B_{12} absorption)

POUCHITIS

What is it?

Inflammation of the pouch of an ileoanal pull-through anastomosis (usually after a colectomy for ulcerative colitis)

What are the signs/ symptoms?

Fever, abdominal cramping, increased frequency of liquid stools

What is the treatment?

Metronidazole PO

AFFERENT LOOP SYNDROME

What is it?

Partial or total obstruction/kink of the afferent limb (draining bile/pancreatic secretions) following a **Billroth II,** with accumulation of bile and pancreatic secretions in the afferent limb

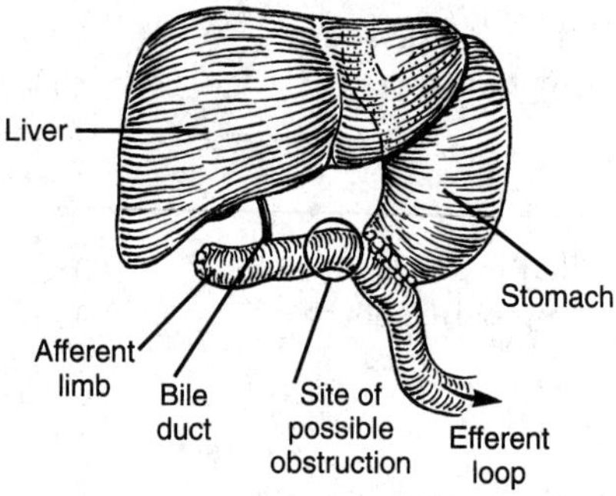

What are the signs/symptoms?

Postprandial right upper quadrant pain and bilious vomiting, anemia, steatorrhea; pain that often resolves suddenly after decompression of afferent limb

When does it present?

Approximately 66% present in the first postoperative week; otherwise it can occur anytime

What are the associated diagnostic findings?

UGI in which the afferent loop will not fill with contrast due to the obstruction or EGD

What is the treatment?

Balloon dilatation, surgical reanastomosis (e.g., Roux-en-Y)

EFFERENT LOOP SYNDROME

What is efferent loop syndrome?

Obstruction of the efferent loop or at the anastomosis of the gastric remnant to the efferent loop (efferent loop drains the stomach remnant)

What are the causes?

Adhesions, volvulus, hernia, omental wrap with fibrosis of the omentum, tight mesocolonic tunnel, anastomotic stricture

Which diagnostic tests are indicated?
Upper GI barium series, EGD

What is the treatment?
Surgical correction of obstruction, balloon dilatation of anastomotic anastomosis

ROUX STASIS SYNDROME

What is it?
Stasis of chyme in a gastric remnant

What is the cause?
Loss of normal jejunal and gastric motility (loss of migration of the normal pacemaker motor waves)

What are the signs/ symptoms?
Abdominal pain, nonbilious vomiting, nausea postprandially

What is the medical treatment?
Cisapride

What is the surgical treatment?
Shorten the Roux limb to 40 cm and perform complete gastrectomy

POSTVAGOTOMY DIARRHEA

What is it?
Diarrhea after a truncal vagotomy

What is the cause?
It is thought that after truncal vagotomy, a rapid transport of bile salts to the colon results in osmotic inhibition of water absorption in the colon, leading to diarrhea

What are the signs/ symptoms?
Diarrhea

What is the medical treatment?
Cholestyramine (binds bile salts)

What is the surgical treatment?
Reversed interposition jejunal segment

ALKALINE REFLUX GASTRITIS

What is it?

Reflux of bile into the stomach after a Billroth I, Billroth II, or pyloroplasty (NOTE: alkaline refers to the alkaline nature of bile in contrast to the more common gastritis due to gastric acidic environment)

What are the signs/ symptoms?

Epigastric burning, abdominal pain, nausea, weight loss, anemia, bilious vomiting

What is the major risk factor for alkaline reflux gastritis?

Billroth II

What are the associated diagnostic findings?

EGD—gastritis/bile
Biliary scan (pooling in stomach remnant)

What is the medical treatment?

H_2 blocker, cholestyramine, metoclopramide (Reglan)

What is the surgical treatment?

Conversion to Roux-en-Y

DUMPING SYNDROME

What is it?

Delivery of **hyperosmotic** chyme to the small intestine causing massive fluid shifts into the bowel (normally the stomach will decrease the osmolality of the chyme prior to its emptying)

With what conditions is it associated?

Any procedure that bypasses the pylorus or compromises its function (i.e., gastroenterostomies or pyloroplasty); thus, "dumping" of chyme into small intestine

What are the signs/ symptoms?

Postprandial diaphoresis, tachycardia, abdominal pain/distention, emesis, increased flatus, dizziness, weakness

How is the diagnosis made?

History; hyperosmolar glucose load will elicit similar symptoms

What is the medical treatment?

Small, multiple, low-fat/carbohydrate meals that are high in protein content; also, **avoidance of liquids** with meals to slow gastric emptying; surgery is a last resort

What is the surgical treatment?

Conversion to Roux-en-Y (+/- reversed jejunal interposition loop)

What is a reversed jejunal interposition loop?

A segment of jejunum is cut and then reversed to allow for a short segment of reversed peristalsis to slow intestinal transit.

ENDOCRINE COMPLICATIONS

DIABETIC KETOACIDOSIS (DKA)

What is it?

Deficiency of body insulin, resulting in hyperglycemia, formation of ketoacids, osmotic diuresis, and metabolic acidosis

What are the signs of DKA?

Polyuria, tachypnea, dehydration, confusion

What are the associated lab values?

Elevated glucose, increased anion gap, hypokalemia, urine ketones, acidosis

What is the treatment?

Insulin drip, IVF rehydration, K^+ supplementation ± bicarbonate IV

What electrolyte must be monitored closely in DKA?

Potassium

THYROID STORM

What is it?

Severe hyperthyroidism

What is the risk factor?

Hyperthyroidism

What events trigger this condition?

Infection, acute abdomen, surgery, trauma, any severe stressor

What are the signs?

Fever, tachycardia, psychosis, delirium/confusion, abdominal pain, nausea and vomiting, diaphoresis, CHF, pulmonary edema, tremors, hypertension, fever

What is the treatment? IVF, propylthiouracil (PTU), propanolol, steroids, (iodide can be administered if the patient is not febrile)

SIADH

What is it? Syndrome of inappropriate antidiuretic hormone (ADH) secretion, which results in excessive fluid retention (think of **inappropriate increase** in antidiuretic hormone secretion)

What are the causes? **Mainly lung/CNS:** CNS trauma, oat-cell lung cancer, pancreatic cancer, duodenal cancer, pneumonia/lung abscess, increased PEEP, stroke (cerebrovascular accident), general anesthesia, idiopathic, postoperative, morphine

What are the associated lab findings? Low sodium, low chloride, low serum osmolality, and increased urine osmolality

What is the treatment? Treat the primary cause and **restrict** fluid intake

DIABETES INSIPIDUS (DI)

What is it? Decreased release of ADH, resulting in massive I's and O's (think: **D**iabetes = **D**ecreased ADH)

What are the risk factors?
Central DI—head trauma, intracranial disorder
Nephrogenic DI—renal disease, electrolyte disorders, medications

What is the treatment? Vasopressin (IV, SQ, or intranasal) to replace the deficiency and massive quantities of IV fluids

ADDISONIAN CRISIS

What is it? Acute adrenal insufficiency in the face of a stressor (i.e., surgery, trauma, or infection); the normal response of increased glucocorticoid release is impaired

What are the signs/ symptoms?
Nausea, vomiting, diarrhea, **abdominal pain,** ± fever, progressive lethargy, **hypotension, eventual hypovolemic shock**

Which lab values are classic?
Decreased sodium, increased K^+ (secondary to decreased aldosterone)

What is the treatment?
IVFs (D5 NS), **hydrocortisone IV,** fludrocortisone PO

CARDIOVASCULAR COMPLICATIONS

What are the arterial line complications?
Infection; thrombosis, which can lead to finger/hand necrosis; death/hemorrhage due to catheter disconnection (remember to perform and document the **Allen test** before inserting an arterial line or obtaining a blood gas sample)

What is an Allen test?
Measures for adequate collateral blood flow to the hand via the ulnar artery: patient clenches fist, then both radial and ulnar arteries are occluded; patient opens the blanched hand. The ulnar artery is released. If the palm has an immediate strong blush, the ulnar artery should be adequate collateral flow if the radial artery thromboses.

What are the common causes of dyspnea following central line placement?
Pneumothorax, pericardial tamponade, carotid puncture (which can cause a hematoma that compresses the trachea), air embolism

What is the differential diagnosis of postoperative chest pain?
MI, atelectasis, pneumonia, pleurisy, esophageal reflux, pulmonary embolism, musculoskeletal pain, subphrenic abscess, aortic dissection, pneumo/chyle/hemothorax, gastritis

What is the differential diagnosis of postoperative atrial fibrillation?
Fluid overload, PE, MI, pain (excess catecholamines), atelectasis, pneumonia, digoxin toxicity, hypoxemia, thyrotoxicosis, hypercapnia, idiopathic, acidosis, electrolyte abnormalities

MYOCARDIAL INFARCTION (MI)

What is the most dangerous period for a postoperative MI following a previous MI?

Six months after an MI

What are the risk factors for postoperative MI?

History of MI, angina, Q's on EKG, S_3, JVD, CHF, aortic stenosis, advanced age, extensive surgical procedure, MI within 6 months, EKG changes

How do postoperative MIs present?

Often without chest pain
New onset **CHF,** new onset **cardiac arrhythmia,** hypotension, chest pain, tachypnea, tachycardia, nausea, vomiting, bradycardia, neck pain, arm pain

What EKG findings are associated with cardiac ischemia/MI?

Flipped T waves, ST elevation, ST depression, Q waves (usually late), arrhythmias (e.g., new onset a fib, PVC, V tach)

Which lab tests are indicated?

Cardiac isoenzymes (elevated CK mb fraction), troponin I

What is the treatment of postoperative MI?

Nitrates (paste or drip), as tolerated
Aspirin
Oxygen
Pain control with IV morphine
β-blocker, as tolerated
Heparin (possibly; thrombolytics are contraindicated in the postoperative patient)
ICU monitoring
(Memory aid for treating cardiac ischemia/MI: **BEMOAN—Be** = **Be**ta blocker [as tolerated], **M** = **M**orphine, **O** = **O**xygen, **A** = **A**spirin, **N** = **N**itrates [IV or paste])

When do postoperative MIs occur?

Two-thirds occur on postoperative days 2 through 5 (often silent and present with **dyspnea** or **arrhythmia**)

MISCELLANEOUS

FAT EMBOLI SYNDROME

What is it?	Embolization of fat particles
What are the risk factors?	Fractures of the long bones, trauma
What are the signs?	**Bergman's triad** (mental status changes, petechiae, and dyspnea); CXR picture similar to ARDS because fat particles cause a pneumonitis
What are the complications?	Respiratory failure, disseminated intravascular coagulation (DIC)
What is the treatment?	Ventilatory support with PEEP as necessary, ± steroids, and treatment of DIC (if it develops)

POSTOPERATIVE RENAL FAILURE

What is it?	Urine output less than 25 ml/hr (30 ml/hr is minimum adult output), increased creatinine, increased BUN
What is the differential diagnosis?	
Prerenal?	Inadequate fluids, hypotension, cardiac pump failure (CHF)
Renal?	Acute tubular necrosis, nephrotoxic dyes or drugs
Postrenal?	Foley catheter obstruction/stone, ureteral/urethral injury, BPH, bladder dysfunction (e.g., medications, spinal anesthesia)
What are the indications for dialysis?	Fluid overload, refractory hyperkalemia, BUN greater than 130, acidosis, uremic encephalopathy

DIC

What is it?	Activation of the coagulation cascade by a substance leading to **thrombosis and consumption** of clotting factors (especially factors V and VIII) and platelets, resulting in bleeding and then activation of fibrinolytic systems, resulting in fibrinolysis
What are the causes?	Tissue necrosis, septic shock, massive large-vessel coagulation, shock, allergic reactions, blood transfusion reaction, cardiopulmonary bypass, cancer, obstetric complications, snakebites, trauma, burn injury, prosthetic material, liver dysfunction
What are the signs/ symptoms?	Acrocyanosis or other signs of thrombosis, then diffuse bleeding from incision sites, venipuncture sites, catheter sites, or mucous membranes
What are the associated lab findings?	Increased fibrin-degradation products, elevated PT/PTT, decreased platelets, decreased fibrinogen (level correlates well with bleeding), presence of schistocytes (fragmented RBCs) increased D-dimer
What is the treatment?	**Removal of the cause;** otherwise supportive: IVFs, O_2, platelets, FFP, cryoprecipitate (fibrin), as needed Use of heparin is controversial, but may be indicated in cases that are predominantly thrombotic (usually early). Antithrombin III supplementation is often useful.

18

Common Causes of Ward Emergencies

What can cause hypotension?

Hypovolemia (iatrogenic, hemorrhage), myocardial infarction, cardiac arrhythmia, hypoxia, false reading (e.g., wrong cuff/arterial line twist or clot), pulmonary embolus, cardiac tamponade (on thoracic service), morphine (histamine release)

What are the common causes of hypertension in a postoperative setting?

Pain (from catecholamine release), anxiety, hypercapnia, hypoxia (which may also cause hypotension), idiopathic origin, preexisting condition

What can cause hypoxia?

Atelectasis, pneumonia, mucous plug, pneumothorax, pulmonary embolus, myocardial infarction/arrhythmia, venous blood in ABG syringe, SAT% machine malfunction/probe malposition, iatrogenic (wrong ventilator settings), severe anemia/hypovolemia, low cardiac output, CHF, ARDS, fluid overload

What can cause mental status change?

Hypoxia until ruled out, hypotension (e.g., cardiogenic shock,), hypovolemia, iatrogenic (narcotics/benzodiazepines), drug reaction, alcohol withdrawal, drug withdrawal, seizure, ICU psychosis, cardiovascular accident, sepsis, metabolic derangements, intracranial bleeding, **urinary retention in the elderly**

What are the signs of alcohol withdrawal?

Confusion, tachycardia/autonomic instability, seizure, hallucinations

What are the causes of tachycardia?

Hypovolemia, pain, alcohol withdrawal, anxiety/agitation, urinary retention, cardiac arrhythmia (e.g., sinoventricular tachycardia, atrial fibrillation with rapid rate), MI, PE, β- blocker withdrawal

What are the causes of decreased urine output?

Hypovolemia, urinary retention, Foley catheter malfunction, cardiac failure, MI, acute tubular necrosis (ATN), ureteral/urethral injury

19 Surgical Nutrition

What is the motto of surgical nutrition?
If the gut works, use it.

What are the normal daily dietary requirements for adults from the following sources:

Protein?
1 g/kg/day

Calories?
35 kcal/kg/day

By how much is basal energy expenditure (BEE) increased or decreased in the following cases:

Severe head injury?
Increased ≈ 1.7×

Severe burns?
Increased ≈ 2–3×

What are the calorie contents and metabolic by-products of the following substances:

Fat?
9 kcal/g; [CO_2 + H_2O]

Protein?
4 kcal/g; [ammonia]

Carbohydrate?
4 kcal/g; [CO_2 + H_2O]

What is the formula for the conversion of nitrogen requirement/loss to protein requirement/loss?
Nitrogen × 6.25 = protein

What is RQ?
Respiratory quotient: the ratio of CO_2 produced to O_2 consumed

What is the normal RQ?
0.8

What can be done to decrease the RQ?
More fat, less carbohydrates

What dietary change can be made to decrease CO_2 production in a patient in whom CO_2 retention is a concern?
Decrease carbohydrate calories and increase calories from fat

What lab tests are used to monitor nutritional status?
Blood levels of:
↓ PREALBUMIN (T ½ ≈ 2–3 days)—acute change determination
↓ Transferrin (T ½ ≈ 8–9 days)
↓ Albumin (T ½ ≈ 14–20 days)—more chronic determination
Total lymphocyte count < 1800
Anergy
↓ Retinol binding protein (T ½ ≈ 12 hours)

Where is iron absorbed?
Duodenum (some in the proximal jejunum)

Where is vitamin B_{12} absorbed?
Terminal ileum

What are the surgical causes of vitamin B_{12} deficiency?
Gastrectomy, excision of terminal ileum, blind loop syndrome

Where are bile salts absorbed?
Terminal ileum

Where are fat-soluble vitamins absorbed?
Terminal ileum

Which vitamins are fat soluble?
K, A, D, E ("KADE")

What are the signs of the following disorders:

Vitamin A deficiency?
Poor wound healing

Vitamin B_{12}/folate deficiency?
Megaloblastic anemia

Vitamin C deficiency?
Poor wound healing, bleeding gums

Vitamin K deficiency?	↓ in the vitamin K–dependent clotting factors (II, VII, IX, and X); bleeding; elevated PT
Chromium deficiency?	Diabetic state, especially in patients with AODM
Selenium deficiency?	Anergy
Zinc deficiency?	Poor wound healing, alopecia, dermatitis, taste disorder
Fatty acid deficiency?	Dry, flaky skin; alopecia
What vitamin increases the PO absorption of iron?	PO vitamin C (ascorbic acid)
What vitamin lessens the deleterious effects of steroids on wound healing?	Vitamin A
What are the common indications for total parenteral nutrition (TPN)?	NPO more than 7 days Enterocutaneous fistulas Short bowel syndrome Pancreatitis
What are the possible complications of TPN?	Line infection, fatty infiltration of the liver, electrolyte/glucose problems, pneumothorax during placement of central line, loss of gut barrier
What are the advantages of enteral feeding?	Keeps gut barrier healthy, thought to lessen translocation of bacteria, not associated with complications of line placement, associated with fewer electrolyte/glucose problems
What is the major nutrient of the gut?	Glutamine
What is "refeeding syndrome"?	Decreased serum **potassium, magnesium, and phosphate** after refeeding (via TPN or enterally) a starving patient

What are the vitamin K–dependent clotting factors?	2,7,9,10 (think: 2 + 7= 9, and then 10)
What is an elemental tube feed?	Very low residue tube feed in which almost all of the tube feed is absorbed
Where is calcium absorbed?	Duodenum (actively) Jejunum (passively)
What is the major nutrient of the colon?	Short-chain fatty acids
What must bind B_{12} for absorption?	Intrinsic factor from the gastric parietal cells
How can serum bicarbonate be increased in patients on TPN?	Increase acetate (which is metabolized into bicarbonate)
What are "trophic" tube feeds?	Very low rate of tube feeds (i.e., approximately 10 cc/hr) is thought to keep mucosa alive and healthy
When should PO feedings be started after a laparotomy?	After flatus or stool PR (usually postoperative days 3–5)

20 Shock

What is the definition of shock?

Inadequate tissue perfusion

What are the different types (5)?

Hypovolemic
Septic
Cardiogenic
Neurogenic
Anaphylactic

What are the signs?

Pale, diaphoretic, cool skin
Hypotension, ↓ mental status
Tachycardia, decreased pulse pressure
Poor capillary refill
Poor urine output, tachypnea

What are the best indicators of tissue perfusion?

Urine output, mental status, capillary refill, blood pressure

What lab tests help assess tissue perfusion?

pH from ABG (acidosis associated with inadequate tissue perfusion), lactic acid (elevated with inadequate tissue perfusion)

HYPOVOLEMIC SHOCK

What is the definition?

Decreased intravascular volume

What are the common causes?

Hemorrhage
Burns
Bowel obstruction
Crush injury
Pancreatitis

What are the signs?

Early—Orthostatic hypotension, mild tachycardia, anxiety, diaphoresis, vasoconstriction (decreased pulse pressure with increased diastolic pressure)
Late—Changed mental status, decreased blood pressure, marked tachycardia

What are the classifications of hypovolemic shock?

Mild (20% or less blood volume loss)—decreased perfusion to nonvital tissues, manifested by pale, cool skin and anxiety
Moderate (20% to 40% blood volume loss)—decreased perfusion to vital tissues (liver, kidneys, intestine), manifested by olig-/anuria and decreased blood pressure, agitation
Severe (40% or greater blood volume loss)—decreased perfusion to brain and heart, manifested by mental status changes and hypotension

What is the treatment?

IVF and blood via one or more IVS; the most effective initial fluid in restoring intravascular volume is **isotonic** crystalloid (normal saline/lactated Ringer's)
As the resuscitation is in progress, the underlying cause of hypovolemia should be identified and treated.

How is the effectiveness of treatment evaluated?

Most useful indicator—urine output
Also useful—central venous pressure, blood pressure, heart rate, Hct, ABG, mental status, capillary refill, wedge pressure, cardiac output, pH, lactic acid level

What usually causes failure of resuscitation?

Persistent massive hemorrhage, requiring emergent surgical procedure

Why does decreased pulse pressure occur with early hypovolemic shock?

Pulse pressure (systolic–diastolic blood pressure) decreases because of vasoconstriction, resulting in an elevated diastolic blood pressure.

What is the most common vital sign change associated with early hypovolemic shock?

Tachycardia

What type of patient cannot mount a tachycardiac response to hypovolemic shock?

Patients on β-blockers
Patients with spinal shock and subsequent loss of sympathetic nervous input
Well-conditioned athletes

SEPTIC SHOCK

What is the definition?	Decreased vascular resistance, decreased intravascular volume (usually due to septicemia) causing increased capillary permeability, microvascular pooling, and, most likely, cardiac dysfunction
What is the specific etiology?	Most common—gram-negative septicemia Less common—gram-positive septicemia
What factors increase the susceptibility to septic shock?	Any mechanism that increases the susceptibility to infection (e.g., trauma, immunosuppression, corticosteroids, hematologic disease, diabetes)
What complications are major risks in septic shock?	Multiple organ failure, DIC, **death**
What are the signs/ symptoms?	Initial—vasodilation, resulting in warm skin and full pulses; normal urine output Delayed—vasoconstriction and poor urine output; mental status changes; hypotension
What percentage of blood cultures are positive in patients with bacterial septic shock?	Only about 50%!
What are the associated findings?	Fever, hyperventilation
Which are the associated lab findings?	Early—hyperglycemia/glycosuria, respiratory alkalosis, hemoconcentration, leukopenia Late—leukocytosis, acidosis, elevated lactic acid Note: It is important to identify organism in order to direct treatment.
What is the treatment?	1. IVFs → blood cultures 2. Antibiotic therapy Versus identified organism Empirical, if origin is unknown

3. Drainage—Surgical drainage of an abscess or focus of infection, because antibiotics will not suffice
4. Pressors PRN

CARDIOGENIC SHOCK

What is the definition?

Cardiac insufficiency; left ventricular failure (usually), resulting in inadequate tissue perfusion

What are the causes?

MI, papillary muscle dysfunction, massive cardiac contusion, cardiac tamponade, tension pneumothorax, cardiac valve failure

What are the signs/ symptoms on exam?

Dyspnea
Rales
Pulsus alternans (increased pulse with greater filling following a weak pulse)
Loud pulmonic component of S_2
Gallop rhythm

What are the associated vital signs/parameters?

Hypotension, decreased cardiac output, elevated CVP/wedge pressure, decreased urine output (low renal blood flow), tachycardia (possibly)

What are the signs on chest x-ray?

Pulmonary venous congestion

What is the treatment?

Based on diagnosis/mechanism:
1. Congestive heart failure: diuretics and vasodilators, with or without pressors
2. Left ventricular failure (myocardial infarction): pressors, afterload reduction

What are the last resort support mechanisms?

Intraaortic balloon pump (IABP), ventricular assist device (VAD)

NEUROGENIC SHOCK

What is the definition?

Inadequate tissue perfusion due to loss of sympathetic vasoconstrictive reflexes

What are the common causes?	Spinal trauma Complete transection of spinal cord Partial cord injury with spinal shock Spinal anesthesia
What are the signs/ symptoms?	Pallor, weakness, lightheadedness, transient **hypotension and bradycardia**
Why are heart rate and blood pressure decreased?	Thought to be because of loss of sympathetic tone (but hypovolemia [e.g., hemoperitoneum] must be ruled out)
What are the associated findings?	Neurologic deficits suggesting cord injury
What is the treatment?	**IV fluids** (vasopressors reserved for those refractory to fluid resuscitation)
What percentage of patients with hypotension and spinal neurologic deficits have hypotension of purely neurogenic origin?	About two-thirds
What is spinal shock?	Complete flaccid paralysis immediately following spinal cord injury; may or may not be associated with circulatory shock
What is the lowest reflex available to the examiner?	Bulbocavernous reflex: checking for contraction of the anal sphincter upon compression of the glans penis or clitoris
What is the lowest level voluntary muscle?	External anal sphincter
What are the classic findings associated with spinal cord shock?	Hypotension Bradycardia or lack of compensatory tachycardia

ANAPHYLACTIC SHOCK

What is the definition?	Inadequate tissue perfusion due to increased vascular permeability; vasodilation; smooth muscle constriction as a result of exposure to an allergen in a previously sensitized individual

What is the most important part of the evaluation?	History (always)
What are the most common causes of anaphylactic death in the United States?	1. Medications (e.g., penicillins) 2. Hymenoptera venom (bee sting) 3. Food/blood transfusions
What are the associated findings?	Skin—urticaria and angioedema Airway—laryngeal edema, resulting in airway obstruction Lungs—Smooth-muscle constriction, resulting in respiratory distress with wheezing Intestines—Mucosal edema causing nausea, vomiting, diarrhea, and crampy abdominal pain
What is the treatment?	1. Establish airway 2. Administer epinephrine 3. Administer diphenhydramine hydrochloride 4. Administer steroids (possibly) 5. Administer aminophylline (possibly)

21

Surgical Infection

What elements are common to surgical infections?

Infectious agent
Susceptible host
Closed unperfused space (ischemic)

What is a superinfection?

A new infection arising while a patient is receiving antibiotics for the original infection at a different site; usually caused by resistant bacteria

URINARY TRACT INFECTIONS (UTIs)

What diagnostic tests are used?

Urinalysis, culture, urine microscopy for WBC

What constitutes a POSITIVE urine analysis?

Positive nitrite (from bacteria)
Positive leukocyte esterase (from WBC)
More than 10 WBC/HPF
Presence of bacteria (supportive)

What number of colony-forming units (CFU) confirm the diagnosis of UTI?

On urine culture, classically 100,000 or 10^5 CFU

What are the associated common organisms?

Escherechia coli, Klebsiella, Proteus (Enterococcus, Staphylococcus aureus)

What is the treatment?

Antibiotics with gram-negative spectrum (e.g., sulfamethoxazole/trimethoprim [Bactrim], gentamicin, ciprofloxacin, aztreonam); check culture and sensitivity

What is the treatment of bladder candidiasis?

1. Remove or change Foley catheter
2. Administer systemic fluconazole or amphotericin bladder washings

CENTRAL LINE INFECTIONS

What are the signs of a central line infection?

Unexplained hyperglycemia, fever, mental status change, hypotension, tachycardia → **shock,** pus and erythema at central line site

What is the treatment? Remove line; administer antibiotics

When should a central line be changed over a wire? **Fever** without obvious external signs (pus, erythema at central line site) of infection; send tip of catheter to the lab for culture

When should a central line changed over a wire be left in place? If culture of previous line returns less than 15 CFU

When should a central line changed over a wire be pulled and a central line placed at a different site? If the previous line culture returns more than 15 CFU

WOUND INFECTION

What is it? Infection in an operative wound

When do these infections arise? Classically, POD 5 to 7

What are the signs/symptoms? **Pain** at incision site, erythema, drainage, induration, warm skin, fever

What is the treatment? Remove skin sutures/staples, perform digital examination to rule out fascial dehiscence, pack wound open, send wound culture, administer antibiotics

What are the most common bacteria found in postoperative wound infections?

Staphylococcus aureus (20%)
Escherichia coli (10 %)
Enterococcus (10%)
Other causes: *Staphylococcus epidermidis*, *Pseudomonas*, anaerobes, other gram-negative organisms, *Streptococcus*

Which bacteria will cause fever and wound infection in the first 24 hours after surgery?

1. *Streptococcus*
2. *Clostridium* (bronze–brown weeping tender wound)

CLASSIFICATION OF OPERATIVE WOUNDS

What is a "clean" wound? Elective, nontraumatic wound without acute inflammation; usually closed primarily without the use of drains

What is the infection rate of a clean wound?	Less than 1.5%
What is a clean contaminated wound?	Operation of the GI or respiratory tract without unusual contamination, or entry into the biliary or urinary tract
Without infection present, what is the infection rate of a clean-contaminated wound?	Less than 3%
What is a contaminated wound?	Acute inflammation present, traumatic wound, GI tract spillage, or a major break in sterile technique
What is the infection rate of a contaminated wound?	Approximately 5%
What is a dirty wound?	Pus present, perforated viscus, or dirty traumatic wound
What is the infection rate of a dirty wound?	Approximately 33%
What are the possible complications of wound infections?	Fistula, sinus tracts, sepsis, abscess, suppressed wound healing, superinfection (i.e., a new infection that develops during antibiotic treatment for the original infection)
What factors influence the development of infections?	Presence of a foreign body (e.g., suture, drains, grafts) Decreased blood flow (poor delivery of PMNs and antibiotics) Strangulation of tissues with excessively tight sutures Presence of necrotic tissue or excessive local tissue destruction (e.g., too much Bovie) Long operations (> 2 hrs) Hematomas or seromas Presence of dead space that prevents the delivery of phagocytic cells to bacterial foci Poor approximation of tissues

Patient factors

Uremia
Hypovolemic shock
Vascular occlusive states
Advanced age
Immunosuppressed states: immunosuppressant treatment, chemotherapy, systemic malignancy, trauma or burn injury, diabetes mellitus, obesity, malnutrition, AIDS, uremia, distant area of infection

What is an abscess?

Localized collection of pus and fibrin surrounded by an area of inflammation (i.e., hyperemia and marked leukocyte infiltration)
CT may aid in the diagnosis
Abscess always requires drainage, which can be either surgical or percutaneous if the anatomic location of the abscess is accessible (except hepatic amebiasis!)

Which lab tests are indicated?

Leukocytosis or leukopenia (as an abscess may act as a WBC sink), blood cultures, imaging studies (i.e., CT to locate an abscess)

What is the treatment?

Incision and drainage—an abscess must be drained (Note: fluctuation is a sign of a subcutaneous abscess. Most abdominal abscesses are drained percutaneously)
Antibiotics

Peritoneal Abscess

What is it?

Abscess within the peritoneal cavity

What are the causes?

Postoperative status after a laparotomy, ruptured appendix, peritonitis, any inflammatory intraperitoneal process, anastomotic leak

What are the sites of occurrence?

Pelvis, Morrison's pouch, subphrenic, paracolic gutters, periappendiceal, lesser sac

What are the signs/ symptoms?
Fever (classically spiking), abdominal pain, mass

How is the diagnosis made?
Abdominal CT (or ultrasound)

When should an abdominal CT be obtained looking for a postoperative abscess?
After POD 7 (otherwise, abscess will not be "organized" and will look like a normal postoperative fluid collection)

What CT findings are associated with abscess?
Fluid collection with fibrous rind, **gas** in fluid collection

What is the treatment?
Percutaneous CT drainage

What is an option for drainage of pelvic abscess?
Transrectal drainage (or transvaginal)

What is cellulitis?
Blanching erythema due to superficial dermal/epidermal bacterial infection (most commonly *Streptococcus*; less commonly *Staphylococcus*)

What is a "stitch" abscess?
Subcutaneous abscess centered around a subcutaneous stitch, which is a "foreign body"; treat with drainage and stitch removal

NECROTIZING FASCITIS

What is it?
Bacterial infection of underlying fascia (spreads rapidly along fascial planes)

What are the causative agents?
Classically, *Streptococcus,* but most often polymicrobial with anaerobes/gram-negative organisms

What are the signs/ symptoms?
Fever, pain, crepitus, cellulitis, skin discoloration, blood blisters (hemorrhagic bullae), weeping skin, increased WBCs, subcutaneous air on x-ray, septic shock

What is the treatment?
IV antibiotics and aggressive early extensive surgical debridement, cultures, tetanus prophylaxis

CLOSTRIDIAL MYOSITIS

What is it?	Clostridial muscle infection
What is another name for this condition?	Gas gangrene
What is the most common causative organism?	*Clostridium perfringens*
What are the signs/ symptoms?	Pain, fever, shock, crepitus, foul-smelling brown fluid, subcutaneous air on x-ray
What is the treatment?	IV antibiotics, aggressive surgical debridement of involved muscle, tetanus prophylaxis

SUPPURATIVE HIDRADENITIS

What is it?	Infection/abscess formation in **apocrine** sweat glands
In what (3) locations does it occur?	Perineum/buttocks, inguinal area, axilla (site of apocrine glands)
What is the most common causative organism?	*Staphylococcus aureus*
What is the treatment?	Antibiotics Incision and drainage (Excision of skin for chronic infections)

PSEUDOMEMBRANOUS COLITIS

What is it?	Antibiotic-induced colonic overgrowth of *C. difficile,* secondary to loss of competitive nonpathogenic bacteria that comprise the normal colonic flora Note: it can be caused by any antibiotic, but especially penicillins, cephalosporins, and clindamycin
What are the signs/ symptoms?	**Diarrhea,** ± fever, ± increased WBCs, ± abdominal cramps, ± abdominal distention
What causes the diarrhea?	Exotoxin released by *C. difficile*

How is the diagnosis made?

Assay stool for exotoxin titer; fecal leukocytes may or may not be present; on colonoscopy, there is an exudate that looks like a membrane (hence, "pseudomembranous")

What is the treatment?

PO vancomycin (97% sensitive) or PO metronidazole (Flagyl; 93% sensitive); discontinuation of causative agent

Never give antiperistaltics.

PROPHYLACTIC ANTIBIOTICS

What are the indications for prophylaxis (IV antibiotics)?

Accidental wounds with heavy contamination and tissue damage

Accidental wounds requiring surgical therapy that has had to be delayed

Injuries in which adequate debridement cannot be performed

Known gross bacterial contamination in any wound

Penetrating injuries of hollow intraabdominal organs

Large bowel resections and anastomosis (PO neomycin plus erythromycin on the day prior to surgery, and cefoxitin preoperatively)

Some clean-contaminated procedures (e.g., common bile duct exploration)

Patient with preexisting valvular heart disease

Cardiovascular surgery with the use of a prosthesis/vascular procedures

Patients with open fractures (start in the ER)

Traumatic wounds occurring more than 8 hours prior to medical attention

What must a prophylactic antibiotic cover for procedures on the large bowel/abdominal trauma?

Anaerobes

What commonly used antibiotics offer anaerobic coverage?

Cefoxitin (Mefoxin), clindamycin, metronidazole (Flagyl), cefotetan, ampicillin-sulbactam (Unasyn)

When is the appropriate time to administer prophylactic antibiotics?	Must be in adequate levels in the blood stream **prior to surgical incision!**

PAROTITIS

What is it?	Infection of the parotid gland
What is the most common causative organism?	*Staphylococcus*
What are the associated risk factors?	Age greater than 65 years, malnutrition, poor oral hygiene, presence of NG tube; NPO, dehydration
What is the most common time of occurrence?	Usually 2 weeks postoperative
What are the signs?	Hot, red, tender parotid gland, and increased WBC
What is the treatment?	Antibiotics, operative drainage as necessary

MISCELLANEOUS

Which bacteria can be found in the stool (colon)?	Anaerobic—*Bacteroides fragilis* Aerobic—*Escherichia coli*
Which bacteria are found in infections from human bites?	*Streptococcus viridans* *Staphylococcus aureus* *Peptococcus* *Eikenella*
What is the most common ICU pneumonia bacteria?	Gram-negative organisms
What antibiotic combination is used to kill *Enterococcus*?	1. Penicillin or vancomycin **and** 2. An aminoglycoside
What is Fournier's gangrene?	Perineal infection starting classically in the scrotum in diabetic patients; treat with triple antibiotics and wide debridement (± colostomy to divert stool from area)

Does adding antibiotics to peritoneal lavage solution lower the risk of abscess formation?	No ("Dilution is the solution to pollution.")
What is the classic finding associated with a *Pseudomonas* infection?	Green exudate and "fruity" smell
What is the most common organism causing osteomyelitis of the foot after a nail puncture through a shoe?	*Pseudomonas*
What are the classic antibiotics for "triple" antibiotics?	Ampicillin, gentamycin, and (metronidazole) Flagyl
Which antibiotic is used to treat ameba infection?	Metronidazole (Flagyl)
Which bacteria commonly infects prosthetic material and central lines?	*Staphylococcus epidermis*
What is the antibiotic of choice for *Actinomyces*?	Penicillin G (exquisitely sensitive)
What is a furuncle?	A staphylococcal abscess that forms in a hair follicle (think: **f**ollicle = **f**uruncle)
What is a carbuncle?	A subcutaneous staphylococcal abscess (usually an extension of a furuncle), most commonly seen in diabetic patients (i.e., rule out diabetes)
What is suppurative hidradenitis?	Infection of an **apocrine** sweat gland (therefore seen in the axilla, perineum, and inguinal distributions)
What microscopic finding is associated with *Actinomyces*?	Sulfur granules
What organism causes tetanus?	*Clostridium tetani*

What are the signs of tetanus?	Lockjaw, muscle spasm, laryngospasm, convulsions, and respiratory failure
What are the appropriate prophylactic steps in tetanus-prone (dirty) injury in the following patients:	
Three previous immunizations?	None (tetanus toxoid only if > 5 years since last toxoid)
Two previous immunizations?	Tetanus toxoid
One previous immunization?	Tetanus immunoglobulin IM and tetanus toxoid IM (at different sites!)
No previous immunizations?	Tetanus immunoglobulin IM and tetanus toxoid IM (at different sites!)
What is Fitz-Hugh-Curtis syndrome?	Right upper quadrant pain due to gonococcal perihepatitis in women
What is bacterial translocation?	Bacteria gain access to lymphatics and blood stream from the colon via compromised mucosal barrier

22 Fever

Define postoperative fever.	Temperature greater than 38.5° C
What are the classic W's of postoperative fever? (5)	**W**ind—atelectasis postoperative day (POD) 1 to 2 **W**ater—urinary tract infection (UTI) **W**ound—wound infection POD 5 to 7 **W**alking—DVT/thrombophlebitis **W**onder drugs—drug fever
What is the most common cause of fever POD 1 to 2?	Atelectasis
What is a "complete" fever work up?	Physical exam (look at wound, etc.) CXR Urinalysis Blood cultures CBC
What are the causes of fever during surgery or immediately after?	Malignant hyperthermia; familial reaction to halothane or succinylcholine; transfusion reaction; drug hypersensitivity; atelectasis; aspiration pneumonia; and endocrine (Addisonian crisis, thyroid storm, pheochromocytoma)
What causes fever before 24 postoperative hours?	Atelectasis, streptococcal, or clostridial wound infections (rare) Note: S.T.A.T. = strep, thyroid, Addisonian crisis, transfusion
What causes fever POD 3 to 5?	UTI, especially after instrumentation/ Foley Pneumonia IV complications: rate of infection is proportional to the duration of IV site (thrombophlebitis/central line sepsis) Wound complications (e.g., leaking anastomosis, hematoma)

What causes fever POD 6 to 10?

Wound infection, pneumonia, abscess, infected hematoma, *C. difficile* colitis, anastomotic leak

Deep venous thrombosis (DVT), abscess, drug fever

Pulmonary embolism, abscess, parotitis

What conditions can cause fever at any time?

Thrombophlebitis
DVT
Drug hypersensitivity
Transfusion reaction
UTI
Central line sepsis

What causes wound infection POD 1 to 2?

Streptococcus
Clostridial (painful bronze–brown weeping wound)

23

Surgical Prophylaxis

What medications provide protection from postoperative GI bleeding?

H_2 blockers (e.g., ranitidine or cimetidine), sucralfate (binds ulcer craters), or antacids

What measures provide protection from postoperative atelectasis/ pneumonia?

Incentive spirometry, coughing, **smoking cessation**

What treatments provide protection from postoperative DVT?

Subcutaneous low-dose heparin and/or sequential compression device (SCD) for lower extremities, support hose

What measures provide protection from wound infection?

Shower the night before surgery with chlorhexidine scrub
Never use a razor for hair removal (electric shavers only)
Adequate skin prep in the OR
Do not close the skin in a contaminated case
Preoperative antibiotics in the bloodstream **before incision**

What treatment provides protection from fungal infection during IV antibiotic treatment?

PO nystatin

What measure provides protection from infection after colon surgery?

Bowel prep: lower bacterial count in colon by catharsis and PO antibiotics (neomycin, erythromycin) preoperatively (and preoperative IV antibiotic with spectrum versus anaerobes (e.g., Cefoxitin)

What treatment provides protection from OPSS after splenectomy?

Immunization versus *H. Influenza, Streptococcus, Meningococcus,* penicillin when illness/fever occurs

What treatment provides protection from endocarditis with faulty heart valve or prosthetic heart valve?	IV antibiotics prior to dental procedure or any surgery
What treatment provides protection from tetanus infection?	Tetanus toxiod and tetanus toxoid (and tetanus immune globulin, if one or no previous toxoid) with dirty wound
What treatment provides protection from ETOH withdrawal?	Chlordiazepoxide (Librium; also consider Rally pack : thiamine, folate, magnesium)

24 Surgical Radiology

What percentage of kidney stones are radiopaque?
Approximately 90%

What percentage of all gallstones are radiopaque?
Approximately 10%

What percentage of patients with acute appendicitis have a radiopaque fecalith?
Approximately 5%

What are the signs of abdominal pathology on abdominal x-ray (AXR)?
Loss of fat stripe, loss of psoas shadow, sentinel loops, cut-off sign, air–fluid levels, free air

What are the radiographic signs of appendicitis?
Fecalith, sentinel loops, scoliosis away from the right due to pain, mass effect (abscess), loss of psoas shadow, loss of preperitoneal fat stripe, and, very rarely, a small amount of free air, if perforated

What is the best x-ray for diagnosing an abdominal aortic aneurysm (AAA)?
Cross-table lateral—reveals AAA in more than two-thirds of cases by eggshell calcifications

What does KUB stand for?
Kidneys, Ureters, and Bladder—commonly used term for a plain film x-ray of the abdomen (abdominal flat plate)

What CXR findings may provide evidence of traumatic aortic injury?
Widened mediastinum (most common)
Apical pleural capping
Central sign of congestion
Pleural fluid
Loss of aortic knob
Inferior displacement of left main bronchus; NG tube displaced to the right, tracheal deviation, hemothorax

What is the "parrot's beak" or "bird's beak" sign?	Evidence of sigmoid volvulus on barium enema; evidence of achalasia on barium swallow
What is a "string" sign?	Contrast GI study that reveals a stricture; contrast appears as a "string" outlining the narrowing
What is the differential diagnosis of retroperitoneal calcification?	Pancreatitis, AAA, generalized aortic calcification, kidney stone, renal cell carcinoma, renal artery aneurysm (phleboliths, if seen in the pelvis), adrenal calcification
What is free air?	Air free within the peritoneal cavity (air normally should be seen only within the bowel or stomach)
What are the differential diagnoses and best positions for the detection of free peritoneal air?	Seen in any intraabdominal viscus perforation; s/p laparotomy, s/p needle biopsy, s/p paracentesis; **upright CXR** air below the diaphragm
If you cannot get an upright CXR, what is the second best plain x-ray for free air?	Left lateral decubitus, because it prevents confusion with gastric air bubble; with free air, **both** sides of the bowel wall can be seen; can detect as little as 1 cc of air
What is the significance of an air–fluid level?	Seen in obstruction or ileus on an upright x-ray; intraluminal bowel diameter increases, allowing for separation of fluid and gas
What is a "cut-off sign"?	Seen in obstruction, bowel distention, and distended bowel that is "cut off" from normal bowel
What are "sentinel loops"?	Distention and/or air–fluid levels near a site of abdominal inflammation (e.g., seen in the RLQ with appendicitis)
What is loss of the psoas shadow?	Loss of the clearly defined borders of the psoas muscle on AXR; loss signifies inflammation or ascites

What is loss of the peritoneal fat stripe (a.k.a. preperitoneal fat stripe)?	Loss of the lateral peritoneal/ preperitoneal fat interface; implies inflammation
What is "thumbprinting"?	Nonspecific colonic mucosal edema that looks like thumb indentations on AXR
What is pneumatosis intestinalis?	Gas within the intestinal wall (usually means dead gut) can be seen in patients with congenital variant or on chronic steroids
How can the small and large bowel be distinguished on AXR?	By the intraluminal folds; the small bowel plicae circulares are complete, whereas the plica semilunares of the large bowel are only partially around the inner circumference of the lumen
How long after a laparotomy can there be free air on AXR?	For 7 to 10 days
What is Chilaiditi's sign?	Transverse colon over the liver simulating free air
How can it be confirmed on CXR that the last hole on a chest tube is in the pleural cavity?	The last hole is through the radiopaque line on the chest tube; thus, look for the break in the radiopaque line to be in the rib cage.
What plain x-rays are used to look for ligamentous C-spine injury?	Lateral flex and extension C-spine films
When should a postoperative abdominal/ pelvic CT looking for a peritoneal abscess be performed?	POD 7 or later, to give time for the abscess to form
How can a loculated pleural effusion be distinguished from a free-flowing pleural effusion?	Ipsilateral decubitus CXR; if fluid is not loculated (or contained) it will layer out

What x-ray should be obtained before feeding via a nasogastric or nasoduodenal tube?

High abdominal x-ray, to make sure the tube is in the GI tract and not in the lung

What x-ray should be obtained after a central line placement?

CXR, to confirm placement and rule out PTX

Classically, how much pleural fluid can be hidden by the diaphragm on upright CXR?

It is said that up to 500 cc can be overshowed by the diaphragm (but probably closer to 200 cc in reality).

What is the best test to evaluate the biliary system and gallbladder?

Ultrasound (U/S)

What diameter common bile duct is considered dilated (with gallbladder present)?

All common bile ducts more than 1 cm are considered dilated (although most radiologists consider > 7 mm dilated)

What U/S findings are associated with acute cholecystitis?

Gallstones, thickened gallbladder wall (> 3 mm), distended gallbladder, pericholecystic fluid

How should a CXR be read?

Check the following:

1. Name
2. Date
3. Penetration (is all of the chest visualized?)
4. Heart size (heart transverse diameter should be ≤ half the transthoracic diameter)
5. Lung fields (e.g., mass, CHF)
6. Bones (ribs/clavicles/spine)
7. Mediastinum (e.g., aortic nob, nodes)
8. Rule out PTX, pleural fluid; check line/endotracheal tube placement

What type of kidney stone is not seen on AXR?

Uric acid (think: **u**ric acid = **un**seen)

25

Anesthesia

Define the following terms:	
Anesthesia	Loss of sensation/pain
Local anesthesia	Anesthesia of a small confined area of the body (i.e., lidocaine for an elbow laceration)
Epidural anesthesia	Anesthetic drugs/narcotics infused into epidural space
Spinal anesthesia	Anesthetic agents injected into the thecal sac
Regional anesthesia	Blocking sensory afferent nerve fibers from a **region** of the body (i.e., radial nerve block)
General anesthesia	Unconsciousness/amnesia (inhalational anesthetics)
GET or GETA	General endotracheal anesthesia
Give examples of the following terms:	
Local anesthetic	Lidocaine, bupivacaine (Marcaine)
Regional anesthetic	Lidocaine, bupivacaine (Marcaine)
General anesthesia	Halothane, isoflurane, enflurane, nitrous oxide
Dissociative agent	Ketamine (children/burn patients)
What is cricoid pressure?	Manual pressure on cricoid cartilage occluding the esophagus and thus decreasing the chance of aspiration of gastric contents

What is "rapid-sequence" anesthesia induction?	1. Short-acting IV barbiturate 2. Muscle relaxant 3. Cricoid pressure 4. Intubation 5. Inhalation anesthetic (rapid: boom, boom, boom → to lower the risk of aspiration during intubation)
What are the contraindications of the depolarizing agent succinylcholine?	Burn patients, neuromuscular diseases/ paraplegia, eye trauma, increased ICP
Why is succinylcholine contraindicated in these patients?	Depolarization in these patients can result in life-threatening **hyperkalemia; also increases intraocular pressure**
What is the side effect of the nonpolarizing neuromuscular blocker pancuronium?	Tachycardia
Why doesn't lidocaine work in an abscess?	Lidocaine does not work in an acidic environment
Why does lidocaine burn on injection and what can be done to decrease the burning sensation?	Lidocaine is acidic, which causes the burning; add sodium bicarbonate to decrease the burning sensation.
Why does some lidocaine come with epinephrine?	Epinephrine is meant to vasoconstrict the small vessels and thus decrease bleeding and washing out of the lidocaine from the area, prolonging its effect.
In what locations is lidocaine with epinephrine contraindicated?	Fingers, toes, penis, etc., because of the possibility of ischemic injury/necrosis due to vasoconstriction
What are the contraindications to nitrous oxide?	Nitrous oxide is poorly soluble in serum and thus expands into any air-filled body pockets; should be avoided in cases with middle ear occlusions, **pneumothorax, small bowel obstruction,** etc.

What is the feared side effect of bupivacaine (Marcaine)?	Cardiac arrhythmia after intravascular injection
What are the side effects of morphine?	Constipation, respiratory failure, hypotension (from histamine release), spasm of sphincter of Oddi (use Demerol in pancreatitis and biliary surgery), decreased cough reflex **Note:** life-threatening side effects can be reversed with **Naloxone**
What are the side effects of meperidine?	Similar to those of morphine, but causes less sphincteric spasm and can cause seizures
What are the side effects of epidural analgesia?	**Orthostatic hypotension,** decreased motor function, urinary retention
What is the advantage of epidural analgesia?	Analgesia without decreased cough reflex
What must be taken out only after the epidural catheter is removed?	The Foley catheter should be removed after the epidural is removed; otherwise, the patient will most likely suffer from urinary retention
What are the side effects of spinal anesthesia?	**Urinary retention** Hypotension (neurogenic shock)
What is the side effect of inhalational (volatile) anesthesia?	Halothane—**hypotension** (cardiac depression, decreased baroreceptor response to hypotension, and peripheral vasodilation), malignant hyperthermia

MALIGNANT HYPERTHERMIA

What is it?	Inherited predisposition to an anesthetic Rxn, causing uncoupling of the excitation–contraction system in skeletal muscle, which in turn causes **malignant hyperthermia;** hypermetabolism will result in death if untreated
What is the incidence?	Very rare

What are the causative agents?
General anesthesia, succinylcholine

What are the signs/ symptoms?
Increased body temperature; hypoxia; acidosis; tachycardia, leading to death if untreated

When does it occur?
Usually soon after the induction of the anesthetic

What is the treatment?
IV dantrolene, body cooling, discontinuation of anesthesia

What are some of the nondepolarizing muscle blockers?
Vecuronium
Pancuronium

What is the antidote to the nondepolarizing neuromuscular blocking agents?
Edrophonium
Neostigmine
Pyridostigmine

Which muscle blocker is depolarizing?
Succinylcholine

What is the duration of action of succinylcholine?
Less than 5 minutes

What is the antidote to reverse succinylcholine?
Time; endogenous blood pseudocholinesterase (patients deficient in this enzyme may be paralyzed for hours!)

At what dose are levels of lidocaine toxic?
Approximately 5 mg/kg

What are the early signs of lidocaine toxicity?
Tinnitus
Perioral/tongue numbness
Blurred vision
Drowsiness

What are the signs of lidocaine toxicity with large overdose (> 10 mcg/ ml)?
Seizures
Loss of consciousness
Apnea

What are the cardiovascular effects of the volatile anesthetics (e.g., halothane)?	Vasodilation Direct cardiac depression Thus, if patients are not well hydrated upon induction of anesthesia, they may become hypotensive.
When should the Foley catheter be removed in a patient with an epidural catheter?	Several hours **after** the epidural catheter is removed
What is a PCA pump?	**P**atient-**C**ontrolled **A**nalgesia; a pump delivers a set amount of pain reliever when the patient pushes a button (e.g., 1 mg of morphine every 6 minutes)
What are the advantages of PCA pump?	Better pain control Patients actually use less pain medication with a PCA! If given a moderate dose without a basal rate, patients should not be able to overdose (they will fall asleep and not be able to push the button!)
What is used to reverse narcotics?	Naloxone (Narcan)
What is used to reverse benzodiazepines?	Flumazenil
What is fentanyl?	Very potent narcotic (number one drug of abuse by anesthesiologists)
What is a Bier block?	Regional anesthesia of an extremity by placing a tourniquet and then infusing local anesthetic into a **vein**

26 Surgical Ulcers

Define the following terms:	
Ulcer	Breakdown of a cell covering (i.e., skin or mucosa)
Peptic ulcer	General term for gastric and duodenal ulcer disease
Duodenal ulcer	Ulcer in the duodenum
Gastric ulcer	Ulcer in the stomach
Curling's ulcer	Gastric ulcer after burn injury
Cushing's ulcer	Peptic ulcer after neurologic insult (think: Cushing = famous neurosurgeon)
Dieulafoy's ulcer	Pinpoint gastric mucosal defect bleeding from underlying arterial vessel malformation
Marjolin's ulcer	Squamous cell carcinoma ulceration overlying chronic osteomyelitis or burn scar
Apthous ulcer	GI tract ulcer seen in Crohn's disease
Marginal ulcer	Mucosal ulcer seen at a site of GI-tract anastomosis
Decubitus ulcer	Skin/subcutaneous ulceration due to pressure necrosis, classically on the buttocks/sacrum
Venous stasis ulcer	Skin ulceration on **medial malleolus** caused by venous stasis of a lower extremity
LE arterial insufficiency ulcer	Skin ulcers usually located on the toes/feet

Section II

General Surgery

27

GI Hormones and Physiology

GASTRIC PHASES

Name the three phases of acid secretion.

1. Cephalic
2. Gastric
3. Intestinal

What stimulates the cephalic phase?

The thought, sight, or smell of food; mediated by the vagus nerve

What stimulates the gastric phase?

Food entering the stomach (i.e., gastric distention, decreased pH); mediated by gastrin

What stimulates the intestinal phase?

The entry of products of digestion into the duodenum

Define the products of the following stomach cells:

Gastric parietal cells

HCl
Intrinsic factor

Chief cells

Pepsinogen (think: "a peppy chief")

G cells

Gastrin (found in the antrum)

Mucous neck cells

Bicarbonate
Mucous

What is pepsin?

A proteolytic enzyme that hydrolyzes peptide bonds

What is intrinsic factor?

A protein secreted by the parietal cells that combines with vitamin B_{12} and allows for absorption in the terminal ileum

Name three receptors on the parietal cell that stimulate HCl release.
1. Histamine
2. Acetylcholine
3. Gastrin

What is the enterohepatic circulation?
Circulation of bile acids from the liver to the gut and back to the liver via the portal vein

Where are most of the bile acids absorbed?
The terminal ileum

How many times is the entire bile acid pool circulated during a typical meal?
Two times

What are the stimulators of gallbladder emptying?
Cholecystokinin
Vagal input

What are the inhibitors of gallbladder emptying?
Somatostatin
Sympathetics (it is impossible to flee and digest food at the same time)
VIP

CHOLECYSTOKININ

What is its source?
Duodenal mucosal cells

What stimulates its release?
Fat, protein, amino acids, HCl

What inhibits its release?
Trypsin and chymotrypsin

What are its actions?
Empties gallbladder
Opens ampulla of Vater
Slows gastric emptying
Stimulates pancreatic acinar cell growth and release of exocrine products

SECRETIN

What is its source?
Duodenal cells (specifically the argyrophil S cells)

What stimulates its release?
pH less than 4.5 (acid)
Fat in the duodenum

What inhibits its release?	High pH in the duodenum
What are its actions?	Releases pancreatic bicarbonate/ enzymes/H_2O Releases bile/bicarbonate Decreases LES Decreases gastric acid release

GASTRIN

What is its source?	Gastric antrum G cells
What stimulates its release?	Stomach peptides/amino acids Vagal input Calcium
What inhibits its release?	pH less than 3.0 Somatostatin
What are its actions?	Release of HCl from parietal cells Trophic effect on mucosa of the stomach and small intestine

SOMATOSTATIN

What is its source?	Pancreatic D cells
What stimulates its release?	Food
What are its actions?	Globally inhibits GI function

MISCELLANEOUS

What is the purpose of the colon?	Reabsorption of H_2O and storage of stool
What is the main small bowel nutritional source?	Glutamine
What is the main nutritional source of the colon?	Short-chain fatty acids
Where is calcium absorbed?	Duodenum actively, jejunum passively

Where is iron absorbed?	Duodenum
Where is vitamin B_{12} absorbed?	Terminal ileum
Which hormone primarily controls gallbladder contraction?	CCK
What supplement does a patient need after removal of the terminal ileum or stomach?	B_{12}
Name the main constituents of bile.	Water, phospholipids (lecithins), bile acids, cholesterol, and bilirubin
What are the majority of gallstones made of?	Cholesterol
How do opiates affect the bowel?	Opiates stimulate sodium absorption and inhibit secretion in the ileum, as well as decreasing GI motility by incoordinated peristalsis. Therefore, place patients on stool softeners when dispensing pain medication.
Which type of muscle fibers, smooth or striated, does the esophagus contain?	Both Upper third—striated muscle control of motor nerves Middle third—mixed Lower third—smooth muscle, primarily under the control of vagal motor fibers
Which electrolytes does the colon actively absorb?	Na^+, Cl^-
Which electrolytes does the colon actively secrete?	HCO_3 (plays a role in diarrhea causing the patient to have a normal anion gap acidosis)
Which electrolytes does the colon passively secrete?	K^+

What is the gastrocolic reflex?	Increased secretory and motor functions of the stomach result in increased colonic motility
What is the blood supply to the liver?	Seventy-five percent from the portal vein, rich in products of digestion Twenty-five percent from the hepatic artery, rich in O_2 (but each provide for 50% of oxygen)
What are Peyer patches?	Nodules of lymphoid tissue with B and T lymphocytes in the small intestine that selectively sample lumenal antigens found in the terminal ileum

28

Acute Abdomen and Referred Pain

What is an "acute abdomen"?

Acute abdominal pain so severe that the patient seeks medical attention (not the same as a "surgical abdomen," because most cases of acute abdominal pain do not require surgical treatment)

What are peritoneal signs?

Signs of peritoneal irritation, including extreme tenderness, rebound tenderness, voluntary guarding, motion pain, **involuntary** guarding/rigidity (late)

Define the following terms:

Rebound tenderness

Pain upon releasing the palpating hand pushing on the abdomen

Motion pain

Abdominal pain upon moving, pelvic rocking, moving of stretcher, or heel strike

Voluntary guarding

Abdominal muscle contraction with palpation of the abdomen

Involuntary guarding

Rigid abdomen as the muscles "guard" involuntarily

What is the most common cause of acute abdominal surgery in the United States?

Acute appendicitis (7% of the population will develop acute appendicitis sometime during their lives)

What important questions should be asked when obtaining the history of a patient with an acute abdomen?

"Have you had this pain before?"
"On a scale from 1 to 10, what would you rank this pain?"
"Fevers/chills?"
"Duration?"
"Quality (sharp vs. dull)?"

"Does anything make the pain better or worse?"
"Migration?"
"Point of maximal pain?"
"Urinary symptoms?"
"Nausea, vomiting, or diarrhea?"
"Constipation?"
"Last bowel movement?"
"Any change in bowel habits?"
"Any relation to eating?"
"Last menses?"
"Last meal?"
"Vaginal discharge?"
"Melena?"
"Hematochezia?"
"Hematemesis?"
"Medications?"
"Allergies?"
"Past medical history?"
"Past surgical history?"

What should acute abdomen physical exam include?

Inspection (e.g., surgical scars, distention)
Auscultation (e.g., bowel sounds, bruits)
Palpation (e.g., tenderness, R/O hernia, CVAT, rectal, pelvic exam, rebound,voluntary guard, motion tenderness)
Percussion (e.g., liver size, spleen size)

What is the classic position of a patient with peritonitis?

Motionless (often with knees flexed)

What is the classic position of a patient with a kidney stone, ovarian torsion, or testicular torsion?

Cannot stay still; writhing in pain

What lab tests are used to evaluate the patient with an acute abdomen?

CBC with **differential,** chem-10, amylase, type and screen, urinalysis, ± ABG, ± LFT

What is a "left shift" on CBC differential?

Sign of inflammatory response:
1. Immature neutrophils (bands)
2. More than 80% of WBC as neutrophils

What lab test should every woman of childbearing age with an acute abdomen receive?

Human chorionic gonadotropin (β-hCG) to rule out pregnancy/ectopic pregnancy

Which x-rays are used to evaluate the patient with an acute abdomen?

Upright chest x-ray, upright abdominal film, supine abdominal x-ray, (if patient is unable to stand, left lateral decubitus abdominal film)

How is free air ruled out if the patient is unable to stand?

Left lateral decubitus—free air collects over the liver and does not get confused with the gastric bubble

If a patient has peritoneal signs, who must be called?

A **general surgeon!**

What diagnosis must be considered in every patient with an acute abdomen?

Appendicitis!

What are the differential diagnoses by quadrant?

RUQ

Cholecystitis, hepatitis, PUD, perforated ulcer, pancreatitis, liver tumors, gastritis, hepatic abscess, choledocholithiasis, cholangitis, pyelonephritis, nephrolithiasis, appendicitis (**especially during pregnancy**); thoracic causes (e.g., pleurisy/pneumonia), PE, pericarditis, MI (especially inferior MI)

LUQ

PUD, perforated ulcer, gastritis, splenic disease or rupture, abscess, reflux, dissecting aortic aneurysm, thoracic causes (as previously described), pyelonephritis, nephrolithiasis, hiatal hernia (strangulated paraesophageal hernia), Boerhaave's syndrome, Mallory-Weiss tear

LLQ

Diverticulitis, sigmoid volvulus, perforated colon, colon cancer, urinary tract infection, small bowel obstruction, inflammatory bowel disease, nephrolithiasis, pyelonephritis, fluid accumulation from aneurysm or perforation, referred hip pain;

	gynecologic causes (e.g., ectopic pregnancy), PID, mittelschmerz, ovarian cyst, fibroid degeneration, endometriosis, gynecologic tumor, torsion of cyst or fallopian tube
RLQ	Same as LLQ, especially **appendicitis,** also mesenteric lymphadenitis, cecal diverticulitis, Meckel's diverticulum, intussusception
What is the differential diagnosis of gynecologic pain?	Ovarian cyst, ovarian torsion, PID, tubo-ovarian abscess, fibroid, necrotic fibroid, pregnancy, ectopic pregnancy, endometritis, cancer of the cervix/uterus/ovary
What is the differential diagnosis of thoracic causes of abdominal pain?	MI (especially inferior), pneumonia, dissecting aorta, aortic aneurysm, empyema, esophageal rupture/tear, PTX, esophageal foreign body
What is the differential diagnosis of scrotal causes of lower abdominal pain?	Testicular torsion, epididymitis, orchitis, inguinal hernia
What are the causes of diffuse abdominal pain?	Uremia, porphyria, diffuse peritonitis, gastroenteritis, IBD, DKA, early appendicitis, SBO, sickle cell crisis, ischemic mesenteric disease, aortic aneurysm, lead poisoning, black widow spider bite, pancreatitis, perforated viscus
What are the possible causes of suprapubic pain?	Cystitis, colonic pain, gynecologic causes
What causes pain limited to specific dermatomes?	Early zoster before vesicles erupt
What is referred pain?	Pain felt at a site distant from a disease process; caused by the convergence of multiple pain afferents in the posterior horn of the spinal cord

What is gastroenteritis?	Viral or bacterial infection of the GI tract, usually with vomiting and diarrhea, pain (usually **after** vomiting), nonsurgical
What is classically stated to be the "great imitator"?	Constipation can cause nonsurgical abdominal pain
Name the classic locations of referred pain:	
Cholecystitis	Right subscapular pain (also epigastric)
Appendicitis	Early: periumbilical Rarely: testicular pain
Diaphragmatic irritation (from spleen, perforated ulcer, or abscess)	Shoulder pain (on the left a + Kehr's sign)
Pancreatitis/cancer	Back pain
Rectal disease	Pain in the small of the back
Nephrolithiasis	Testicular pain/flank pain
Rectal pain	Midline small of back pain
Small bowel	Periumbilical
Uterine pain	Midline small of back pain
Give the classic diagnosis for the following cases:	
Abdominal pain out of proportion to exam	Rule out mesenteric ischemia
Hypotension and pulsatile abdominal mass	Ruptured AAA; go to the OR
Fever, left lower quadrant pain, and change in bowel habits	Diverticulitis
Give the test of choice for the following conditions:	
Cholelithiasis	Ultrasound (U/S)

Bile duct obstruction	U/S
Mesenteric ischemia	Mesenteric A-gram
Ruptured abdominal aortic aneurysm	OR
AAA	Abdominal CT or U/S
Abdominal abscess	Abdominal CT or U/S
Severe diverticulitis	Abdominal CT

What is the most common cause of right upper quadrant pain?

Cholelithiasis

What is the most common cause of surgical right lower quadrant pain?

Acute appendicitis

What is the most common cause of GI tract left lower quadrant pain?

Diverticulitis

29 Hernias

What is a hernia?

The protrusion of an organ or tissue out of the body cavity in which it normally lies; fascial defect

What is the incidence?

Between 5% and 10% lifetime incidence; 50% are indirect inguinal, 25% are direct inguinal, and approximately 15% are femoral

What are the precipitating factors?

Increased intraabdominal pressure: straining at defecation or urination (rectal cancer, colon cancer, prostatic enlargement, constipation), obesity, pregnancy, ascites, valsavagenic (coughing) COPD; the presence of an abnormal congenital anatomic route (i.e., patent processus vaginalis)

Why should hernias be repaired?

To avoid complications of incarceration/strangulation, bowel necrosis, small bowel obstruction, pain

What is more dangerous: a small or large hernia defect?

A small defect is more dangerous because a tight defect is more likely to strangulate if incarcerated

Define the following descriptive terms:

Reducible

The ability to return the displaced organ or tissue/hernia contents to their usual anatomic site

Incarcerated

Swollen or fixed within the hernia sac (incarcerated = imprisoned); may or may not cause intestinal obstruction (i.e., an irreducible hernia)

Strangulated

Incarcerated hernia with resulting ischemia; will result in signs and symptoms of ischemia and intestinal obstruction or bowel necrosis (think: strangulated = choked)

Complete	Hernia sac and its contents protrude all the way through the defect
Incomplete	Defect present without sac or contents protruding completely through it

Define the following types of hernias:

Sliding hernia	The hernia sac is partially formed by the wall of a viscus (i.e., bladder/cecum)
Littre's hernia	Hernia involving a Meckel's diverticulum
Spigelian hernia	Hernia through the linea semilunaris (or spigelian fascia); also known as spontaneous lateral ventral hernia
Internal hernia	Hernia into or involving intraabdominal structure
Obturator hernia	Hernia through obturator canal (females ≥ males)
Lumbar hernia	Petit's hernia or Grynfeltt's hernia
Petit's hernia	(Rare) hernia through Petit's triangle (AKA inferior lumbar triangle) (Think: petit = small = inferior)
Grynfeltt's hernia	Hernia through Grynfeltt-Lesshaft triangle (superior lumbar triangle)
Pantaloon hernia	Hernia sac exists as **both a direct and indirect** hernia straddling the inferior epigastric vessels and protruding through the floor of the canal as well as the internal ring (two sacs separated by the inferior epigastric vessels [the pant crouch] like a pair of pantaloon pants)
Incisional hernia	Hernia through an incisional site; most common cause is a wound infection
Ventral hernia	Incisional hernia in the ventral abdominal wall

Richter's hernia — Incarcerated or strangulated hernia involving only **one sidewall of the bowel,** which can spontaneously reduce, resulting in gangrenous bowel and perforation within the abdomen without signs of obstruction

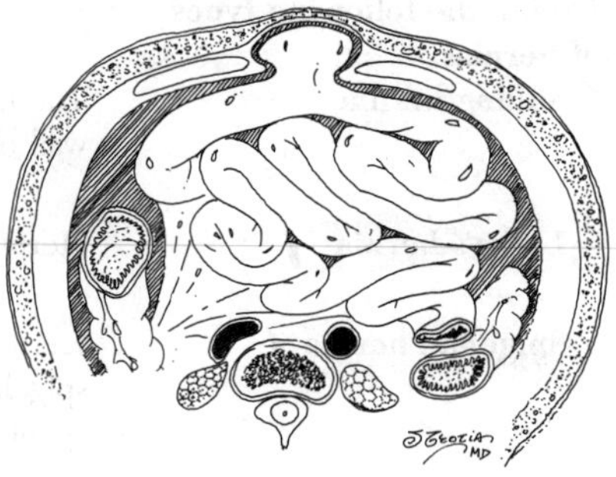

Epigastric hernia — Hernia through the linea alba above the umbilicus

Umbilical hernia — Hernia through the umbilical ring, associated with ascites, pregnancy, and obesity

Intraparietal hernia — Hernia in which abdominal contents migrate between the layers of the abdominal wall

Femoral hernia — Hernia medial to femoral vessels (under inguinal ligament)

Hesselbach's hernia — Hernia under inguinal ligament **lateral** to femoral vessels

Bochdalek's hernia — Hernia through the posterior diaphragm, usually on the left (think: Boch de lek = back to the left on the diaphragm)

Morgagni's hernia — Anterior parasternal diaphragmatic hernia

Properitoneal hernia — Intraparietal hernia between the peritoneum and the transversalis fascia

Cooper's hernia — Hernia through the femoral canal and tracking into the scrotum or labia majus

Indirect inguinal — Inguinal hernia lateral to Hesselbach's triangle

Direct inguinal — Inguinal hernia within Hesselbach's triangle

Hiatal hernia — Hernia through the esophageal hiatus

What are the boundaries of Hesselbach's triangle?

1. Inferior epigastric vessels
2. Inguinal ligament (Poupart's)
3. Lateral border of the rectus sheath

What are the boundaries of Petit's triangle (A.K.A. inferior lumbar triangle)?

Think of a petit white L.I.E.:
Posteriorly—**L: Latissimus dorsi**
Inferiorly—**I: Iliac crest**
Anteriorly—**E: External oblique**
Floor consists of internal oblique and the transversus abdominis muscle

What are the boundaries of Grynfeltt-Lesshaft's triangle (superior lumbar triangle)?

Superiorly—**12th rib**
Anteriorly—**internal oblique**
Floor—**quadratus lumborum**

What are the layers of the abdominal wall?

Skin
Subcutaneous fat
Scarpa's fascia
External oblique
Internal oblique
Transversus abdominous
Transversalis fascia
Preperitoneal fat
Peritoneum
Note: all three muscle layer aponeuroses form the anterior rectus sheath, with the posterior rectus sheath being deficient below the arcuate line

What are the contents of the spermatic cord?

Vas deferens, spermatic vessels, genital branch of the genitofemoral nerve, cremasteric vessels

DIRECT INGUINAL HERNIA

What is it?

A hernia within the floor of Hesselbach's triangle, i.e., the hernia sac does not traverse the internal ring (think of **directly** through the abdominal wall)

What is the cause?	Acquired defect from mechanical breakdown over the years
What is the incidence?	Approximately 1% of all men, with frequency increasing with advanced age
What nerve runs with the spermatic cord in the inguinal canal?	Ilioinguinal nerve

INDIRECT INGUINAL HERNIA

What is it?	Hernia through the internal ring of the inguinal canal, traveling down toward the external ring; it may enter the scrotum upon exiting the external ring (i.e., if complete); think of the hernia sac traveling **indirectly** through the abdominal wall from the internal ring to the external ring
What is the cause?	Patent processus vaginalis (i.e., congenital)
What is the incidence?	Approximately 5% of all men; most common hernia in both men **and** women
How is an inguinal hernia diagnosed?	Relies mainly on history and physical exam with index finger invaginated into the external ring and palpation of hernia; examine the patient standing up if diagnosis is not obvious **Note:** if swelling occurs below the inguinal ligament, it is possibly a femoral hernia
What is the differential diagnosis of an inguinal hernia?	Inguinal lymphadenopathy, femoral lymphadenopathy, psoas abscess, ectopic testis, hydrocele of the cord, saphenous varix, lipoma, varicocele
What is the risk of strangulation?	Higher with indirect than direct inguinal hernia, but highest in femoral hernias
What is the treatment?	Emergent herniorrhaphy is indicated if strangulation is suspected or acute incarceration present; otherwise, elective herniorrhaphy is indicated to prevent the chance of incarceration/strangulation.

CLASSIC INTRAOPERATIVE INGUINAL HERNIA QUESTIONS

From what abdominal muscle layer is the cremaster muscle derived?
Internal oblique muscle

From what abdominal muscle layer is the inguinal ligament (AKA Poupart's ligament) derived?
External oblique muscle

To what does the inguinal (Poupart's) ligament attach?
Anterior superior iliac spine to the pubic tubercle

Which nerve travels on the spermatic cord?
Ilioinguinal nerve

What is in the spermatic cord (5)?
1. Cremasteric muscle fibers
2. Vas deferens
3. Testicular artery
4. Testicular pampiniform venous plexus
5. ± hernia sac

What is the hernia sac made of?
Basically peritoneum or a patent processus vaginalis

What attaches the testicle to the scrotum?
The gubernaculum

What is the most common organ in an inguinal hernia sac in men?
Small intestine

What is the most common organ in an inguinal hernia sac in women?
Ovary/fallopian tube

What lies in the inguinal canal in the female instead of the VAS?
Round ligament

Where in the inguinal canal does the hernia sac lie in relation to the other structures?
Anteriomedially

What is a "cord lipoma"?
Preperitoneal fat on the cord structures (pushed in by the hernia sac); not a real lipoma; remove surgically, if feasible

What is a small outpouching of testicular tissue off of the testicle?
Testicular appendage (AKA the appendix testes); remove with electrocautery

What action should be taken if a suture is placed through the femoral artery or vein during an inguinal herniorrhaphy ?
Remove the suture as soon as possible and apply pressure (i.e., do not tie the suture down!)

What nerve is found on top of the spermatic cord?
Ilioinguinal nerve

What nerve travels within the spermatic cord?
The genital branch of the genitofemoral nerve

What is Hesselbach's triangle?
1. Epigastric vessels
2. Inguinal ligament
3. Lateral border of the rectus sheath

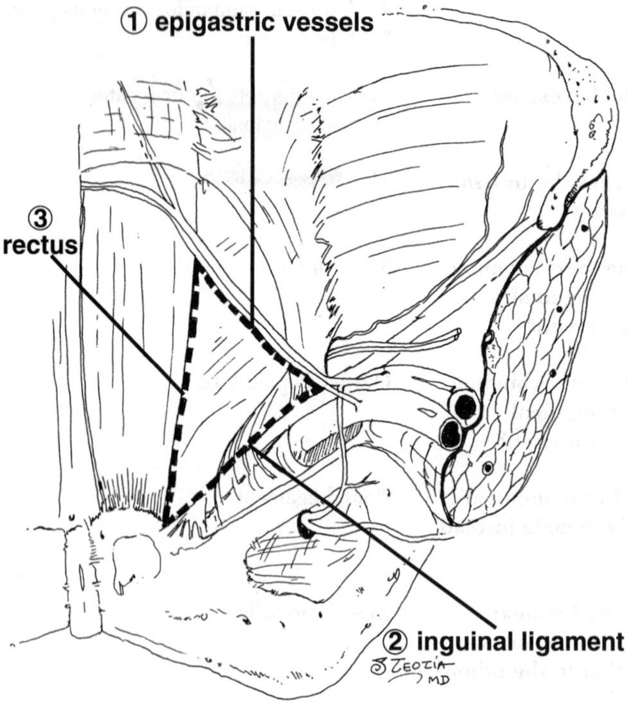

What type of hernia goes through Hesselbach's triangle?

A direct hernia due to a weak abdominal floor

What is a "relaxing incision"?

Incision(s) in the rectus sheath to relax the conjoint tendon so that it can be approximated to the reflection of the inguinal ligament without tension

What is the conjoint tendon?

The aponeurotic attachments of the transversus abdominis to the pubic tubercle (the classic conjoining of the aponeurosis of the internal oblique and transversus aponeurosis attaching to the tubercle is actually very rare [< 4%])

Define inguinal anatomy.

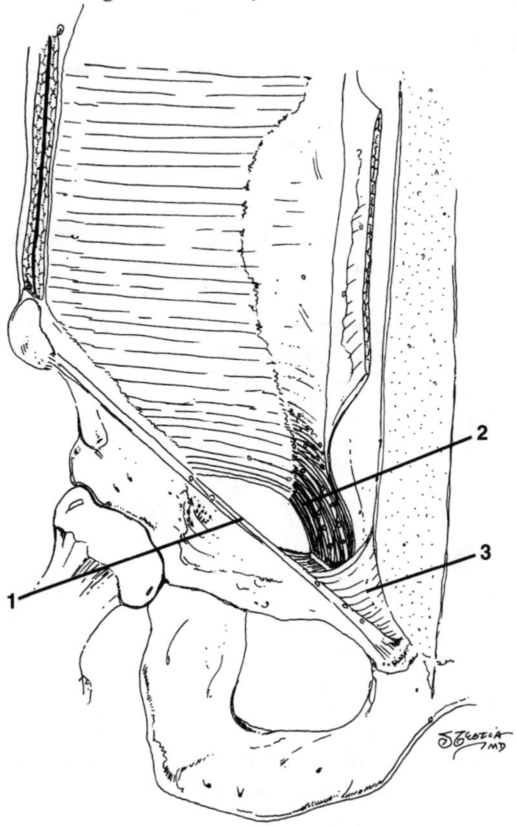

1. Inguinal ligament (Poupart's ligament)
2. Transversus aponeurosis
3. Conjoint tendon

FEMORAL HERNIA

What is it?	Hernia traveling beneath the inguinal ligament down the femoral canal medial to the femoral vessels
What factors are femoral hernias associated with?	Women, pregnancy, and exertion
What is the incidence?	Greater in females than males, but indirect inguinal is still the most common in females
What are the complications?	Approximately one-third incarcerate (due to narrow, unforgiving neck)
What is the most common hernia in females?	Indirect inguinal hernia

ESOPHAGEAL HIATAL HERNIAS

What are the types?

1. Paraesophageal
2. Sliding

PARAESOPHAGEAL HIATAL HERNIA

What is it?

Herniation of all or part of the stomach through the esophageal hiatus into the thorax without displacement of the gastroesophageal junction; also known as type II hiatal hernia

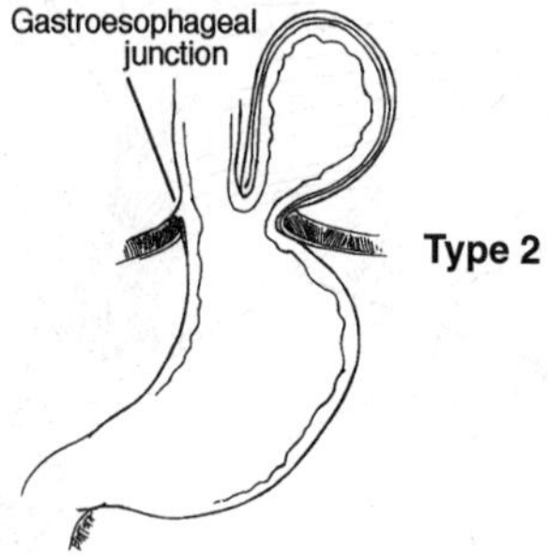

What is the incidence?	Less than 5% of all hiatal hernias (rare)
What are the symptoms?	Derived from mechanical obstruction—dysphagia, stasis gastric ulcer, and strangulation; many cases are asymptomatic and not associated with reflux because of a relatively normal position of the GE junction

What are the complications?

Hemorrhage, incarceration, obstruction, and strangulation

What is the treatment?

Surgical, because of frequency and severity of potential complications

SLIDING ESOPHAGEAL HIATAL HERNIA

What is it?

Both the stomach and the GE junction herniate into the thorax via the esophageal hiatus; also known as type I hiatal hernia

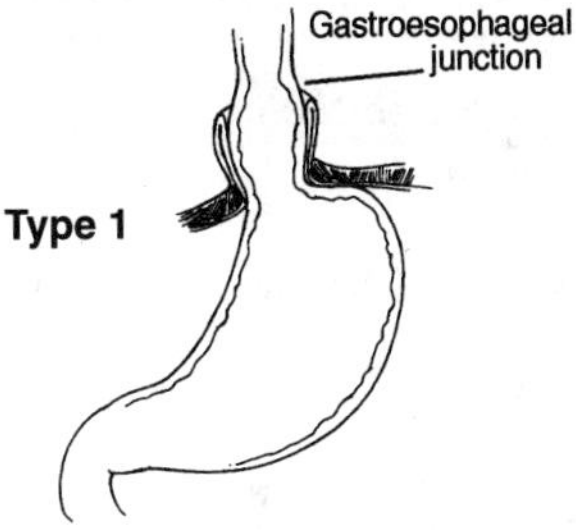

What is the incidence?

More than 90% of all hiatal hernias

What are the symptoms?

The majority of patients are asymptomatic, but the condition can cause **reflux,** dysphagia (from inflammatory edema), esophagitis, and pulmonary problems secondary to aspiration.

Reflux is due to the displacement of the GE junction into the thorax, resulting in loss of the normal contribution from intraabdominal pressure to the competency of the LES because the intrathoracic pressure is 10 to 15 mm Hg lower

How is it diagnosed?

UGI series, manometry, EGD with biopsy for esophagitis

What are the complications?

Reflux → esophagitis → Barrett's esophagus → cancer and stricture formation; aspiration pneumonia; it can also result in UGI bleeding from esophageal ulcerations

What is the treatment?
Eighty-five percent of cases are treated medically with antacids, head elevation after meals, small meals, and no food prior to sleeping; fifteen percent of cases require surgery for persistent symptoms despite adequate medical treatment; Nissen fundoplication involves wrapping the fundus around the LES and suturing it in place, thus maintaining the LES intraabdominally and helping to buttress the sphincter

HERNIA REVIEW QUESTIONS

What is the most common hernia in females?
Indirect inguinal hernia

Should elective TURP or elective herniorrhaphy be performed first?
TURP

Which type of esophageal hiatal hernia is associated with GE reflux?
Sliding esophageal hiatal hernia

How can an incarcerated hernia be reduced in the ER?
1. Apply ice to the incarcerated hernia
2. Sedate
3. Use the Trendelenburg position for inguinal hernias
4. Apply steady manual pressure
5. Admit and observe for signs of necrotic bowel after reduction
6. Perform surgical herniorrhaphy ASAP

What is the major difference in repairing a pediatric indirect inguinal hernia and the repair of an adult inguinal hernia?
In babies and children it is rarely necessary to repair the inguinal floor; repair with "high ligation" of the hernia sac.

What is the Howship-Romberg sign?
Pain along the medial aspect of the proximal thigh due to nerve compression caused by an obturator hernia

What is the "silk glove" sign?
The inguinal hernia sac in an infant/toddler feels like a finger of a silk glove when rolled under the examining finger

30 Laparoscopy

What is laparoscopy?

Minimally invasive surgical technique using gas to insufflate the peritoneum and instruments manipulated through ports introduced through small incisions with video camera guidance

What gas is used and why?

CO_2 because of better solubility in blood and, thus, less risk of gas embolism

Which operations are performed with the laparoscope?

Frequently—cholecystectomy; appendectomy; hernia repair; liver biopsy; many gynecologic operations, including tubal ligation and laparoscopic-assisted vaginal hysterectomy; many urologic procedures, including retroperitoneal lymphadenectomy; Nissen fundoplication

Infrequently—bowel resection, colostomy, surgery for PUD (PGV), colectomy

What are the contraindications?

Absolute—hypovolemic shock, severe cardiac decompensation

Relative—peritonitis, multiple previous surgical procedures, diaphragmatic hernia, COPD

What are the associated complications?

Pneumothorax, bleeding, perforating injuries, infection, intestinal injuries, solid organ injury, vascular injury, **CO_2 embolus,** increased end-tide CO_2, decreased venous return, bladder injury

What are the advantages over laparotomy?

Shorter hospitalization, less pain and scarring, lower cost, decreased ileus

What are the steps in laparoscopic cholecystectomy?

1. Dissection of peritoneum overlying the cystic duct and artery
2. Clipping of cystic artery and cannulation of cystic duct
3. Intraoperative cholangiogram, if necessary

4. Division of cystic duct between clips
5. Dissection of gallbladder from the liver bed
6. Cauterization; irrigation; suction, to obtain hemostasis of the liver bed
7. Removal of the gallbladder through the umbilical trocar site

What are the steps in laparoscopic appendectomy (lap appy)?

1. Identify the appendix
2. Staple the mesoappendix (or coagulate)
3. Staple and transect the appendix at the base (or use Endoloop® and cut between)
4. Remove the appendix from the abdomen
5. Irrigate and aspirate until clear

What are the indications for laparoscopic inguinal hernia repair?

1. Bilateral inguinal hernias
2. Recurring hernia
3. Need to resume full activity as soon as possible (e.g., college football player)

What are the steps in a laparoscopic hernia?

1. Identify the inguinal anatomy/hernia
2. Open investing peritoneum over the internal inguinal ring
3. Staple mesh to abdominal wall over the hernia site
4. Staple the overlying peritoneum shut

What is the Veress needle?

Needle with spring loaded, retractable, blunt inner protective tube that protrudes from the needle end when it enters peritoneal cavity; used for blind entrance and then insufflation of CO_2 through the Veress needle

How can it be verified that the Veress needle is in the peritoneum?

Syringe of saline; saline should flow freely without pressure through the needle "drop test"

If the Veress needle is not in the peritoneal cavity, what happens to the CO_2 flow/pressure?

Flow decreases and pressure is way up

What is the Hasson technique?

No Veress needle—cut down and place trocar under **direct visualization**

What is the cause of postlaparoscopic shoulder pain?

Referred pain from CO_2 on diaphragm and diaphragm stretch

What is a laparoscopic-assisted procedure?

Laparoscopic dissection; then, part of the procedure is performed through an open incision

What is FRED®?

Fog **R**eduction **E**limination **D**evice; sponge with antifog solution used to coat the camera lens

Give some tips for "driving" the camera during laparoscopy.

1. Keep the camera centered on the action
2. Watch all trocars as they enter the peritoneal cavity (and the tissues beyond, so they can be avoided!)
3. Watch all instruments as they come through the trocars (unless directed otherwise)
4. Ask if you want to come out and clean and re-FRED the lens
5. Look outside the body at the trocars and instrument angles to reorient yourself
6. Keep the camera oriented at all times (i.e., up and down); usually the camera cord is on the bottom of the camera—orient yourself to the camera before entering the abdomen
7. You may clean the camera lens at times by lightly touching the lens to the liver or peritoneum
8. Never let the camera lens come into contact with the bowel because it may get very hot and you can burn a hole in the bowel!
9. Put your helmet on (i.e., expect to get yelled at!)
10. Never act agitated when the surgeons are a little abrupt (e.g., "Center—center the camera!")
11. Always watch the trocars as they are removed from the abdominal wall for bleeding from the site and view the layers of the abdominal wall looking for bleeding as you pull the camera trocar out at the end of the case

31 Trauma

What widely accepted protocol does trauma care in the United States follow?

The Advanced Trauma Life Support (ATLS) precepts of the American College of Surgeons

What are the three main elements of the ATLS protocol?

1. Primary survey/resuscitation
2. Secondary survey
3. Definitive care

How and when should the patient history be obtained?

Should be obtained while completing the primary survey; often the rescue squad, witnesses, and family members must be relied upon

PRIMARY SURVEY

What are the five steps of the primary survey?

A—Airway (and C-spine control)
B—Breathing
C—Circulation
D—Disability
E—Exposure and **E**nvironment
(You **must** know these!)

What principles are followed in completing the primary survey?

Life-threatening problems discovered during the primary survey are **always** addressed **before** proceeding to the next step.

AIRWAY

What are the goals during assessment of the airway?

Securing the airway and protecting the spinal cord

In addition to the airway, what MUST be considered during the airway step?

Spinal immobilization

What comprises spinal immobilization?

Use of a full backboard and rigid cervical collar

In an alert patient, what is the quickest test for an adequate airway?	Ask a question; if the patient can speak, the airway is intact.
What is the first maneuver used to establish an airway?	Chin lift and/or jaw thrust; if successful, often an oral or nasal airway can be used to temporarily maintain the airway
If these methods are unsuccessful, what is the next maneuver used to establish an airway?	Endotracheal intubation, either nasal or oral (oral if the patient is not breathing with inline C-spine traction)
When is nasotracheal intubation contraindicated?	Patients with maxillofacial fracture, apnea
If all other methods are unsuccessful, what is the definitive airway?	Cricothyroidotomy (by surgical placement of a tube through the cricothyroid membrane ["surgical airway"])
What must always be kept in mind during difficult attempts at establishing an airway?	Spinal immobilization and adequate oxygenation; if at all possible, patients must be adequately ventilated with 100% oxygen using a bag and mask before any attempt at establishing an airway

BREATHING

What are the goals in assessing breathing?	Securing oxygenation and ventilation Treating life-threatening thoracic injuries
What comprises adequate assessment of breathing?	Inspection—for air movement, respiratory rate, cyanosis, tracheal shift, jugular venous distention, asymmetric chest expansion, use of accessory muscles of respiration, open chest wounds Auscultation—for upper airway sounds (stridor, wheezing, or gurgling) and for lower airway sounds present over both lung fields Percussion—hyperresonance or dullness over either lung field Palpation—presence of subcutaneous emphysema, flail segments

What are six life-threatening conditions that MUST be diagnosed and treated during the breathing step?

Airway obstruction, tension pneumothorax, open pneumothorax, flail chest, cardiac tamponade, massive hemothorax

Pneumothorax

What is it?

Injury to the lung, resulting in release of air into pleural space between the normally apposed parietal and visceral pleura

How is it diagnosed?

Tension pneumothorax is a clinical diagnosis: dyspnea, jugular venous distention, tachypnea, anxiety, pleuritic chest pain, unilateral decreased or absent breath sounds, tracheal shift away from the affected side, hyperresonance on the affected side

What is the treatment of a tension pneumothorax?

Immediate decompression by **needle thoracostomy** in the second intercostal space midclavicular line, followed by **tube thoracostomy** placed in the anterior/midaxillary line in the fourth intercostal space (level of the nipple in men)

How is open pneumothorax, also known as sucking chest wound, diagnosed and treated?

Diagnosis: usually obvious, with air movement through a chest wall defect
Treatment in the ER: +/- intubation with positive-pressure ventilation, tube thoracostomy (chest tube), dressing

Flail Chest

How is it diagnosed?

The classic picture consists of four or more multiply fractured ribs, resulting in a flail segment of chest wall that moves **paradoxically** and results in hypoventilation

What is the treatment?

Intubation with positive pressure ventilation and PEEP prn

Cardiac tamponade

What is it?

Bleeding into the pericardial sac, resulting in constriction of heart

How is it diagnosed?

Beck's triad of decreased heart sounds, jugular venous distention, and decreased blood pressure

Also, tachycardia, pulsus paradoxus, Kussmaul's sign

Hypotension due to tamponade implies imminent cardiac collapse

What is the treatment?

Immediate IV fluid bolus; **with pericardiocentesis, subsequent surgical exploration is mandatory**

Massive Hemothorax

How is it diagnosed?

Hypotension; unilaterally decreased or absent breath sounds; dullness to percussion; obvious appearance on CXR if massive (but remember, up to 500 ml of blood can be hidden by the diaphragm on upright CXR)

What is the treatment?

Volume replacement

Tube thoracostomy (chest tube)

Use of cell saver, if available

Removal of the blood (which will allow apposition of the parietal and visceral pleura, sealing the defect and slowing the bleeding)

If bleeding continues (> 200 cc per hour), perform exploratory thoracotomy.

CIRCULATION

What are the goals in assessing circulation?

Securing adequate tissue perfusion; treatment of external bleeding

What is the initial test for adequate circulation?

Palpation of pulses:

As a rough guide, if a radial pulse is palpable, then systolic pressure is at least 80 mm Hg, and if a femoral or carotid pulse is palpable, then systolic pressure is at least 60 mm Hg.

What comprises adequate assessment of circulation?

Heart rate, blood pressure, peripheral perfusion, urinary output, mental status, capillary refill (normal < 2 seconds), exam of skin: cold, clammy = hypovolemia

Beware of relying only on the blood pressure. Especially in the young, autonomic tone can maintain blood pressure until cardiovascular collapse is imminent

Which patients may not mount a tachycardic response to hypovolemic shock?

Those with concomitant spinal cord injuries
Those on β-blockers
Well-conditioned athletes

How are sites of external bleeding treated?

By direct pressure; avoid tourniquets and blind clamping of bleeding sites (both lead to increased limb loss)

What is the best and preferred intravenous access in the trauma patient?

"Two large-bore IVS" (14–16 gauge) intravenous catheters in the upper extremities (peripheral IV access)

What are alternate sites of intravenous access?

Percutaneous and cutdown catheters in the lower leg saphenous (cutdown) and femoral veins (percutaneous); avoid subclavian and jugular lines if possible because of their increased morbidity in the trauma patient (e.g., PTX)

For a femoral vein catheter, how can the anatomy of the right groin be remembered?

Navel:
N—nerve
A—artery
V—vein
E—extralymphatic material
L—lymphatics
Thus, the vein is medial to the femoral artery pulse

What is the resuscitation fluid of choice?

Lactated Ringer's (LR) solution (isotonic, and the lactate helps buffer the hypovolemia-induced metabolic acidosis)

What types of decompression must the trauma patient receive?

Gastric decompression with an NG tube and Foley catheter bladder decompression **after normal rectal exam**

What are the contraindications to placement of a Foley?

Signs of urethral injury:
Severe pelvic fracture in men
Blood at the urethral meatus (penile opening)
"High-riding" prostate (loss of urethral tethering)
Scrotal/perineal injury/ecchymosis

What test should be obtained prior to placing a Foley catheter if uretheral injury is feared?

A retrograde urethrogram (RUG; dye in penis retrograde to the bladder and x-ray looking for extravasation of dye)

How is gastric decompression achieved with a maxillofacial fracture?

Not with an NG tube because the tube may perforate from the cribriform plate into the brain; place an **oral**-gastric tube (OGT), not an NG tube

DISABILITY

What are the goals in assessing disability?

Determination of neurologic injury (think: neurologic disability)

What comprises adequate assessment of disability?

Mental status—Glasgow coma scale (GCS)
Pupils—a blown pupil reflects ipsilateral brain mass (blood) as the CN III is compressed by herniation of the brain
Motor/sensory—screening exam for lateralizing extremity movement, sensation deficit

Describe the GCS scoring system?

Eye opening (E)
4—Opens spontaneously
3—Opens to voice (command)
2—Opens to painful stimulus
1—Does not open eyes
(think: eyes = "four eyes")
Motor response (M)
6—Obeys commands
5—Localizes painful stimulus
4—Withdraws from pain
3—Decorticate posture
2—Decerebrate posture
1—No movement
(think: motor = 6 "cylinder motor")

Verbal response (V)
5—Appropriate and oriented
4—Confused
3—Inappropriate words
2—Incomprehensible sounds
1—No sounds
(think: verbal 5 = "Jackson 5")

What is the GCS score for a dead man?
GCS 3

What is the GCS score for a patient in a "coma"?
GCS < 8

How does scoring differ if the patient is intubated?
The verbal evaluation is omitted and replaced with a "T"; thus, the highest score for an intubated patient is 10T.

EXPOSURE

What are the goals in obtaining adequate exposure?
Complete disrobing to allow a thorough visual inspection and digital palpation of the patient during the secondary survey

What is the "environment" of the E?
Keep a warm **E**nvironment (i.e., keep the patient warm; a hypothermic patient can become acidotic, arrhythmic, and coagulopathic).

Secondary Survey

What principle is followed in completing the secondary survey?
Complete physical examination, including all orifices: ears, nose, mouth, vagina, rectum

Why look in the ears?
Hemotympanum is a sign of basilar skull fracture, otorrhea is a sign of basilar skull fracture

Examination of what part of the trauma patient's body is often forgotten?
The patient's back (logroll the patient and examine!)

What are typical signs of basilar skull fracture?
Raccoon eyes, Battle's sign, clear otorrhea or rhinorrhea, hemotympanum

What diagnosis with blood in the anterior chamber must not be missed on the eye exam?

Traumatic hyphema

What potentially destructive lesion must not be missed on the nasal exam?

Nasal septal hematoma
The hematoma must be evacuated; if not, it can result in pressure necrosis of the septum!

What is the best indication of a mandibular fracture?

Dental malocclusion; tell the patient to "bite down" and ask:
"Does that feel normal to you?"

What signs of thoracic trauma are often found on the neck exam?

Crepitus or subcutaneous emphysema from tracheobronchial disruption/PTX; tracheal deviation from tension pneumothorax; jugular venous distention from cardiac tamponade; carotid bruit heard with seatbelt neck injury resulting in carotid artery injury

What is the best exam for broken ribs or sternum?

Lateral and anterior–posterior compression of the thorax to elicit pain/instability

What physical signs are diagnostic for thoracic great vessel injury?

None; diagnosis of great vessel injury requires a high index of suspicion based on the mechanism of injury, associated injuries, and CXR/radiographic findings (e.g., widened mediastinum)

What must be considered in every penetrating injury of the thorax at or below the level of the nipple?

Concomitant injury to the abdomen; remember, the diaphragms go up to the level of the nipples in the male on full expiration

What is the significance of subcutaneous air?

Indicates PTX, until proven otherwise

What is the proper technique for examining the thoracic and lumbar spine?

Logrolling the patient to allow complete visualization of the back and palpation of the spine to elicit pain over fractures

What conditions must exist to pronounce an abdominal physical exam negative?	An alert patient without any evidence of head/spinal cord injury or drug/ETOH intoxication (and even then, the abdominal exam is not 100% accurate)
What physical signs may indicate intraabdominal injury?	Tenderness; guarding, plus rebound tenderness and other signs of peritoneal irritation; progressive distention (always use a gastric tube for decompression of air)
What must be documented from the rectal exam?	Sphincter tone (as an indication of spinal cord injury); presence of blood (as an indication of colon or rectal injury); prostate position (as an indication of urethral injury)
What is the best physical exam technique to test for pelvic fractures?	Lateral compression of the iliac crests and greater trochanters and anterior–posterior compression of the symphysis pubis to elicit pain/instability
What physical signs indicate possible urethral injury, thus contraindicating placement of a Foley catheter?	**High-riding ballotable prostate** on rectal exam; presence of blood at the meatus; scrotal or perineal ecchymosis
What must be documented from the extremity exam?	Any fractures or joint injuries; any open wounds; motor and sensory exam, particularly distal to any fractures; distal pulses; peripheral perfusion
What complication that must be treated immediately to save the lower extremity is seen after prolonged ischemia to an extremity?	Compartment syndrome
What is that treatment?	Four-compartment fasciotomy
What injuries must be suspected in a trauma patient with a progressive decline in mental status?	Epidural hematoma, subdural hematoma, brain swelling with rising intracranial pressure But **hypoxia/hypotension must be ruled out!**

TRAUMA STUDIES

During evaluation of blunt trauma, radiographic films are usually obtained sometime during the primary survey in the ER. What films are required?

The trauma triple:
1. Lateral cervical spine film
2. AP (anterior-to-posterior) chest film
3. AP pelvis film

Also during the primary survey, specimens are sent for laboratory analysis. Which specimens are usually sent?

Blood for complete blood count, chemistries, amylase, liver function tests, lactic acid, coagulation studies, and **type and crossmatch**

Blood is often spun in the emergency department for a quick estimate of hematocrit

Urine for urinalysis

What films are required to evaluate for possible cervical spinal injury?

Lateral spine, AP spine, open-mouth odontoid

What vertebral bodies must be seen to adequately evaluate a lateral cervical spine film?

C_1 to T1

What view is used for seeing these vertebrae beyond the normal lateral spine film?

Swimmer's view can help visualize C_7 to T1

Which x-rays are used for evaluation of cervical spine LIGAMENTOUS injury?

Lateral flexion and extension C-spine films

What findings on chest film are suggestive of thoracic great vessel injury?

Widened mediastinum (most common finding), apical pleural capping, loss of aortic contour/KNOB/a–p window, depression of left main stem bronchus, nasogastric tube/tracheal deviation, pleural fluid

What study is used to rule out thoracic great vessel injury?

Thoracic arch aortogram (gold standard)

What percentage of thoracic aortograms will reveal an aortic injury?

Only about 10% of studies are positive

What studies are available to evaluate for intraabdominal injury?

Diagnostic peritoneal lavage (DPL) and CT scan (laparoscopy and ultrasound are being evaluated for use in trauma)

What are the respective advantages of these studies?

Peritoneal lavage (DPL) is a sensitive and specific test for intraperitoneal blood and can be rapidly completed in the emergency room, operating room, or even in the CT scanner while the head is being studied. But DPL does not evaluate the retroperitoneum.

CT scanning can detect retroperitoneal injury and can better localize and characterize an injury, thus giving the option of nonoperative therapy (e.g., liver laceration/spleen laceration). But CT misses small bowel injury.

What injuries does a DPL miss?

Retroperitoneal injury (e.g., contained kidney lacertion)

What injuries does abdominal CT miss?

Small bowel injuries
Diaphragmatic injuries

What is the indication for abdominal CT in blunt trauma?

Stable vital signs with abdominal pain/ tenderness

What is the indication for DPL in blunt trauma?

Unstable vital signs

How is a DPL performed?

Place a catheter below the umbilicus (in patients without a pelvic fracture) into peritoneal cavity
Aspirate for blood and if less than 10 cc are aspirated, infuse 1 L of saline or LR
Drain the fluid (by gravity) and analyze

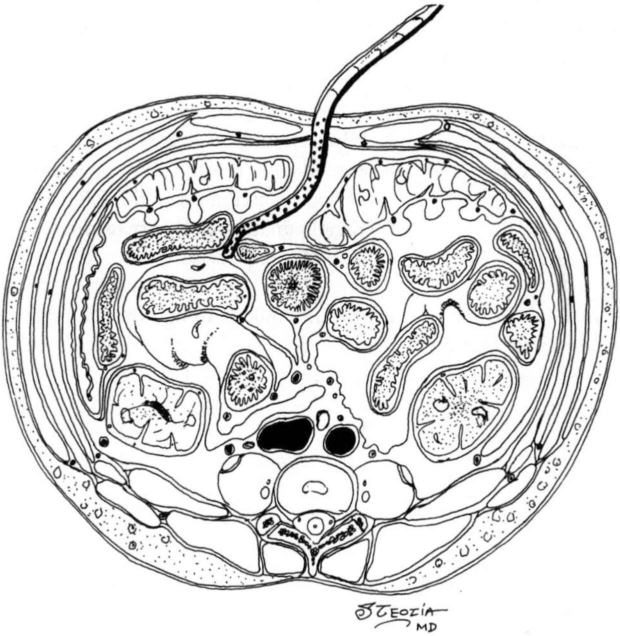

Where should the DPL catheter be placed in a patient with a pelvic fracture?

Above the umbilicus
A common error—if you go below the umbilicus, you may get into a pelvic hematoma tracking between the fascia layers and thus obtain a false-positive DPL

What are the indicators of a positive peritoneal lavage?

Classic: inability to read newsprint through lavaged fluid
RBC $\geq$ 100,000/mm^3
WBC $\geq$ 500/mm^3 (Note: mm^3, **not** mm^2)
Lavage fluid (LR/NS) drained from chest tube, Foley, NG tube
Less common:
Bile present
Bacteria present
Feces present

	Vegetable matter present Elevated amylase level
What must be in place before a DPL is performed?	NG tube and Foley catheter (to remove the stomach and bladder from the firing line!)
What study is used to evaluate the urethra in cases of possible disruption due to blunt trauma?	Retrograde urethrogram (RUG)
What are the most emergent orthopaedic injuries?	1. **Hip dislocation**—must be reduced immediately (on the x-ray table or during resuscitation in the ER) 2. Exsanguinating **pelvic fracture** (external fixator)
What depth of neck injury must be further evaluated?	Pentrating injury through the platysma

Define the anatomy of the neck by trauma zones:

Zone III — Angle of the mandible and up

Zone II — Angle of the mandible to the cricoid cartilage

Zone I — Below the cricoid cartilage (think of the zone Roman numerals piled in anatomic order: III, II, I and thus, forming the shape of a face)
Note: the zones are in the same anatomic order as the LeFort facial fractures (III, II, I!)

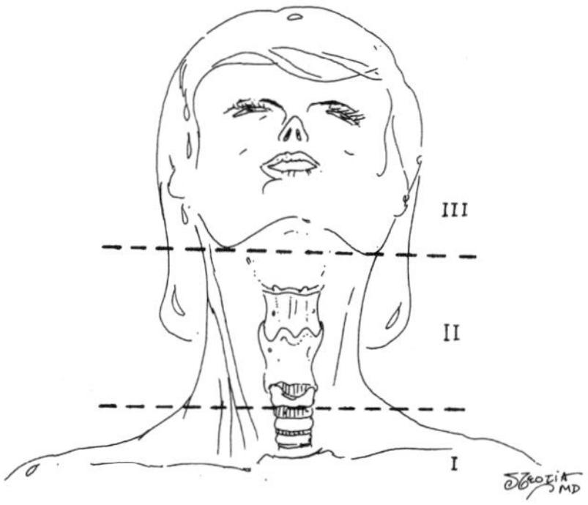

How do most surgeons treat penetrating (that penetrate the platysma) neck injuries by neck zone:

Zone III — A-gram first

Zone II — Surgical exploration

Zone I — A-gram first

What films are typically obtained to evaluate extremity fractures? — Complete views of the involved extremity, including the joints above and below the fracture

MISCELLANEOUS TRAUMA FACTS

What is the "3-for-1" rule? — The trauma patient in hypovolemic shock acutely requires 3 L of crystalloid (LR) for every 1 L of blood loss

What is the minimal urine output for an adult trauma patient?	50 ml/hr
What findings would require a celiotomy in a blunt trauma victim?	Peritoneal signs, free air on AXR/CT, positive DPL, massive injury on CT scan
What is the treatment of a gunshot wound to the belly?	Exploratory laparotomy
What is the treatment of a stab wound to the belly?	If there are peritoneal signs, heavy bleeding, shock, omentum or bowel sticking out the wound, unstable vital signs, perform exploratory laparotomy. Otherwise, many surgeons observe the asymptomatic stab wound patient **closely.**
What constitutes a positive peritoneal tap?	Prior to starting a peritoneal lavage, the DPL catheter should be aspirated. If more than 10 ml of blood or enteric contents are aspirated, then this constitutes a positive tap and requires laparotomy.
How much blood can be lost into the thigh with a closed femur fracture?	Up to 3 L of blood, or more than half the patient's blood volume!
Can an adult lose enough blood in the skull from a brain injury to cause hypovolemic shock?	Absolutely **not!** But infants can lose enough blood from a brain injury to cause shock.
What is the brief ATLS history?	An "AMPLE" history: A—Allergies M—Medications P—PMH L—Last meal (when) E—Events (of injury, etc.)
In what population is a surgical cricothyroidotomy not recommended?	Any patient less than 12 years old; instead perform needle cricothyroidotomy

What is the treatment of subcutaneous emphysema?	Nothing (unless there is external compression by the emphysema of the upper airway [rare]; rule out PTX)
What is a massive hemothorax?	More than 1500 ml of blood from the chest tube (treat initially by IVF and chest tube)
What are the signs of a laryngeal fracture?	Subcutaneous emphysema in neck Altered voice Palpable laryngeal fracture
What is the treatment of rectal penetrating injury?	**Diverting proximal colostomy;** closure of perforation (if easy, and definitely if intraperitoneal); and **presacral drainage**
What is the treatment of extraperitoneal minor bladder rupture?	Catheter bladder (Foley) drainage and observation. Intraperitoneal or large bladder rupture requires operative closure in three layers.
What intraabdominal injury is associated with seatbelt use?	Small bowel injuries, (L2 fracture, pancreatic injury)
What is the treatment of a pelvic fracture?	± MAST trousers until the external fixator is placed; IVF/blood, supraumbilical DPL; and A-gram to embolize bleeding pelvic vessels Do not enter pelvic hematoma in the OR for positive DPL unless there is major arterial injury
If a patient has a laceration through an eyebrow, should you shave the eyebrow prior to suturing it closed?	No; 20% of the time, the eyebrow will not grow back if shaved!
What is the treatment of extensive irreparable duodenal and pancreatic head injury?	Trauma Whipple

What is the most common intraabdominal organ injured with penetrating trauma?	Small bowel
How high up do the diaphragms go?	To the nipples (intercostal space # 4); thus, intraabdominal injury with penetrating injury below the nipples must be ruled out
Classic trauma question: "If you have only one vial of blood from a trauma victim to send to the lab, what test should be ordered?"	Type and cross (for blood transfusion)
What is the treatment of penetrating injury to the colon?	If the patient is unstable and/or there is abundant fecal soilage, resection and colostomy If the patient is stable and there is minimal fecal soilage, the trend is primary repair, +/- resection
What is the treatment of small bowel injury?	Primary closure or resection and primary anastomosis
What is the treatment of minor pancreatic injury?	Drainage (e.g., JP drains)
What comprises the workup/treatment of a parasternal chest gun shot/ stab wound?	1. CXR 2. Chest tube, OR for subxiphoid window; if blood returns, then sternotomy to assess for cardiac injury

BLUNT TRAUMA ALGORITHM

OUTLINE BASIC WORK UP FOR A SEVERE BLUNT TRAUMA VICTIM:

IN E.R.:

Airway, physical exam.IV X 2, 2 L LR, labs, spun HCT, type & cross
OGT/NGT, Foley, +/– chest tube
X-rays:CXR, Pelvis, cross-table C-spine, Femur (if femur fracture is suspected)

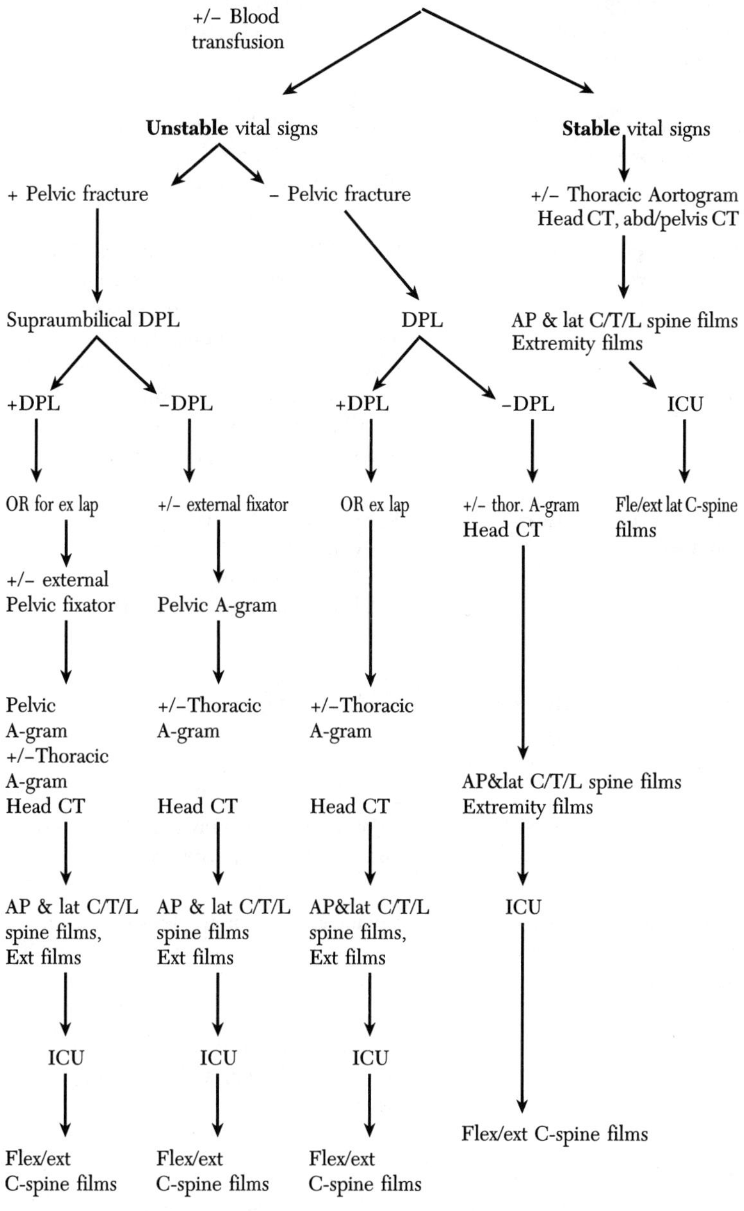

(NOTE: +/– Thoracic aortogram = if Aortic injury suspected on CXR = widened mediastinum)

32 Burns

What consideration besides temperature affects the severity of thermal burns?

Heat capacity; moist heat has a much higher heat capacity (e.g., steam), and thus capacity to burn, than dry heat

Are acid or alkali chemical burns more serious?

In general, alkali burns because the body cannot buffer the alkali, thus allowing them to burn for much longer

Why are electrical burns so dangerous?

Most of the destruction from electrical burns is internal because the route of least electrical resistance follows nerves, blood vessels, and fascia. Injury is usually far worse than external burns at entrance and exit sites would indicate. **Cardiac arrhythmias,** myoglobinuria, acidosis, and renal failure are common.

How is myoglobinuria treated?

To avoid renal injury:
- Hydration with IV fluids
- Mannitol diuresis
- Alkalization of urine with IV bicarbonate

Which skin structures *do* first degree burns involve?

Epidermis only

How do they present?

Painful, dry, red areas that do not form blisters (think of **sunburn**)

Which skin structures do second degree burns involve?

Epidermis and varying levels of dermis

How do they present?

Painful, hypersensitive, swollen, mottled areas with **blisters** and open weeping surfaces

Which skin structures do third degree burns involve?

All layers of the skin, including skin appendages, blood vessels, and nerve endings (think: "getting the third degree")

How do they present?

Painless, insensate, swollen, dry, mottled white, and charred areas

What is the major clinical difference between second and third degree burns?

Third degree burns are painless and second degree burns are very painful (laudable pain)

By which measure is burn severity determined?

Depth of burn and total body surface area (TBSA) affected by second and third degree burns

TBSA is calculated by the "rule of nines" in adults and by a modified rule in children to account for the disproportionate size of the head and trunk

What is the "rule of nines"?

In an adult, the total body surface area that is burned can be estimated by the following:

- Each upper limb = 9%
- Each lower limb = 18%
- Anterior and posterior trunk = 18% each
- Head and neck = 9%
- Perineum and genitalia = 1%

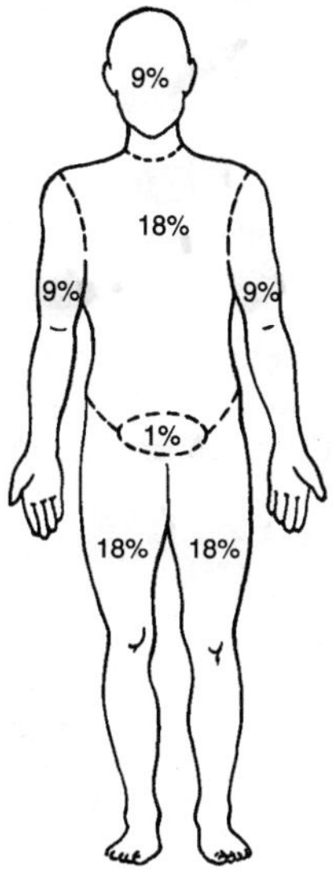

What technique can be used to estimate TBSA in small or discontinuous burns?	The "rule of the palm": the surface area of the patient's palm is approximately 1% of the TBSA
What are the hospitalization criteria for burn patients?	Second degree burns greater than 20% TBSA Third degree burns greater than 10% TBSA Any burns greater than 10% TBSA in children and the elderly Any burns involving the face, hands, feet, or perineum Any burns with inhalation injury Any burns with associated trauma Any electrical burns
What is the first treatment step for any burn?	Stop the burning process; immediately remove all clothes, remove hot and adherent substances such as grease and tar, and copiously irrigate all chemical burns with water; chemical eye burns require prolonged (up to 8 hours) flushing
What is the treatment of third degree burns?	Excision of eschar and split-thickness skin grafting
What is the treatment of second degree burns?	Remove blisters; apply antibiotic ointment and dressing; most second degree burns do not require skin grafting (epidermis grows from hair follicles and from margins)
What is the treatment of first degree burns?	Keep clean
What principles guide the initial assessment and resuscitation of the burn patient?	Airway, breathing, circulation, disability, and exposure (same as for the trauma patient)
What are the signs of smoke inhalation?	Smoke and soot in sputum/mouth/nose; nasal/facial hair burns, carboxyhemoglobin, throat/mouth erythema, history of loss of consciousness/explosion/fire in small enclosed area, dyspnea, low O_2 saturation, confusion, headache, coma

What lab value assesses smoke inhalation?

Carboxyhemaglobin level (a carboxyhemoglobin level of more than 60% is associated with a 50% mortality); treat with 100% O_2 and time

How should the airway be managed in the burn patient with an inhalational injury?

With a low threshold for **intubation;** oropharyngeal swelling may so occlude the airway that intubation is impossible, either very rapidly or slowly and progressively over 24 to 48 hours; 100% oxygen should be administered immediately and continued until significant carboxyhemoglobin is ruled out

What is the "Parkland formula"?

Formula widely used to estimate the volume (V) of crystalloid necessary for the initial resuscitation of the burn patient; half of the calculated volume is given in the **first 8 hours,** the rest in the next 16 hours

V = Total Body Surface Area (%) x Weight (kg) x 4 **(know this formula!)**

How is the crystalloid given?

Through two large-bore peripheral venous catheters introduced through unburned skin

Why is glucose-containing IVF contraindicated in burn patients in the first 24 hours postburn?

The patient's serum glucose will be elevated on its own because of the stress response

What fluid is used after the first 24 hrs postburn?

Colloid; use D5W **and** 5% albumin at 0.5 cc/kg/% burn surface area over 4 to 8 hours

Why should D5W IV be administered after 24 hours postburn?

Because of the massive sodium load in the first 24 hrs of LR infusion and because of the massive evaporation of H_2O from the burn injury, the patient will need free water; after 24 to 36 hours, the capillaries begin to work and then the patient can usually benefit from **albumin** IV (i.e., colloid)

How is volume status monitored in the burn patient?	Blood pressure, heart rate, peripheral perfusion, mental status, and **urinary output;** Foley catheter is mandatory, and may be supplemented by central venous pressure and pulmonary capillary wedge pressure monitoring
Why is it important to monitor temperature closely in the burn patient?	Temperature tends to be very labile due to exposure, fluid losses with evaporation, administration of large volumes of hypothermic fluids, and central temperature instability; hypothermia predisposes patients to cardiac irritability and coagulopathy.
Why do most severely burned patients require nasogastric decompression?	Patients with greater than 20% TBSA burns usually develop a paralytic **ileus** → vomiting→ aspiration risk→ pneumonia
What stress prophylaxis must be given to the burn patient?	H_2 blocker to prevent burn stress ulcer (Curling's ulcer)
What are the clinical signs of burn wound infection?	Fever (possibly), increased WBC with left shift, **discoloration of burn eschar** (most common sign), green pigment, necrotic skin lesion in unburned skin, edema, ecchymosis tissue below eschar, second degree burns that turn into third degree burns
What are the common organisms found in burn wound infections?	*Staphylococcus aureus, Pseudomonas, Streptococcus, Candida albicans*
How is a burn wound infection diagnosed?	Send burned tissue in question to the lab for quantitative burn wound bacterial count. If the count is more than 10^5/g, infection is present and IV antibiotics should be administered.
How are minor burns dressed?	Gentle cleaning with nonionic detergent and debridement of loose skin and broken blisters; the burn is dressed with a topical antibacterial (e.g., neomycin) and covered with a sterile dressing

How are major burns dressed?	Cleansing and application of topical antibacterial agent
Why are systemic IV antibiotics contraindicated?	The bacteria live in the eschar, which is avascular (the systemic antibiotic will not be delivered to the eschar); thus, apply topical antimicrobial agents.
Note some advantages and disadvantages of the following topical antibiotic agents:	
Silver nitrate	Broad spectrum, painless, and inexpensive, but has very poor eschar penetration and may cause **electrolyte imbalances**
Silver sulfadiazine (Silvadene)	Painless, does not cause electrolyte imbalances, does not require occlusive dressing, but little eschar penetration, misses *Pseudomonas,* and has idiosyncratic **neutropenia;** agent of choice for small burns
Mafenide	Penetrates eschars, broad spectrum (but misses *Staphylococcus*), but causes pain and burning on application; triggers allergic reaction in 7% of patients; may cause **acid-base imbalances** (think: **MA**fenide = **M**etabolic **A**cidosis); agent of choice in already-contaminated burn wounds
Betadine	Very poor eschar penetration; use on small, thin eschar burns
Are prophylactic systemic antibiotics administered to burn patients?	**No.** Prophylactic antibiotics have not been shown to reduce the incidence of sepsis, but rather have been shown to select for resistant organisms. IV antibiotics are reserved for established wound infections, pneumonia, urinary tract infections, etc.
Circumferential, full-thickness burns to the extremities are at risk for what complication?	Distal neurovascular impairment similar to compartment syndrome

How is it treated?

Escharotomy: full-thickness longitudinal incision through the eschar with scalpel or electrocautery; incision must extend into healthy fat

What is the major infection complication (other than wound infection) in burn patients?

Pneumonia, central line infection (change central lines prophylactically every 3 to 4 days)

Is tetanus prophylaxis required in the burn patient?

Yes; mandatory in all patients except those actively immunized within the past 12 months (with complete immunization: toxoid x3)

What is the most common failure in the care of burn patients?

Delay in treatment; many complications of severe burns, including renal failure and sepsis, are severely aggravated by inadequate or delayed fluid resuscitation

From which burns is water evaporation highest?

Third degree

Can infection convert a partial-thickness injury into a full-thickness injury?

Yes!

How is carbon monoxide inhalation overdose treated?

100% O_2 ($\pm$ hyperbaric O_2)

Which electrolyte must be closely followed acutely after a burn?

Na^+ (sodium)

When should central lines over a wire be changed in the burn patient?

Every 3 to 4 days **(only in the burn patient)**

What is the name of the gastric/duodenal ulcer associated with burn injury?

Curling's ulcer (think: curling iron burn = Curling's burn ulcer)

What is a better bed for a skin graft: fat or fascia?

Fascia (better blood supply)

33

Upper GI Bleeding

What is it?

Bleeding into the lumen of the proximal GI tract, usually proximal to the ligament of Trietz

What are the signs/ symptoms?

Hematemesis, melena, syncope, shock, fatigue, coffee-ground emesis, hematochezia, epigastric discomfort, epigastric tenderness, signs of hypovolemia, guaiac-positive stools

Why is it possible to have hematochezia?

Blood is a cathartic and usually indicates a vigorous rate of bleeding from the UGI source.

Are stools melenic or melanotic?

Melenic (melanotic is not a word in the English language)

What are the risk factors?

Alcohol, cigarettes, liver disease, burn/ trauma, aspirin/NSAIDs, vomiting, sepsis, steroids, previous UGI bleeding, history of peptic ulcer disease (PUD), esophageal varices, portal hypertension, splenic vein thrombosis, abdominal aortic aneurysm repair (aortoenteric fistula), burn injury, trauma

What is the most common cause of significant UGI bleeding?

Duodenal ulcer (25%)

What are the other possible causes?

Gastric ulcer (20%)
Acute gastritis (15%)
Esophageal varices
Mallory-Weiss tear
Also: gastric cancer, esophagitis, hemobilia, duodenal diverticula, gastric volvulus, Boerhaave's syndrome, aortoenteric fistula, paraesophageal hiatal hernia, epistaxis, NGT irritation, Dieulafoy's ulcer, angiodysplasia

Which diagnostic tests are useful?	History, NGT aspirate, abdominal x-ray, endoscopy (EGD)
What is the diagnostic test of choice with UGI bleeding?	EGD
What are the treatment options with the endoscope during an EGD?	Coagulation, injection of epinephrine (for vasoconstriction), injection of sclerosing agents
Which lab tests should be performed?	Chem-7, bilirubin, LFTs, CBC, **type & cross,** PT/PTT, amylase
Why is BUN elevated?	Because of absorption of blood by the GI tract
What is the initial treatment?	1. **IVFs** (16 G or larger peripheral IVS x 2), **Foley** catheter (monitor fluid status) 2. **NGT** suction (determine rate and amount of blood) 3. Water lavage (use warm H_2O—will remove clots, facilitating esophagogastroduodenoscopy) 4. **EGD:** Endoscopy (determine etiology/location of bleeding and possible treatment—coagulate bleeders)
What test may help identify the site of massive UGI bleeding when there is failure to diagnose cause with EGD and continued blood per NGT?	Selective mesenteric angiography
What are the indications for surgical intervention in UGI bleeding?	Refractory or recurrent bleeding and site known
What percentage of patients require surgery?	Approximately 20%
What percentage of patients spontaneously stop bleeding?	Approximately 80% to 85%

What is the mortality of acute UGI bleeding?	Clasically stated as 10% (approximately 8% mortality in patients less than 60 years old and approximately 13% mortality in patients more than 60 years old)
What are the risk factors for death following UGI bleed?	Age greater than 60 years Shock More than 5 units of PRBC transfusion Concomitant health problems (e.g., heart disease)

PEPTIC ULCER DISEASE (PUD)

What is it?	Includes gastric and duodenal ulcers
What is the incidence in the United States?	Approximately 10% of all Americans will suffer from PUD during their lifetime!
What are the possible consequences of PUD?	Pain, hemorrhage, perforation, obstruction
Which bacteria are associated with PUD?	*Helicobacter pylori*
What is the treatment?	Treat *H. pylori* with **M**etronidazole, **O**meprazole, **C**larithromycin **(MOC)** regimen.

DUODENAL ULCERS

In which age group are these ulcers most common?	Between 40 and 65 years old (younger than gastric ulcer patients)
What is the ratio of male to female patients?	Men > women (2 to 1)
What is the incidence?	More common than gastric ulcer
What is the most common location?	Majority are within 2 cm of the pylorus in the duodenal bulb
What is the cause?	Increased gastric acid production

What are the associated risk factors?	Male gender, smoking, aspirin and other NSAIDs, uremia, Zollinger-Ellison syndrome, *H. pylori,* trauma, burn injury
What are the symptoms?	Epigastric pain—burning or aching, usually several hours after a meal (pain is initially relieved by food, milk, or antacids) Back pain Nausea, vomiting, and anorexia ↓ appetite
What are the signs?	Tenderness in epigastric area (possibly), guaiac-positive stool, melena, hematochezia, hematemesis
What is the differential diagnosis?	Acute abdomen, pancreatitis, cholecystitis, **all causes of UGI bleeding,** Zollinger-Ellison syndrome, gastritis, MI, gastric ulcer
How is the diagnosis made?	History, PE, EGD, UGI series **(if patient is not actively bleeding)**
What EGD finding is associated with rebleeding?	Visible vessel in the ulcer crater (90% rebleed rate)
How is it prevented?	Avoid aspirin (NSAIDs), cigarettes, and alcohol
What is the medical treatment?	**H_2 receptor antagonists**—heal ulcers in 4 to 6 weeks in most cases **Antacids**—control gastric pH, promote healing **Sucralfate**—coats ulcer **Omeprazole**—↓ acid production by stopping H^+–K^+ ion pump; used for refractory ulcers and ulcers associated with Zollinger-Ellison syndrome
What is the most common cause of death from a duodenal ulcer?	Exsanguination

When is surgery indicated?

The acronym I HOP:
I—intractability

H—hemorrhage (massive or relentless)
O—obstruction (gastric outlet obstruction)
P—perforation

What is the goal of surgery?

Decrease gastric acid secretion and fix IHOP

TYPES OF SURGERIES

Define the following terms:

Graham patch

For treatment of duodenal perforation in poor operative candidates/unstable patients
Place viable omentum over perforation and tack into place with sutures.

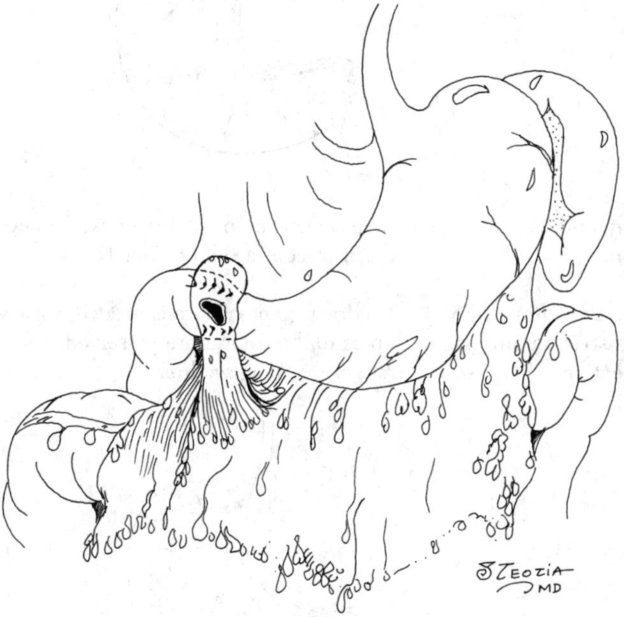

Truncal Vagotomy

Resection of a 1- to 2-cm segment of each vagal **trunk** as it enters the abdomen on the distal esophogus, decreasing gastric acid secretion **and** gastric emptying; also selective vagotomies

What other procedure must be performed along with a truncal vagotomy?

A **"drainage procedure"** (pyloroplasty, antrectomy, or gastrojejunostomy), because vagal fibers provide relaxation of the pylorus and if you cut them the pylorus will not open

Vagotomy and pyloroplasty

Pyloroplasty performed with vagotomy to compensate for decreased gastric emptying

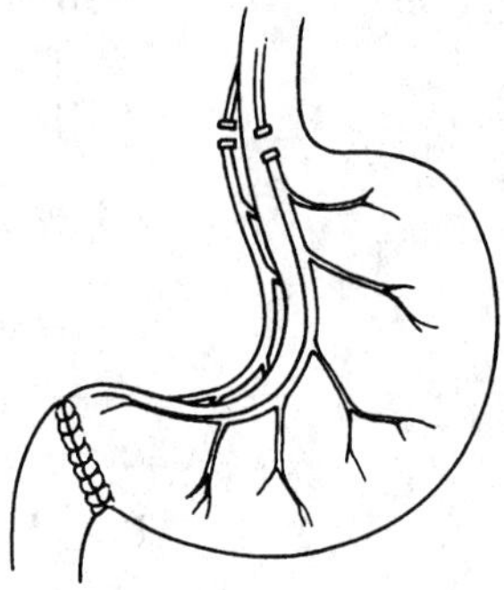

Vagotomy and antrectomy

Remove antrum in addition to vagotomy; reconstruct as a Billroth I or II

What is the advantage of proximal gastric vagotomy (highly selective vagotomy)?

No drainage procedure is needed; vagal fibers to the pylorus are preserved; low rate of dumping syndrome

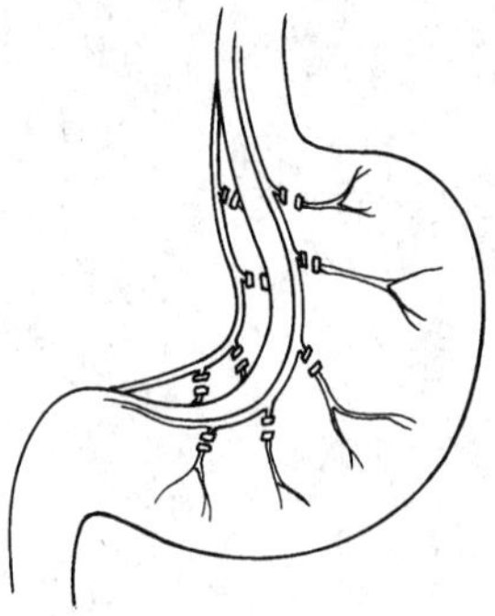

What is a Billroth I (BI)?

Truncal vagotomy, antrectomy, and gastroduodenostomy (think: BI = one limb off of the stomach remnant)

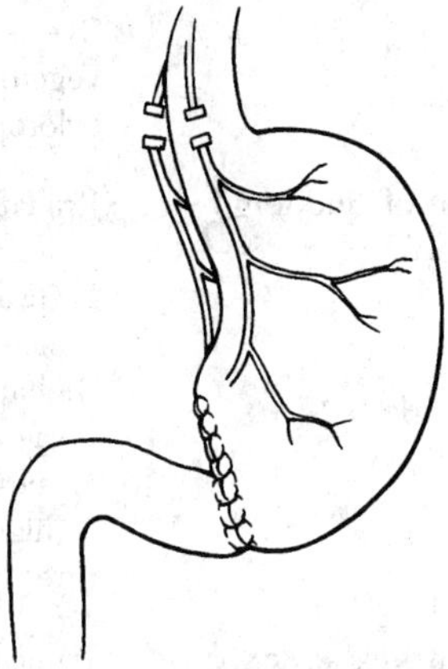

What is a Billroth II (BII)?

Truncal vagotomy, antrectomy, and gastrojejunostomy (think: BII = two limbs off of the stomach remnant)

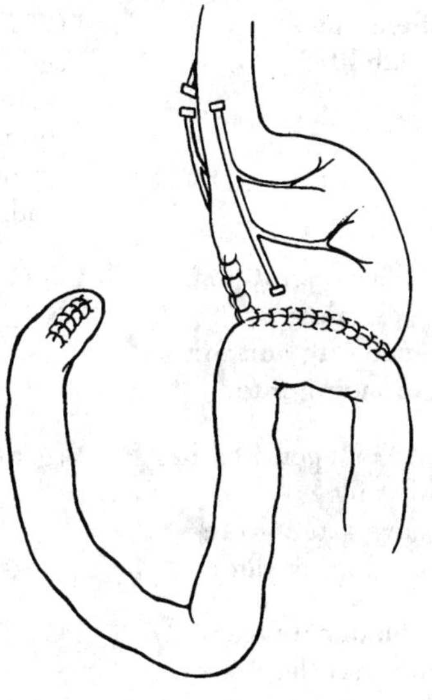

What are the common surgical options for the following conditions:

Correction of a bleeding duodenal ulcer?	Opening of the duodenum through the pylorus Oversewing of the bleeding vessel Vagotomy Pyloroplasty
Treatment of duodenal perforation?	Graham patch (poor candidates, shock, prolonged perforation) Truncal vagotomy and pyloroplasty incorporating ulcer Graham patch and highly selective vagotomy Truncal vagotomy and antrectomy (higher mortality rate, but lowest recurrence rate)
Treatment of duodenal obstruction due to duodenal ulcer scarring (gastric outlet obstruction)?	Truncal vagotomy, antrectomy, and gastroduodenostomy (BI or BII) Truncal vagotomy and drainage procedure (gastrojejunostomy)
Duodenal ulcer intractability?	PGV (highly selective vagotomy) Vagotomy and pyloroplasty Vagotomy and antrectomy BI or BII (especially if there is a coexistent pyloric/prepyloric ulcer) but associated with a higher mortality

Which ulcer operation has the highest ulcer recurrence rate and the lowest dumping rate?

PGV (proximal gastric vagotomy)

Which ulcer operation has the lowest ulcer recurrence rate and the highest dumping rate?

Vagotomy and antrectomy

Which duodenal ulcer operation has the lowest mortality rate?

PGV (1/200 mortality), truncal vagotomy and pyloroplasty (1–2/200), vagotomy and antrectomy (1%–2% mortality)

Thus, PGV is the operation of choice for intractable duodenal ulcers with the cost of increased risk of ulcer recurrence.

What are the relative contraindications for PGV for duodenal ulcers?

Concomitant pyloric or prepyloric ulcer (one-third of patients will have a recurrent ulcer if treated with a PGV)

What is a "kissing" ulcer?

Two ulcers, each on opposite sides of the lumen so that they can "kiss"

Why may a duodenal rupture be painless?

Fluid can be sterile with a nonirritating pH of 7.0 initially

Why may a perforated duodenal ulcer present as lower quadrant abdominal pain?

Fluid from stomach/bile drains down paracolic gutters to lower quadrants and causes localized irritation.

GASTRIC ULCERS

In which age group are these ulcers most common?

Between 40 and 70 years old (older than the duodenal ulcer population)
Rare in patients less than 40 years old

How does the incidence in men compare with that of women?

Men > women

Which is more common overall: gastric or duodenal ulcers?

Duodenal ulcers are more than twice as common as gastric ulcers.

What is the cause?

Decreased cytoprotection or gastric protection (i.e., decreased bicarbonate/ mucous production)

Is gastric acid production high or low?

Nl or low gastric acid production!

What type of gastric ulcers are associated with INCREASED gastric acid?

Prepyloric
Pyloric
Coexist with duodenal ulcers

What are the associated risk factors?

Smoking, alcohol, burns, trauma, CNS tumor/trauma, NSAIDs, steroids, shock, severe illness, male gender, advanced age

What are the symptoms?

Epigastric pain
- Most often transiently relieved by food/antacids (but food can make pain worse in some cases)
- Associated with vomiting, anorexia, and nausea

How is the diagnosis made?

History, PE, **EGD** with multiple biopsy (looking for gastric cancer)

What is the most common location?

Approximately 70% arc on a lesser curvature; 5% are on a greater curvature

When and why should biopsy be performed?

With all gastric ulcers, to rule out gastric cancer

If the ulcer does not heal in 6 weeks after medical treatment **rebiopsy** (biopsy in OR also) must be performed

What is the medical treatment?

Similar to that of duodenal ulcer (e.g., H_2 blockers)

What are the indications for surgery?

The acronym I CHOP
- **I**—intractability
- **C**—cancer (rule out)
- **H**—hemorrhage (massive or relentless)
- **O**—obstruction (gastric outlet obstruction)
- **P**—perforation

(Surgery is indicated if gastric cancer cannot be ruled out.)

What is the common operation for hemorrhage, obstruction, and perforation?

Distal gastrectomy with excision of the ulcer **without** vagotomy unless there is duodenal disease (i.e., BI or BII)

What are the options for concomitant duodenal and gastric ulcers?

BI, BII, and **truncal vagotomy**

What is a common option for surgical treatment of a pyloric gastric ulcer?

Truncal vagotomy and antrectomy (i.e., BI or BII)

What is a common option for a poor operative candidate with a perforated gastric ulcer?	Graham patch
What must be performed in every operation for gastric ulcers?	Biopsy looking for gastric cancer
What is the recurrence rate?	~ up to two-thirds in 2 years with medical treatment alone (usually recur within 6 months of the first event)
Define the following terms:	
Cushing's ulcer	PUD/gastritis associated with **CNS** trauma or tumor (think, Dr. Cushing = neurosurgeon)
Curling's ulcer	PUD/gastritis associated with major **burn** injury (think: curling iron burn)
Marginal ulcer	Ulcer at the margin of a GI anastomosis
Dieulafoy's ulcer	Pinpoint gastric mucosal defect bleeding from an underlying vascular malformation

PERFORATED PEPTIC ULCER

What are the symptoms?	**Acute** onset of upper abdominal pain
What causes pain in the lower quadrants?	Passage of perforated fluid along colic gutters
What are the signs?	Decreased bowel sounds, tympanic sound over the liver (air), peritoneal signs, tender abdomen
What are the signs of posterior duodenal erosion/perforation?	Bleeding from gastroduodenal artery (and acute pancreatitis)
What sign indicates anterior duodenal perforation?	Free air (anterior perforation is more common than posterior)

What is the differential diagnosis?

Acute pancreatitis, acute cholecystitis, perforated acute appendicitis, colonic diverticulitis, MI, any perforated viscus

Which diagnostic tests are indicated?

X-ray: free air under diaphragm or in lesser sac in an upright CXR (if upright CXR is not possible, then left lateral decubitus can be performed because air can be seen over the liver and not confused with the gastric bubble)

What are the associated lab findings?

Leukocytosis, high amylase serum (secondary to absorption into the blood stream from the peritoneum)

What is the initial treatment?

NGT (↓ contamination of the peritoneal cavity)
IVF/Foley catheter
Antibiotics
Surgery

What is a Graham patch?

A piece of omentum incorporated into the suture closure of perforation

What are the surgical options for treatment of a duodenal perforation?

Graham patch
Truncal vagotomy and pyloroplasty incorporating ulcer
Graham patch and highly selective vagotomy

What are the surgical options for perforated gastric ulcer?

Antrectomy incorporating perforated ulcer or Graham patch in unstable/poor operative candidates

What is increased mortality associated with?

↑ age, female gender, gastric perforation

What is the significance of hemorrhage and perforation with duodenal ulcer?

May indicate two ulcers (kissing); posterior is bleeding and anterior is perforated with free air

What type of perforated ulcer may present just like acute pancreatitis?

Posterior perforated duodenal ulcer into the pancreas (i.e., epigastric pain radiating to the back; high serum amylase)

STRESS GASTRITIS

What is it?	**Superficial** mucosal erosions in the stressed patient
What are the risk factors?	Sepsis, intubation, trauma, shock
What is the prophylactic treatment?	H_2 blockers, antacids, sucralfate
What are the signs/ symptoms?	NGT blood (usually), painless (usually)
How is it diagnosed?	EGD, if bleeding is significant
What is the disadvantage of H_2 blockers and antacids in ICU patients?	Loss of acidic environment of stomach acid and bacterial overgrowth associated with higher rates of pneumonia from aspiration of stomach contents

MALLORY-WEISS SYNDROME

What is it?	Post-retching, postemesis longitudinal tear (submucosa and mucosa) of the stomach near the GE junction; approximately three-fourths are in the stomach
What are the causes of a tear?	Increased gastric pressure, often aggravated by hiatal hernia
What are the risk factors?	Retching, alcoholism (50%), more than 50% of patients have hiatal hernia
What are the symptoms?	Epigastric pain, thoracic substernal pain, emesis, hematemesis
What are the signs?	Post-retching hematemesis
How is the diagnosis made?	History, PE, EGD
What is the "classic" history?	Alcoholic patient after binge drinking—first, vomit food and gastric contents, followed by forceful retching and bloody vomitus

What is the treatment?	Room temperature water lavage (90% of patients stop bleeding), electrocautery, arterial embolization, or surgery for refractory bleeding
Can you use the Sengstaken-Blakemore tamponade balloon for treatment of Mallory-Weiss tear bleeding?	No; makes bleeding worse Use the balloon only for bleeding from esophageal varices

ESOPHAGEAL VARICEAL BLEEDING

What is it?	Bleeding from formation of esophageal varices from back-up of portal pressure via the coronary vein to the submucosal esophageal venous plexi secondary to portal hypertension from liver cirrhosis
What is the "rule of two-thirds" of esophageal variceal hemorrhage?	Two-thirds of patients with portal hypertension develop esophageal varices Two-thirds of patients with esophageal varices bleed
What are the signs/symptoms?	Liver disease, portal hypertension, hematemesis, caput medusa, ascites, etc.
How is the diagnosis made?	EGD (very important because only 50% of UGI bleeding in patients with known esophageal varices are bleeding from the varices and the other 50% have bleeding from ulcers, etc.)
What is the medical treatment?	Lower portal pressure with vasopressin (give nitroglycerin to protect coronary blood flow) or somatostatin
What is the definitive treatment?	Sclerotherapy via endoscope Sengstaken-Blakemore balloon tamponade, if bleeding is massive Liver transplant Warren shunt (distal splenorenal shunting of portal blood to vena cava), other shunts

What is the problem with shunts?	Decreased portal pressure, but increased encephalopathy

BOERHAAVE'S SYNDROME

What is it?	Postemetic esophageal rupture (all layers), does not bleed profusely very frequently
What is the most common location?	Posterolateral aspect of the esophagus (on the left), 3 to 5 cm above the GE junction
What is the cause of rupture?	Increased intraluminal pressure, usually caused by violent retching and vomiting
What is the associated risk factor?	Esophageal reflux disease (50%)
What are the symptoms?	Pain postemesis (may radiate to the back, dysphagia)
What are the signs?	Left pneumothorax, Hamman's sign, left pleural effusion, subcutaneous/ mediastinal emphysema, fever, tachypnea, tachycardia, signs of infection by 24 hours, neck crepitus, widened mediastinum on CXR
What is Hamman's sign?	"Mediastinal crunch," produced by the heart beating against air-filled tissues
How is the diagnosis made?	History, physical examination, CXR, esophagram with water-soluble contrast
What is the treatment?	Surgery within 24 hours to drain the mediastinum and surgically close the perforation and placement of pleural patch; broad-spectrum antibiotics
What is the mortality rate in less than 24 hours until surgery?	Approximately 25% (10%–30%)
What is the mortality rate in more than 24 hours until surgery?	Approximately 60%

34 The Stomach

ANATOMY

Identify the parts of the stomach:

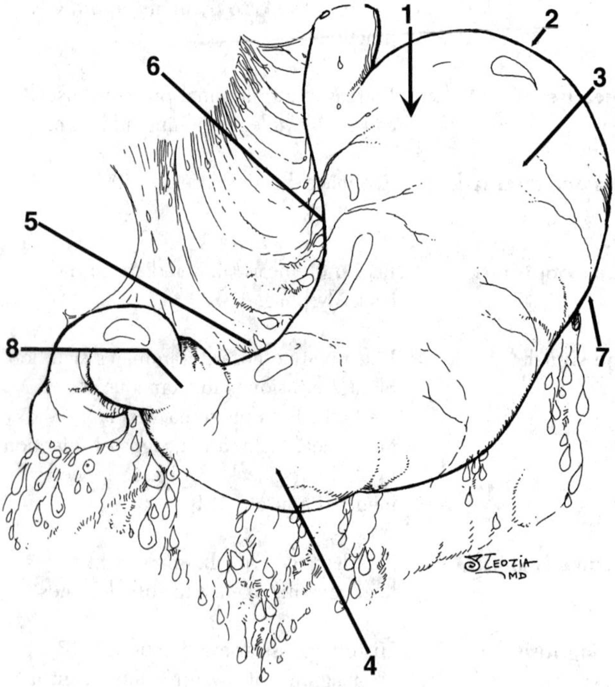

1. Cardia
2. Fundus
3. Body
4. Antrum
5. Incisura angularis
6. Lesser curvature
7. Greater curvature
8. Pylorus

Identify the blood supply to the stomach:

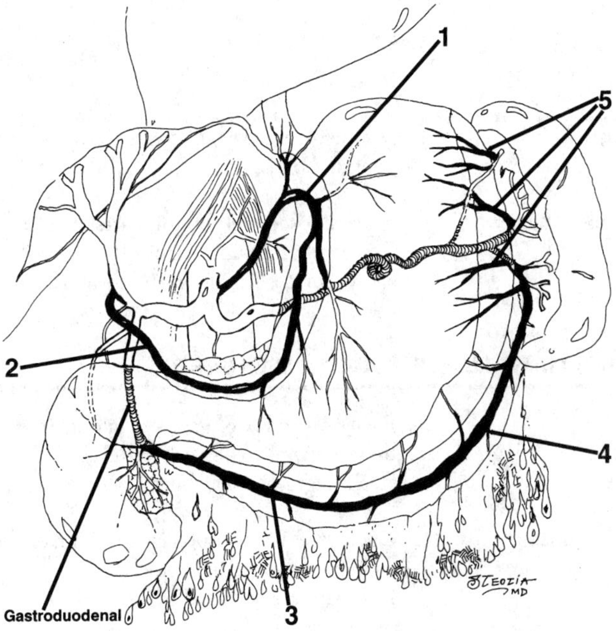

1. Left gastric artery
2. Right gastric artery
3. Right gastroepiploic artery
4. Left gastroepiploic artery
5. Short gastrics (from spleen)

What space lies behind the stomach?

The lesser sac; the pancreas lies behind the stomach

What is the opening into the lesser sac?

Foreman of Winslow

What are the folds of gastric mucosa called?

Rugae

GASTRIC PHYSIOLOGY

Define the products of the following stomach cells:

Gastric parietal cells

HCl
Intrinsic factor

Chief cells	Pepsinogen (think: "a peppy chief")
G cells	Gastrin (found in the antrum)
Mucous neck cells	Bicarbonate Mucus

What is pepsin?
A proteolytic enzyme that hydrolyzes peptide bonds

What is intrinsic factor?
A protein secreted by the parietal cells that combines with vitamin B_{12} and allows for absorption in the terminal ileum

GASTROESOPHAGEAL REFLUX DISEASE (GERD)

What is it?
Excessive reflux of gastric contents into the esophagus (everyone refluxes to a small degree); "heartburn"

What are the causes?
Decreased lower esophageal sphincter (LES) tone (> 50% of cases)
Decreased esophageal motility to clear refluxed fluid
Gastric outlet obstruction
Hiatal hernia

What are the signs/ symptoms?
Heartburn, regurgitation, respiratory problems/pneumonia from aspiration of refluxed gastric contents; substernal pain

What disease must be ruled out when the symptoms of GERD are present?
Coronary artery disease

What tests are included in the workup?
EGD
UGI contrast study
Twenty-four hour acid analysis (pH probe in esophagus)
Manometry

What is the medical treatment?
Small meals
H_2 blockers or omeprazole
Cisapride
Elevation of the head at night and no meals prior to sleeping

What are the indications for surgery?

Intractability (failure of medical treatment)
Respiratory problems due to reflux and aspiration of gastric contents (e.g., pneumonia)
Severe esophageal injury (e.g., ulcers, hemorrhage, stricture, ± Barrett's esophagus)

What is Barrett's esophagus?

Columnar metaplasia due to chronic irritation from reflux

Define the following surgical options for severe GERD:

Nissen

360° fundoplication (may be done laparoscopically)

Belsey mark IV

240° to 270° fundoplication

Hill

Arcuate ligament repair and gastropexy to diaphragm

GASTRIC CANCER

What is the incidence?

Rare in the United States (higher in Japan)

What are the associated risk factors?

Diet—smoked meats, high nitrates, low fruits and vegetables, alcohol, tobacco
Environment—raised in high-risk area, poor socioeconomic status, atrophic gastritis, male gender, blood type A, previous partial gastrectomy, pernicious anemia

What is the average age at the time of discovery?

More than 60 years old

What is the ratio of male to female patients?

3:2

Which blood type is associated with gastric cancer?

Blood type A

What are the symptoms?

Asymptomatic in early stages; possible postprandial, epigastric pain/discomfort, anorexia/weight loss, dysphagia, burping, hematemesis, melena, dyspepsia, nausea/vomiting

What are the signs?

Anemia, melena, heme occult, epigastric mass (in advanced disease), hepatomegaly, coffee-ground emesis, Blumer's shelf, Virchow's node, enlarged ovaries, axillary adenopathy

What is a Blumer's shelf?

A solid peritoneal deposit anterior to the rectum, forming a "shelf," palpated on **rectal examination**

What is a Virchow's node?

Metastatic gastric cancer to the nodes in the left supraclavicular fossa

What is Sister Mary Joseph's sign?

Periumbilical lymph node gastric cancer metastases; presents as periumbilical mass

What is a Krukenberg's tumor?

Gastric cancer (or other adeno cancer) that has metastasized to the ovary

What is "Irish's" node?

Left axillary adenopathy from gastric cancer metastasis

Which diagnostic tests should be performed?

UGI series, EGD (remember: biopsy all gastric ulcers at surgery and at EGD), endoscopic ultrasound to evaluate the level of invasion

What is the histology?

The majority are adenocarcinoma

What is the morphology?

Ulcerative (25%)—ulcer through all layers
Polyploid (25%)
Superficial spreading (10%)—early cancer, through mucosa/submucosa
Linitis plastica (10%)— "leather bottle" due to early spread through all layers

What is the treatment?

Surgical resection with wide (> 5 cm) margins (total or subtotal gastrectomy) and lymph node dissection, with or without chemotherapy

When should splenectomy be performed?	Most experts would perform splenectomy during resection for gastric cancer when the tumor directly invades the spleen/splenic hilum, or with splenic hilar adenopathy.
Define "extended lymph node dissection."	Extensive lymph node dissection, usually one group past the lymph node group with positive metastases (The Japanese have popularized an extensive lymph node dissection with great results)
What percentage of patients are inoperable at presentation?	Approximately 10%
What is the 5-year survival rate for gastric cancer?	Only 10% of patients are alive 5 years after diagnosis in the United States (in Japan, 50% are alive at 5 years because of aggressive screening, it is believed)
What is the differential diagnosis of gastric tumors?	Adenocarcinoma, leiomyoma, leiomyosarcoma, lymphoma, carcinoid, ectopic pancreatic tissue, gastrinoma, benign gastric ulcer, polyp

35

Bariatric Surgery

What is it?

Weight reduction surgery for the morbidly obese

Define morbid obesity.

More than 100 lbs over ideal body weight

What medical conditions are associated with morbid obesity?

Coronary artery disease, pulmonary disease, diabetes mellitus, venous stasis ulcers, arthritis, infections, sex-hormone abnormalities

What are the current options for surgery?

Gastric bypass
Vertical banded gastroplasty

Define gastric bypass.

Stapling off of small gastric pouch
Roux-en-Y limb to gastric pouch

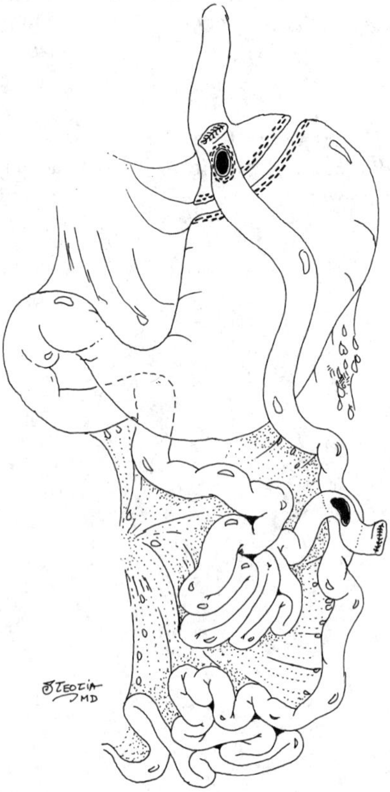

Define vertical-banded gastroplasty.

Vertical stapled small gastric pouch
Placement of silastic ring **band**

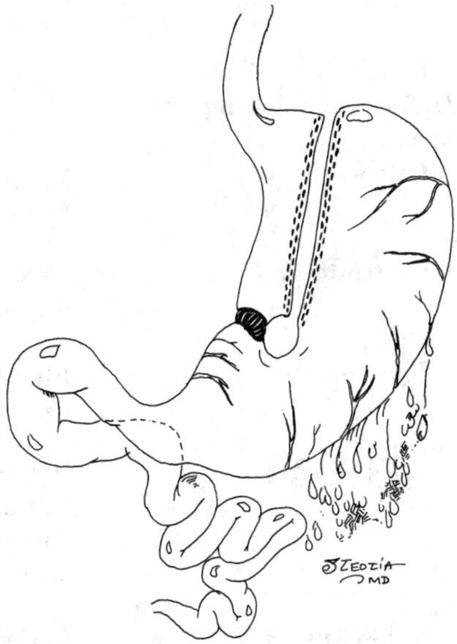

How does vertical-banded gastroplasty work?

Decreased gastric reservoir and early satiety

How can patients "beat" vertical-banded gastroplasty?

By eating sweets and high-calorie liquids

How does the gastric bypass work?

Small gastric reservoir
Dumping symptoms when too much food or high-calorie foods are eaten and the food is "dumped" into the Roux-en-Y limb

What are the possible postoperative complications after weight-reduction surgery?

Gallstones (if gallbladder in situ), anastomotic leak, marginal ulcer, stenosis of pouch/anastomosis, malnutrition, incisional hernia

36

Ostomies

Define the following terms:

Ostomy	Connection of the GI tract to abdominal wall skin; a manmade fistula
Gastrostomy	G-tube through the abdominal wall to the stomach for drainage or feeding
Jejunostomy	J-tube through the abdominal wall to the jejunum for feeding
Kock pouch	"Continent ileostomy" Pouch is made of several ileal loops Patient must access pouch with a tube intermittently
Colostomy	Connection of colon mucosa to the abdominal wall skin for stool drainage
End colostomy	Proximal end of colon brought to the skin for stool drainage
Mucus fistula	Distal end of transected colon brought to the skin for decompression; the mucosa produces mucus, a colostomy is a fistula, and, hence, the term **mucus fistula** (proximal colon brought up as a colostomy or, if the proximal colon is removed, an ileostomy)
Hartmann's pouch	Distal end of transected colon stapled and dropped back into the peritoneal cavity, resulting in a blind pouch; mucus is decompressed through the anus (proximal colon is brought up as an end colostomy or, if proximal colon is removed, an end ileostomy)
Double-barrel colostomy	End colostomy and a mucus fistula (i.e., two barrels brought up to the skin)

Loop colostomy

A loop of large bowel is brought up to the abdominal wall skin and a plastic rod is placed underneath the loop. The colon is then opened and sewn to the abdominal wall skin as a colostomy.

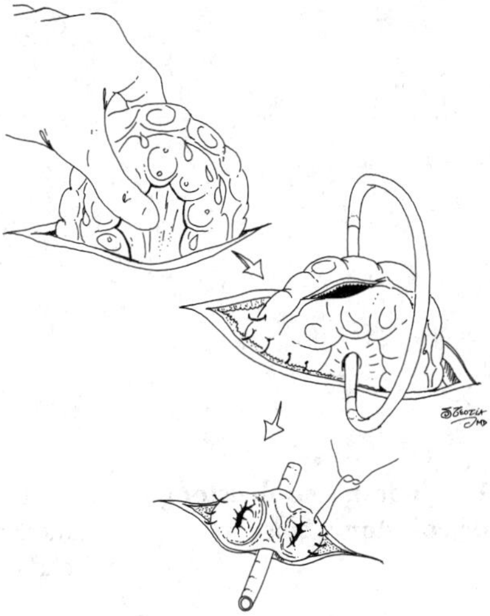

Ileal conduit

Loops of stapled-off ileum made into a pouch, anastomosed to the ureters, and then brought to the abdominal wall skin to allow drainage of urine in patients who undergo removal of the bladder (cystectomy)

Brooke ileostomy

Ileostomy folded over itself to provide clearance from skin

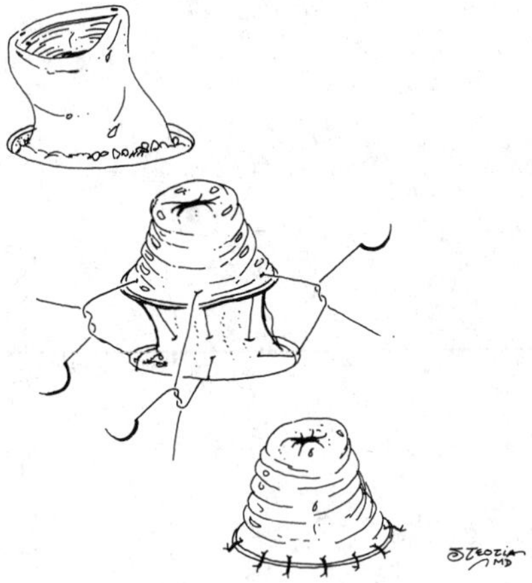

Why doesn't an ileostomy or colostomy close?

Epithelialization (mucosa to skin) from the acronym FRI**E**ND (see Fistula chapter)

Why doesn't a gastrostomy close?

Foreign body (the plastic tube) from the acronym **F**RIEND

If the plastic tube, G-tube, or J-tube is removed, how fast can the hole to the stomach or jejunum close?

In a matter of hours! (Thus, if it comes out inadvertently, it must be replaced immediately)

What is a "tube check"?

A gastrografin contrast study to confirm that a G-tube or J-tube is within the lumen of the stomach or jejunum, respectively

37 Small Intestine

SMALL BOWEL

ANATOMY

What comprises the small bowel?	Duodenum, jejunum, and ileum
What provides blood supply to the small bowel?	Branches of the superior mesenteric artery
What does the small bowel do?	Major site of digestion and absorption
What are the plicae circulares?	Plicae means folds, circulares means circular; thus, the circular folds of mucosa (A.K.A., valvulae conniventes) in the small bowel lumen
What are the major structural differences between the jejunum and the ileum?	Jejunum—long vasa rectae, large plicae circulares, thicker wall Ileum—shorter vasa rectae, smaller plicae circulares, thinner wall (think: **I**leum = **I**nferior vasa rectae, **I**nferior plicae circulares, and **I**nferior wall)
What is absorbed by the terminal ileum?	B_{12}, fatty acids, bile salts

SMALL BOWEL OBSTRUCTION

What is small bowel obstruction (SBO)?	Mechanical obstruction to the passage of intraluminal contents
What are the signs/ symptoms of SBO?	Abdominal discomfort, cramping, and nausea Abdominal distention Emesis High-pitched bowel sounds

What lab tests are performed with SBO?
Electrolytes, CBC, type and screen, urinalysis

What must be ruled out on physical exam in patients with SBO?
Incarcerated hernia (also look for surgical scars)

What major AXR findings are associated with SBO?
Distended loops of small bowel
Air–fluid levels on upright film

Define complete SBO.
Complete obstruction of the lumen; usually paucity or no colon gas

What is the danger of complete SBO?
Closed loop strangulation of the bowel

Define partial SBO.
Incomplete SBO; some colon gas

What is the initial management of all patients with SBO?
NGT, IVF, Foley (to monitor urine output)

What are the causes of SBO?
Peritoneal adhesions, hernias, tumors, intussusception, gallstone ileus, inflammatory process, bowel-wall hematoma (patients on warfarin [Coumadin]), Crohn's disease, Meckel's diverticulum, radiation enteritis, abscess

What are the A,B,Cs of SBO?
Causes of SBO:
1. **A**dhesions
2. **B**ulge (hernias)
3. **C**ancer and tumors

What is the treatment of complete SBO?
Laparotomy

What is the treatment of incomplete SBO?
Initially, conservative treatment with close observation

Intraoperatively, how can the level of obstruction be determined in patients with SBO?
Transition from dilated bowel proximal to the transition to decompressed bowel distal to the obstruction

What is the most common indication for abdominal surgery in patients with Crohn's disease?

SBO

Can a patient have complete SBO and bowel movements and flatus?

Yes; the bowel distal to the obstruction can clear out gas and stool

After a small bowel resection, why should the mesenteric defect always be closed?

To prevent an internal hernia

What is the number one cause of SBO in adults?

Postoperative adhesions

What is the number one cause of SBO in children?

Hernias

What are the signs of strangulated bowel with SBO?

Fever, severe/continuous pain, hematemesis, **shock,** gas in the bowel wall or portal vein, abdominal free air, **peritoneal signs, acidosis** (increased lactic acid)

What are the clinical parameters that will lower the threshold to operate on a partial SBO?

Increasing **WBC**
Fever
Tachycardia/tachypnea

What is an absolute indication for operation with partial SBO?

Peritoneal signs

What classic saying is associated with complete SBO?

"Never let the sun set or rise on complete small bowel obstruction"

What condition commonly mimics SBO?

Paralytic ileus (AXR reveals gas distention throughout, including the colon)

What is the differential diagnosis of paralytic (nonobstructive) ileus?

Postoperative ileus after abdominal surgery (normally resolves in 3–5 days)
Electrolyte abnormalities (hypokalemia is most common)
Medications (anticholinergic, narcotics)
Inflammatory intraabdominal process

Sepsis/shock
Spine injury/spinal cord injury
Retroperitoneal hemorrhage

SMALL BOWEL TUMORS

What is the differential diagnosis of benign tumors of the small intestine?
Leiomyoma, lipoma, lymphangioma, fibroma, adenomas, hemangiomas

What is the most common benign small bowel tumor?
Leiomyoma

What is the most common malignant small bowel tumor?
Adenocarcinoma

What is the differential diagnosis of malignant tumors of the small intestine?
1. Adenocarcinoma (50%)
2. Carcinoid (25%)
3. Lymphoma (20%)
4. Sarcomas

MECKEL'S DIVERTICULUM

What is it?
Remnant of the omphalomesenteric duct/vitelline duct, which connects the yolk sac with the primitive midgut in the embryo

What is its claim to fame?
Most common small bowel congenital abnormality

What is the usual location?
Within approximately 2 feet of the ileocecal valve on the **antimesenteric** border of the bowel

What is the major differential diagnosis?
Appendicitis

Is it a true diverticulum?
Yes; all layers of the intestine are found in the wall

What is the incidence?
Approximately 2% of the population at autopsy

What is the gender ratio?
Two times more common in **men**

What is the average age at onset of symptoms?	Most frequently in the first **2 years of life,** but can occur at any age
What are the possible complications?	**Intestinal hemorrhage** (painless)—50%; accounts for half of all lower GI bleeding in patients younger than 2 years Bleeding is due to ectopic gastric mucosa secreting acid → ulcer → bleeding **Intestinal obstruction**—25%; most common complication in adults; includes volvulus and intussusception **Inflammation** (± perforations)—20%
What are the signs/ symptoms?	Painless lower GI bleeding, with or without abdominal pain or SBO
What is the most common complication of Meckel's diverticulum in adults?	Intestinal obstruction
In what percentage of cases is heterotopic tissue found in the diverticulum?	More than 50%
What heterotopic tissue type is most often found?	**Gastric mucosa** (85%), but duodenal, pancreatic, and colonic mucosa are also found
What is the "rule of 2s"?	2% of patients are **symptomatic** Found approximately **2 feet** from the ileocecal valve Found in **2%** of the population Majority of symptoms occur before age **2** years Ectopic tissue will be present in 1 of **2** patients Most diverticula are approximately **2** inches long **2** to 1 male : female ratio
What is the role of incidental Meckel's diverticulectomy (surgical removal upon finding asymptomatic diverticulum)?	Most experts would remove in children (very controversial in adults)

What is a Meckel's scan?	Scan for ectopic gastric mucosa in Meckel's diverticulum; uses **technetium pertechnetate** IV, which is preferentially taken up by gastric mucosa
What is the treatment of a Meckel's diverticulum that is causing bleeding and obstruction?	Surgical resection, with or without small bowel resection
What is the name of the hernia associated with incarcerated Meckel's diverticulum?	Littre's hernia
In patients with guaiac-positive stools and a negative upper- and lower-GI workup, what must be ruled out?	A small bowel tumor; evaluate with enteroclysis (small bowel contrast study)

38 The Appendix

What vessel provides blood supply to the appendix?

Appendiceal artery

Name the mesentery of the appendix.

Mesoappendix (contains the appendiceal artery)

How can the appendix be located if the cecum has been identified?

Follow the taenia coli down to the appendix. The taeniae converge on the appendix.

APPENDICITIS

What is it?

Inflammation of the appendix caused by **obstruction** of the appendiceal lumen, producing a closed loop with resultant inflammation that can lead to necrosis and perforation

What are the causes?

Fecalith (A.K.A. appendolith); **lymphoid hyperplasia**
Rare—parasite, foreign body, tumor (e.g., carcinoid)

What is the lifetime incidence of acute appendicitis in the United States?

Approximately 7%!

What is the most common cause of emergent abdominal surgery in the United States?

Acute appendicitis

How does it present?

Onset of referred **periumbilical pain** followed by **anorexia,** nausea, and vomiting
(**Note:** Unlike gastroenteritis, pain precedes vomiting.) Pain then migrates to the RLQ, where it becomes more intense and localized due to local peritoneal irritation. The

presentation may vary, depending on the anatomic location of the appendix. Anorexia is almost always present; if the patient is hungry and can eat, seriously question the diagnosis of appendicitis.)

Why does periumbilical pain occur?

Referred pain

Why does right lower quadrant pain occur?

Peritoneal irritation

How is the diagnosis made?

History and physical examination

What are the signs/ symptoms?

Signs of peritoneal irritation may be present: guarding, muscle spasm, rebound tenderness, obturator and psoas signs, low-grade fever (high-grade if perforation occurs)

Define the following terms:

Obturator sign

Pain upon internal rotation of the leg with the hip and knee flexed; seen in patients with appendicitis/pelvic abscess

Psoas sign

Pain elicited by extending the hip with the knee in full extension or by flexing the hip against resistance; seen with appendicitis and psoas inflammation

Rovsing's sign

Palpation or rebound pressure of the left lower quadrant results in pain in the right lower quadrant; seen in appendicitis

McBurney's point

Point one-third from the anterior iliac spine to the umbilicus (often the point of maximal tenderness)

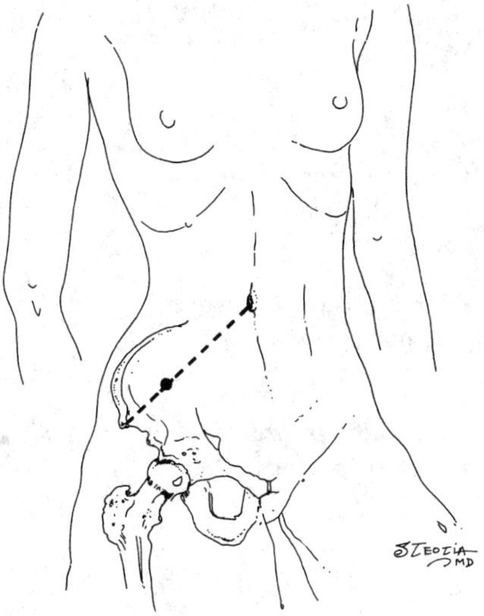

What is the differential diagnosis?

Meckel's diverticulum; Crohn's disease; ovarian torsion, cyst, or tumor; perforated ulcer; pancreatitis; pelvic inflammatory disease; ruptured ectopic pregnancy; mesenteric lymphadenitis; mittelschmerz; constipation; gastroenteritis; intussusception; volvulus; tumors; urinary tract infection (e.g., cystitis); pyelonephritis

What lab tests should be performed?

CBC: increased WBC (> 10,000 per mm^3 in > 90% of cases), most often with a "left shift"
Urinalysis: to evaluate for pyelonephritis or renal calculus
(Note: Mild hematuria and pyuria are common in appendicitis with pelvic inflammation resulting in inflammation of the ureter)

What additional tests can be performed if the diagnosis is not clear?

AXR
Ultrasound (may see a large, noncompressible appendix or fecalith)

	Barium enema may help if the entire appendix is seen, but will not fill in many normal appendixes
What is the "hamburger" sign?	Ask patients with suspected appendicitis if they would like a hamburger or their favorite food; if they can eat, seriously question the diagnosis.
In acute appendicitis, what classically precedes vomiting?	Pain (in gastroenteritis, the pain classically follows vomiting)
Does a positive urinalysis rule out appendicitis?	No; abnormal urinalysis can be due to ureteral inflammation caused by the periappendiceal inflammation
What radiographic studies are often performed?	CXR: to rule out RML or RLL pneumonia AXR: abdominal films are usually nonspecific, but calcified fecaliths present in about 5% of cases
What are the radiographic signs of appendicitis on AXR?	Fecalith, sentinel loops, **scoliosis** away from the right due to pain, mass effect (abscess), loss of psoas shadow, loss of preperitoneal fat stripe, and (very rarely) a small amount of free air, if perforated
With acute appendicitis, what percentage of the time will there be a radiopaque fecalith on AXR?	Only approximately 5% of the time!
What are the preoperative medications/preparation?	1. Rehydration with **IV fluids** (LR) 2. Preoperative **antibiotics** with anaerobic coverage (appendix is considered part of the colon); cefoxitin (Mefoxin) is most often used
What is a lap appy?	Laparoscopic appendectomy; used in most cases in adults and older children
How does treatment differ for nonperforated and perforated appendicitis?	Nonperforated—prompt appendectomy (prevents perforation), 24 hours of antibiotics Perforated—fluid resuscitation and prompt appendectomy; all pus is drained and cultures obtained, with

postoperative antibiotics continued for 5 to 7 days; wound is left open in most cases of perforation after closing the fascia (heals by secondary intention or delayed primary closure)

How is an appendiceal abscess treated?

Usually by drainage of the abscess, antibiotic administration, and elective appendectomy approximately 6 to 8 weeks later (A.K.A., interval appendectomy)

If a normal appendix is found upon exploration, what must be examined/ ruled out?

Terminal ileum: Meckel's diverticulum, Crohn's disease, intussusception
Gynecologic causes: ovarian cysts, etc.

How long after removal of a NONRUPTURED appendicitis should the antibiotics be continued postoperatively?

For 24 hours

What is the risk of perforation?

Approximately 25% after 24 hours from onset of symptoms, approximately 50% by 36 hours, and approximately 75% by 48 hours

What is the most common general surgical abdominal emergency in pregnancy?

Appendicitis (about 1/1750; **appendix may be in the RUQ due to the enlarged uterus)**

What are the possible complications of appendicitis/ appendectomy?

Abscess, free perforation, liver abscess, wound infection, appendiceal stump abscess, wound/inguinal hernia, minor bleeding, portal pylethrombophlebitis (very rare)

What percentage of the population has a retrocecal, retroperitoneal appendix?

Approximately 15%

What percentage of negative appendectomies is acceptable?

Up to 20%; it is better to take out some normal appendixes than to miss a case of acute appendicitis that goes on to rupture.

Who is at risk of dying from acute appendicitis?	Very old and very young patients
What bacteria is associated with "mesenteric adenitis"?	*Yersinia*

APPENDICEAL TUMORS

What is the most common appendiceal tumor?	Carcinoid tumor
What is the treatment of an appendiceal carcinoid less than 2 cm?	Appendectomy (if not through the bowel wall)
What is the treatment of an appendiceal carcinoid larger than 2 cm?	Right hemicolectomy
What percentage of appendiceal carcinoids are malignant?	Less than 5%
What are the differential diagnoses of appendiceal tumor?	Carcinoid, adenocarcinoma, malignant mucoid adenocarcinoma
What type of appendiceal tumor can cause the dreaded pseudomyxoma peritonei if the appendix ruptures?	Malignant mucoid adenocarcinoma

39

Carcinoid Tumors

What is a carcinoid tumor?	Tumor arising from neuroendocrine cells (APUDomas), A.K.A. **Kulchitsky cells;** basically, a tumor that secretes **serotonin**
What is the incidence?	Approximately 25% of all small bowel tumors
What are the common sites of occurrence?	1. **Appendix (most common)** 2. Ileum 3. Rectum 4. Bronchus Other sites: jejunum, stomach, duodenum, colon, ovary, testicle, pancreas, thymus
What are the signs/ symptoms?	Depends on the location; most are asymptomatic; also can present with small bowel obstruction, abdominal pain, bleeding, weight loss, diaphoresis, **pellagra skin changes,** intussusception, or carcinoid syndrome
What is carcinoid syndrome?	Syndrome of symptoms caused by release of substances from a carcinoid tumor
What are the symptoms of carcinoid syndrome?	Acronym **B FDR:** **B**ronchospasm **F**lushing (skin) **D**iarrhea **R**ight-sided heart failure (due to valve failure)
What is the incidence of carcinoid SYNDROME in patients who have a carcinoid TUMOR?	Approximately 10%

What released substances cause carcinoid syndrome?

Serotonin and vasoactive peptides

How does the liver prevent carcinoid syndrome?

By degradation of serotonin and the other vasoactive peptides when the **tumor drains into the portal vein**

Why does carcinoid syndrome occur in some tumors and not others?

It occurs when **venous drainage from the tumor gains access to the systemic circulation** (i.e., the serotonin and other vasoactive substances escape hepatic degradation) in the following scenarios:

- **Liver metastases**
- Retroperitoneal disease draining into paravertebral veins
- Primary tumor outside the GI tract and/or portal venous drainage (e.g., ovary, **testicular,** bronchus)

To what does the liver break down the serotonin?

5-hydroxyindoleacetic acid **(5-HIAA)**

What are the associated diagnostic lab findings?

Elevated urine 5-HIAA, as well as urine and blood **serotonin** levels

What is 5-HT?

Serotonin

What stimulation test can often elevate serotonin levels and cause symptoms of carcinoid syndrome?

Pentagastrin stimulation

What radiologic studies should be performed?

Barium enema, upper GI series with small bowel follow-through (or enteroclysis: barium instilled into the intestine via a tube from above for a better evaluation of the small bowel), colonoscopy, abdominal CT or arteriography for liver metastasis

Note: abdominal CT is usually not helpful for locating primary tumors because they are small and slow growing

What is the surgical treatment?

Excision of the primary tumor and single or feasible metastasis in the liver (liver transplant is an option with unresectable liver metastasis); chemotherapy for advanced disease

What is the medical treatment?	Medical therapy for palliation of the carcinoid syndrome (serotonin antagonists, somatostatin analogue [**octreotide**])
How effective is octreotide?	Shown to relieve diarrhea and flushing in more than 85% of cases
What is a common antiserotonin drug?	**Cyproheptadine**
What is the overall prognosis?	Two-thirds of patients are alive at 5 years
What is the prognosis of patients with liver metastasis?	Half the patients are alive at 3 years
What does carcinoid tumor look like?	Usually intramural bowel mass; appears as **yellow**ish tumor upon incision
For appendiceal carcinoid, when is a right hemicolectomy indicated versus an appendectomy?	If the tumor is **more than 2 cm,** right **hemicolectomy** is indicated; if there are no signs of serosal involvement and tumor is less than **2 cm, appendectomy** should be performed (controversial; some experts state 1.5 cm)
Which primary site has the highest rate of metastasis?	Ileal primary tumor
Can a carcinoid tumor be confirmed malignant by looking at the histology?	No; metastasis must be present to diagnose malignancy
What is the correlation between tumor size and malignancy potential?	The vast majority of tumors less than 2 cm are benign In tumors more than 2 cm, malignancy potential is significant

40

Fistulas

What is a fistula?

An abnormal **communication** between two hollow organs or a hollow organ and the exterior (i.e., two epithelial cell layers)

What are the predisposing factors and conditions that maintain patency of a fistula?

The acronym **FRIEND:**

- **F**oreign body (e.g., G tube)
- **R**adiation
- **I**nfection
- **E**pithelization (e.g., colostomy)
- **N**eoplasm
- **D**istal obstruction

Note: increased flow and steroids may inhibit closure, but usually will not maintain a fistula

SPECIFIC TYPES OF FISTULAS

ENTEROCUTANEOUS

What is it?

A fistula from the GI tract to the skin (enterocutaneous = **bowel to skin)**

What are the causes?

Anastomotic leak, trauma/injury to the bowel/colon, Crohn's disease, abscess, diverticulitis, inflammation/infection

What are the possible complications?

High-output fistulas, malnutrition, skin problems, and patient discomfort

What is the treatment?

NPO; TPN; rule out and correct FRIEND; may feed distally (or if fistula is distal, feed elemental diet to decrease residue)

Half will close spontaneously, but the other half require operation and resection of the involved bowel segment

Which enterocutaneous fistula closes faster: a short or a long fistula?	A long fistula

COLONIC FISTULAS

What are they?	Include colovesical, colocutaneous, colovaginal, and coloenteric fistulas
What are the most common causes?	**Diverticulitis** (most common cause), cancer, IBD, foreign body, and irradiation
What is the most common type?	**Colovesical fistula,** which often presents with recurrent urinary tract infections Other signs include pneumaturia, dysuria, and fecaluria
How is the diagnosis made?	Via BE and cystoscopy
What is the treatment?	Surgery: segmental colon resection and primary anastomosis; repair/resection of the involved organ (may require temporary colostomy)
What is a cholecystenteric fistula?	Connection between gallbladder and duodenum or other loop of small bowel due to large gallstone erosion, often resulting in SBO as the gallstone lodges in the ileocecal valve (gallstone ileus)
What are the common causes of a gastrocolic fistula?	Penetrating ulcers, **gastric** or **colonic cancer,** and Crohn's disease
What are the possible complications of gastrocolic fistula?	Malnutrition and severe **enteritis** due to reflux of colonic contents into the stomach and small bowel with subsequent bacterial overgrowth

FISTULA IN ANO

What is it?	Anal fistula, from the rectum to the perianal skin
What are the causes?	Usually due to anal crypt/gland infection

What are the signs/ symptoms?

Perianal drainage, perirectal abscess, recurrent perirectal abscess, "diaper rash," itching

What disease should be considered with fistula in ano?

Crohn's disease (also consider ulcerative colitis, but fistulas are much less likely)

How is the diagnosis made?

Exam, proctoscope

What is Goodsall's rule?

Fistulas originating **anterior** to a transverse line through the anus will course **straight** ahead and exit anteriorly, whereas those exiting **posteriorly** have a **curved** tract.

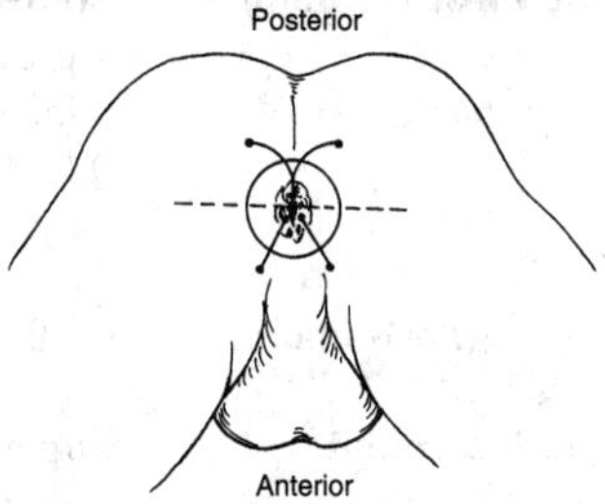

How can Goodsall's rule be remembered?

Think of a dog with a **straight** nose (anterior) and a **curved** tail (posterior)

What is the management of anorectal fistulas?

Define the pathoanatomy
Marsupialization of fistula tract (i.e., fillet tract open)
Wound care: routine Sitz baths and dressing changes
Seton placement if fistula is through the sphincter muscle

What is a Seton?

A thick suture placed through fistula tract to allow slow transection of sphincter muscle; the scar tissue formed will hold the sphincter muscle in place and allow for continence after transection

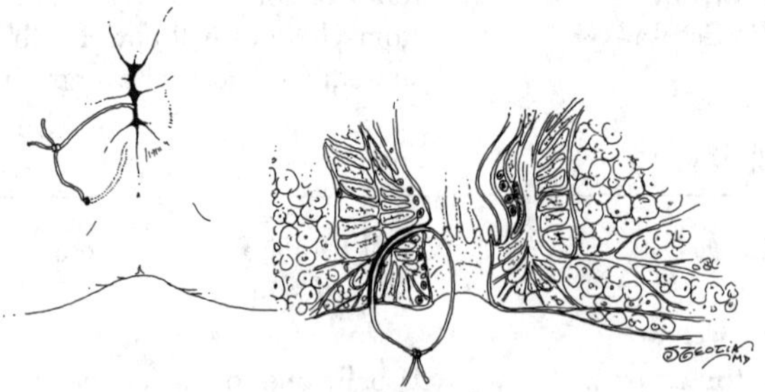

What percentage of patients with a perirectal abscess develop a fistula in ano after drainage?

Approximately 50%

PANCREATIC ENTERIC FISTULA

What is it?

Decompression of a **pseudocyst** or **abscess** into an adjacent organ (a **rare** complication); usually done surgically or endoscopically to treat a pancreatic pseudocyst

EXTERNAL PANCREATIC FISTULA

What is it?

Pancreaticocutaneous fistula; drainage of pancreatic exocrine secretions through to the abdominal skin (usually through a drain tract/wound)

What is the treatment?

NPO, TPN, skin protection, **octreotide**

What is a "refractory" pancreatic fistula?

Pancreaticocutaneous fistula that does not resolve with conservative medical management (the minority of cases)

What is the diagnostic test for "refractory" pancreatic fistulas?

ERCP to define site of fistula tract (i.e., tail versus head of pancreas)

How is refractory tail of a pancreas fistula treated?

Resection of the tail of the pancreas and the fistula

How is refractory head of a pancreas fistula treated?

Pancreaticojejunostomy

BLADDER FISTULAS

What are the specific types?

Vesicoenteric (50% due to sigmoid diverticulitis)

Vesicovaginal (most are secondary to gynecologic procedures; signs include urinary leak through the vagina, and it is diagnosed by IVP or instilling the bladder with methylene blue and monitoring the vagina for the appearance of dye)

41

Colon and Rectum

ANATOMY

Identify the arterial blood supply to the colon:

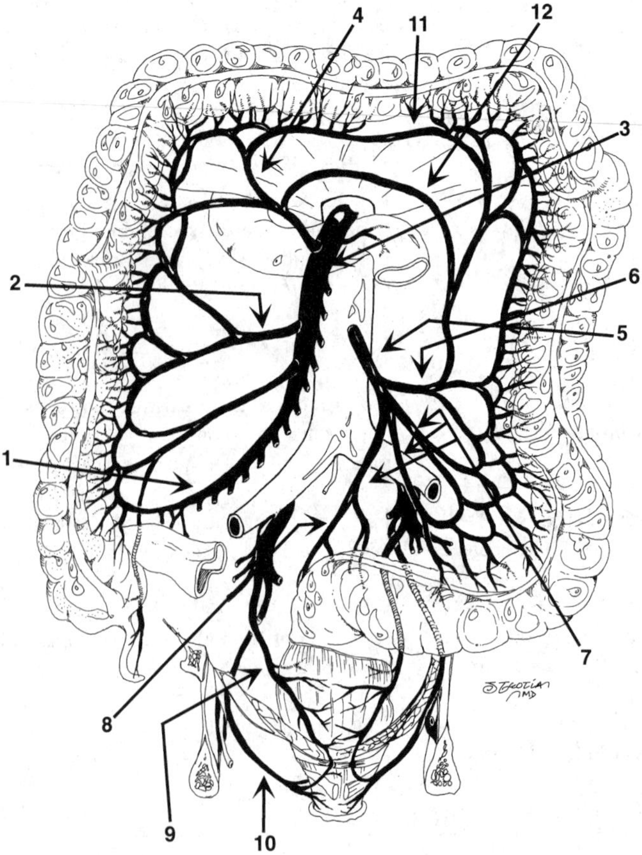

1. Ileocolic artery
2. Right colic artery
3. Superior mesenteric artery (SMA)
4. Middle colic artery
5. Inferior mesenteric artery
6. Left colic artery
7. Sigmoidal artery
8. Superior hemorrhoidal artery (superior rectal)
9. Middle hemorrhoidal artery
10. Inferior hemorrhoidal artery
11. Marginal artery of Drummond
12. Meandering artery of Gonzalez

What are the white lines of Toldt?	The lateral peritoneal reflections of the ascending and descending colon
What part of the GI tract does not have a serosa?	Esophagus Middle and distal **rectum**
What are the major anatomic differences between the colon and the small bowel?	The colon has taenia coli, haustra, and appendices epiploicae (fat appendages), whereas the small intestine is smooth
What is the blood supply to the rectum?	**Proximal:** superior hemorrhoidal (or superior rectal) from the IMA **Middle:** middle hemorrhoidal (or middle rectal) from the hypogastric (int. iliac) **Distal:** Inferior hemorrhoidal (or inferior rectal) from the pudendal artery (the pudendal is a branch of the hypogastric artery)
What is the venous drainage of the rectum?	**Proximal:** via the IMV to the splenic vein, then to **the portal vein** **MIDDLE:** via the iliac vein to the **IVC** **DISTAL:** via the iliac vein to the **IVC**
What is the main purpose of the colon?	H_2O absorption

COLORECTAL CARCINOMA

What is it?	Adenocarcinoma of the colon or rectum
What is the incidence?	Most common GI cancer Second most common cancer in the United States Incidence increases with age starting at age 40, and peaks at 70 to 80 years
How common is it as cause of cancer deaths?	Second most common cause of cancer deaths
What is the male to female ratio?	Approximately 1:1

What are the risk factors?

Dietary: low-fiber, high-fat diets correlate with increased rates
Genetic: family history is important when taking history
IBD: ulcerative colitis > Crohn's disease
Other: Obesity, sedentary lifestyle, age, previous colon cancer, radiation

What are current ACS recommendations for colorectal screening without family (first-degree) history of colorectal cancer?

Annual digital rectal exam starting at age 40 (remember that approximately 10% of tumors are palpable by rectal exam!)
Annual test for fecal occult blood starting at age 40
Sigmoidoscopy at age 50, repeated every 3 to 5 years thereafter

What are the current ACS recommendations for colorectal cancer screening if there is a history of colorectal cancer in a first-degree relative?

For patients with a family history of colorectal cancer, a more aggressive approach is needed: colonoscopy or BE every 5 years starting at age 35 to 40.

What percentage of adults will have a guaiac-positive stool test?

Approximately 2%

What percentage of patients with a guaiac-positive stool test will have colon cancer?

Approximately 10%

What signs/symptoms are associated with the following conditions:

Right-sided lesions?

Right side of the bowel has a large luminal diameter, so a tumor may attain a large size before causing problems.
Microcytic anemia, occult/melena > hematochezia PR, postprandial discomfort, right-sided mass
Obstruction and change in bowel habits are uncommon, but liquid stools/ electrolyte losses, nausea, and vomiting are possible.

Left-sided lesions?	Left side of the bowel has smaller lumen and semisolid contents. Change in bowel habits (small-caliber stools), signs of obstruction, abdominal mass, heme(+) or gross blood, with or without small clots (Bleeding is rarely massive.) Nausea and vomiting, constipation
From which site is melena more common?	Right-sided cancer
From which site is hematochezia more common?	Left-sided cancer
What is the incidence of rectal cancer?	Comprises 20% to 30% of all colorectal cancer
What are the signs/ symptoms of rectal cancer?	Most common symptom is hematochezia (or passage of red blood ± stool) or mucus; also tenesmus, feeling of incomplete evacuation of stool (due to mass), rectal mass
What is the differential diagnosis of a colon tumor/ mass?	Adenocarcinoma, carcinoid tumor, lipoma, liposarcoma, leiomyoma, leiomyosarcoma, lymphoma, diverticular disease, ulcerative colitis, Crohn's disease, polyps
Which diagnostic tests are helpful?	History and physical exam (**Note: approximately 10% of cancers are palpable on rectal exam**), heme occult, CBC, barium enema, sigmoid/ colonoscopy **Remember:** with rectal bleeding in middle-aged and older individuals, even in the presence of hemorrhoids, cancer must be ruled out
What disease does microcytic anemia signify until proven otherwise in a man or a postmenopausal woman?	Colon cancer

What tests help find metastases?

CXR (lung metastases), LFTs (liver metastases), abdominal CT (liver metastases), other tests based on history and physical exam (e.g., head CT for left arm weakness looking for brain metastasis)

What is the preoperative workup for colorectal cancer?

History, physical exam, LFTs, CEA, CBC, Chem 10, PT/PTT, type and cross 2 u PRBCs, CXR, U/A, abdominal CT (add pelvic CT for rectal cancer)

What are the means by which the cancer spreads?

Direct extension: circumferentially and then through the bowel wall to later invade other abdominoperineal organs
Hematogenous: Portal circulation to the liver; lumbar/vertebral veins to lungs
Lymphogenous: Regionally
Transperitoneal
Intraluminal

Is CEA useful?

Not for screening, but it is useful for baseline and recurrence surveillance (but offers no proven survival benefit)

What unique diagnostic test is helpful in patients with rectal cancer?

Endorectal ultrasound (probe is placed transanally and depth of invasion and nodes are evaluated)

How are tumors classified?

Dukes' Astler-Coller modified staging system

Give the modified Dukes' staging (simplified):

A? 90%

Limited to **muscularis mucosa**

B? 70%

Into the submucosa /**muscularis propria** (B1), through the entire bowel wall (B2), or through the bowel wall and into adjacent tissues (B3) (think: past muscularis mucosa without node metastasis)

C? 40%

Positive regional **lymph nodes**

D? 5%

Distant metastasis

What is the approximate survival rate at 5 years for the following Dukes' stages:

A?

90%

B?	70%
C?	40%
D?	5%
Define the preoperative "bowel preparation."	Preoperative preparation for colon/rectal resection: 1. Golytely colonic lavage until clear effluent per rectum or phosphasoda cathartics 2. PO antibiotics (1 gm neomycin and 1 gm erythromycin x 3 doses) Patient should also receive preoperative and 24-hr IV antibiotics (i.e., cefoxitin or cefotetan; clindamycin/aztreonam for severe penicillin allergy)
What are the treatment options?	Resection: wide surgical resection of lesion and its regional lymphatic drainage
What decides Low Anterior Resection (LAR) versus Abdominal Perineal Resection (APR)?	**Distance from the anal verge** General rule: tumors less than 8 cm from the anal verge = APR Tumors more than 8 cm from the anal verge = LAR
What surgical margins are needed for colon cancer?	Traditionally more than 5 cm, but actual margins are usually more than 5 cm and based on blood/lymphatic supply to the colon segment to be removed. Margins must be at least 2 cm.
What is the minimal surgical margin for rectal cancer?	2 cm
What is the adjuvant treatment of Dukes' C colon cancer?	5-FU and levamisole chemotherapy if there are nodal metastasis
What is the adjuvant treatment of rectal cancer with positive nodal metastasis or transmural extension?	**Radiation therapy** and 5-FU chemotherapy as a "radiosensitizer" (for local control; may be used preoperatively or postoperatively) **Note** that there is no role for radiation in Dukes' C colon cancer

What is the most common site of distant (hematogenous) metastasis from colorectal cancer?
Liver

What is the treatment of liver metastases from colorectal cancer?
Resect with 1 to 2 cm margins and administer chemotherapy

What is the 5-year survival rate after resection of liver colorectal metastases?
Approximately 25% if resected with 1 to 2 cm margins (0% survive 5 years without resection)

What is the appropriate postoperative follow-up at 3 months?
Physical exam, stool guaiac, CEA (every 3 months for 3 years, then every 6 months for 2 years)

Why is follow-up so important the first 3 postoperative years?
Approximately 90% of colorectal recurrences occur within 3 years after surgery.

For what tumor was the Dukes' classification originally described?
Rectal cancer

What is the most common cause of colonic obstruction in the adult population?
Colon cancer (number two is diverticular disease, number three is colonic volvulus)

POLYPS

POLYPS OF THE COLON AND RECTUM

What are they?
Tissue growth into the bowel lumen, usually consisting of mucosa and/or submucosa

How are they anatomically classified?
Sessile (flat)
Pedunculated (on a stalk)

What are the histologic classifications of the following types:

Inflammatory (pseudopolyp)?
As in Crohn's disease or ulcerative colitis

Hamartomatous?
Normal tissue in abnormal configuration; most common is juvenile polyp, which has no malignant potential

Hyperplastic?
Benign with no malignant potential, but significant because they often occur in areas of neoplastic polyps; must rule out neoplasm

Neoplastic?
Proliferation of undifferentiated cells; often premalignant or have malignant cells

What are the subtypes of neoplastic polyps?
Tubular adenomas (usually pedunculated)
Tubulovillous adenomas
Villous adenomas (usually sessile and look like broccoli heads)

What determines malignant potential of an adenomatous polyp?
Size
Histologic type
Atypia of cells

What is the correlation between size and malignancy?
Polyps larger than 2 cm have a high risk of carcinoma (33%–55%)

What about histology and cancer potential of an adenomatous polyp?
Villous polyps have a higher risk of carcinoma than tubulovillous, which have a higher risk than tubular (**think: VILL**ous = **VILL**ain)

What is the approximate percentage of carcinomas found in the following polyps:

Tubular adenoma less than 1 cm?
1%

Tubulovillous adenoma less than 1 cm?
5%

Villous adenoma less than 1 cm?	10%
Tubular adenoma 1 to 2 cm?	10%
Tubulovillous adenoma 1 to 2 cm?	10%
Villous adenoma 1 to 2 cm?	10%
Tubular adenoma more than 2 cm?	33%
Tubulovillous adenoma more than 2 cm?	45%
Villous adenoma more than 2 cm?	55%

Which neoplastic polyp is most common?
Tubular adenoma (A.K.A. adenomatous polyp)

Where are most polyps found?
Rectosigmoid

What are signs/symptoms?
Bleeding (red or dark blood), change in bowel habits, mucus per rectum, electrolyte loss, totally asymptomatic

What are the diagnostic tests?
Fecal occult blood, CBC, BE, endoscope, all suspect tissue should be biopsied or excised (snare) and sent to pathology

What is the treatment?
Endoscopic resection (snared) if polyps are small; large sessile villous adenomas should be removed with bowel resection

POLYPOSIS SYNDROMES

FAMILIAL POLYPOSIS

What is another name for this condition?
Familial adenomatous polyposis or familial polyposis coli

What are the characteristics?

Hundreds of adenomatous polyps within the rectum and colon that begin developing at puberty; all undiagnosed; untreated patients develop cancer by the age of 40 to 50

What is the inheritance pattern?

Autosomal dominant (i.e., 50% of offspring)

What is the treatment?

Total protocolectomy and ileostomy
Total colectomy and rectal mucosal removal (mucosal proctectomy) and ileoanal anastomosis

GARDNER'S SYNDROME

What are the characteristics?

Neoplastic polyps of **the small bowel** and **colon;** cancer by the age of 40 in 100% of undiagnosed patients, as in familial adenomatous polyposis (FAP)

What are the other associated findings?

Desmoid tumors (in the abdominal wall or cavity), **osteomas** of skull (seen on x-ray), **sebaceous** cysts, adrenal tumors, thyroid tumors, and retroperitoneal fibrosis, duodenal and periampullary tumors

How can the findings associated with Gardner's syndrome be remembered?

Think of a Gardener planting **SOD:**
S = **S**ebaceous cysts
O = **O**steomas
D = **D**esmoid tumors

What is a desmoid tumor?

Tumor of the musculoaponeurotic sheath, usually of the abdominal wall; benign, but grows locally; treated by wide resection

What is the inheritance pattern?

Varying degree of penetrance from a gene that is autosomal dominant

What is the treatment of colon polyps in patients with Gardner's syndrome?

Total protocolectomy and ileostomy
Total colectomy and rectal mucosal removal (mucosal proctectomy) and ileoanal anastomosis

PEUTZ-JEGHERS SYNDROME

What are the characteristics?	Hamartomas throughout the GI tract (jejunum/ileum > colon > stomach)
What is the associated cancer risk from polyps?	None
What is the associated cancer risk for women with Peutz-Jeghers?	Ovarian cancer (granulosa cell tumor is most common)
What is the inheritance pattern?	Autosomal dominant
What are the other signs?	Melanotic pigmentation (black/brown) of buccal mucosa (mouth), lips, digits, palms, feet (soles) (Think: **P**eutz = **P**igmented)
What is the treatment?	Removal of polyps, if symptomatic (i.e., bleeding, intussusception or obstruction)
What are juvenile polyps?	Benign hamartomas in the small bowel and colon; not premalignant; also known as "retention polyps"
What is Cronkhite-Canada syndrome?	Diffuse GI hamartoma polyps (i.e., no cancer potential) associated with malabsorption/weight loss, diarrhea and **loss of electrolytes/protein;** signs include **alopecia,** nail atrophy, skin pigmentation
What is Turcot's syndrome?	Colon polyps with malignant CNS tumors (glioblastoma multiforme)

DIVERTICULAR DISEASE OF THE COLON

DIVERTICULOSIS

What is diverticulosis?	A condition in which diverticula can be found within the colon, especially the sigmoid colon; the diverticula are actually **false diverticula** in that only mucosa and submucosa herniate through the bowel musculature; true diverticula involve all layers of the bowel wall and are rare in the colon

Describe the pathophysiology

Weakness in the bowel wall develops at points where nutrient **blood vessels** enter between antimesenteric and mesenteric taenia; increased intraluminal pressures then cause herniation through these areas

What is the incidence?

Approximately 50% to 60% in the United States by age 60, with only 10% to 20% becoming symptomatic

What is the most common site?

Ninety-five percent of people with diverticulosis have **sigmoid** colon involvement

Who is at risk?

People with **low-fiber diets,** chronic constipation, and a positive family history

What are the symptoms/ complications?

Bleeding: may be massive
Diverticulitis: see the following description
Asymptomatic (80% of cases): usually diagnosed incidentally on endoscopy or BE

What is the diagnostic approach?

Bleeding without signs of inflammation (fever, increased WBCs): colon cancer must be ruled out; therefore, colonoscopy and BE should be performed
Diverticulitis with accompanying spasm and infection and/or inflammation: BE and endoscopy should be avoided; usually diagnosed by history, but abdominal and/or pelvic CT may be helpful, especially because it may reveal an abscess; BE or colonoscopy may be done **weeks** after the inflammation resolves

What is the treatment of diverticulosis?

High-fiber diet is recommended

What are the indications for operation with diverticulosis?

Complications of diverticulitis (e.g., abscess, fistula, obstruction, stricture), recurrent episodes of diverticulitis, hemorrhage, suspected carcinoma, prolonged symptoms

DIVERTICULITIS

What is it?	Infection or perforation of a diverticulum, leading to infection/ inflammation of peridiverticular tissue, abscess formation, or generalized peritonitis
What are the signs/ symptoms?	Left lower quadrant pain (cramping or steady), change in bowel habits (**diarrhea**), fever, chills, anorexia, left lower quadrant mass, nausea, vomiting, and dysuria
What are the associated lab findings?	Increased WBCs
What are the associated radiographic findings?	On x-ray: ileus; partially obstructed colon; air-fluid levels; free air if perforated On abdominal/pelvic CT: swollen, edematous bowel wall; particularly helpful in diagnosing an abscess
What are the associated barium enema findings?	Barium enema should be avoided in acute setting
What are the associated colonoscopic findings?	Also should be avoided in acute cases Colonic spasm increases the risk of perforation May be performed (along with BE) after attack subsides
What are the possible complications?	Abscess, peritonitis, fistula (e.g., colovesicular), obstruction
What is the initial therapy?	IV fluids, NPO, broad-spectrum antibiotics with anaerobic coverage, NG suction (as needed)
When is surgery warranted?	Obstruction, fistula, free perforation, abscess not amenable to percutaneous drainage, sepsis
What surgery is usually performed ELECTIVELY for recurrent bouts of diverticulitis?	A one-stage operation: resection of the involved segment and primary anastomosis (with preoperative bowel prep)

What type of surgery is usually performed for an acute case of diverticulitis with a complication of the disease (e.g., abscess, obstruction)?	**A two-staged operation;** resection of the involved segment with an end colostomy and subsequent reanastomosis of the colon (usually after 2–3 postoperative months)
What is the treatment of diverticular abscess?	Percutaneous drainage, transrectal drainage; if abscess is not amenable to percutaneous drainage, then surgical approach for drainage is necessary
How common is massive lower GI bleeding with diverticulitis?	Very **rare!** Massive lower GI bleeding is seen with diverticulosis, not diverticulitis.
What are the most common causes of massive lower GI bleeding in the adult population?	Diverticulosis (especially right-sided), vascular ectasia

COLONIC VOLVULUS

What is it?	**Twisting of the colon on its self** about its mesentery, resulting in obstruction and, if complete, vascular compromise with potential for necrosis and/or perforation
What is the most common type of colonic volvulus?	Sigmoid volvulus (makes sense because the sigmoid is a redundant/"floppy" structure!)

SIGMOID VOLVULUS

What is it?

Volvulus or "twist" in the sigmoid colon

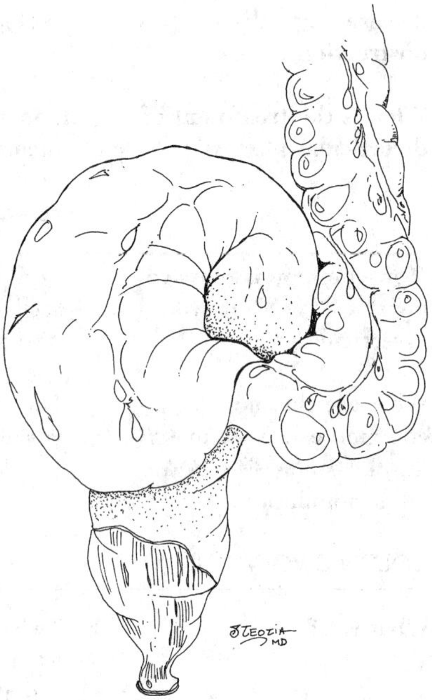

What is the incidence?

Approximately 75% of colonic volvulus cases

What are the etiologic factors?

High-residue diet resulting in bulky stools and tortuous, elongated colon; chronic constipation; laxative abuse; pregnancy; seen most commonly in elderly/bedridden or **institutionalized** patients, many of whom have history of prior abdominal surgery or distal colonic obstruction

What are the signs/ symptoms?

Acute abdominal pain, progressive abdominal **distention,** anorexia, obstipation, cramps, nausea, and vomiting

What findings are evident on abdominal plain film?

Distended loop of sigmoid colon, often in the classic "bent inner tube" or "omega" sign with the loop aiming toward the right upper quadrant

What are the signs of necrotic bowel in colonic volvulus?

Free air, pneumatosis (air in the bowel wall)

How is the diagnosis made?

Sigmoidoscopy or radiographic exam with gastrografin enema

Under what conditions is gastrografin enema useful?

If sigmoidoscopy and plain films fail to confirm the diagnosis; "**bird's beak**" is pathognomonic seen on enema contrast study as the contrast comes to a sharp end

What are the signs of strangulation?

Discolored or hemorrhagic mucosa on sigmoidoscopy, bloody fluid in the rectum, frank ulceration or necrosis at the point of the twist, peritoneal signs, fever, hypovolemia, ↑ WBCs

What is the treatment?

If there is no strangulation, sigmoidoscopic reduction is successful in approximately 80% of cases (i.e., **80%** are treated **nonoperatively** initially)

If unsuccessful, enema study will occasionally reduce

In either case, a colonic tube is inserted to serve as a stent

Most patients undergo subsequent elective sigmoid resection

What is the percentage of recurrence after nonoperative reduction of a sigmoid volvulus?

Approximately 40%!

What are the indications for surgery?

If strangulation is suspected or nonoperative reduction unsuccessful, then laparotomy with formation of a colostomy after resection; most patients should undergo interval resection of the redundant sigmoid after successful nonoperative reduction because of the high recurrence rate (40%)

CECAL VOLVULUS

What is it?

Twisting of the cecum upon itself and upon the mesentery

What is a cecal "bascule" volvulus?	Instead of the more common axial twist, the cecum folds upward (lies on the ascending colon)
What is the incidence?	Approximately 25% of colonic volvulus (i.e., much less common than sigmoid volvulus)
What is the etiology?	Idiopathic poor fixation of the right colon; many patients have history of abdominal surgery
What are the signs/ symptoms?	Acute onset of abdominal pain or a colicky pain beginning in the right lower quadrant and progressing to a constant pain, vomiting, obstipation, abdominal distention, and small bowel obstruction; many patients will have had previous similar episodes
How is the diagnosis made?	Abdominal plain film; dilated, ovoid colon with large air/fluid level in the right lower quadrant often forming the classic **"coffee bean"** sign with the apex aiming toward the left upper quadrant, epigastrium, or left upper quadrant (must rule out gastric dilation with NG aspiration)
What diagnostic studies should be performed?	Colonoscopy or water-soluble contrast study (gastrografin), if diagnosis cannot be made by AXR
What is the treatment?	Treated with emergent surgery If the cecum is viable, **cecopexy** is performed If the cecum has infarcted or perforated, right colectomy with ileostomy and mucus fistula (primary reanastomosis may be performed if conditions are near perfect)
What are the major differences in the emergent management of cecal volvulus versus sigmoid?	Cecal volvulus patients require surgical reduction, whereas the vast majority of patients with sigmoid volvulus undergo endoscopic reduction of the twist

42 The Anus

ANAL CANCER

What is the most common carcinoma of the anus?	Squamous cell carcinoma
What cell types are found in carcinomas of the anus?	1. Squamous cell carcinoma (accounts for two-thirds) 2. Cloacogenic (transitional cell) 3. Adenocarcinoma/melanoma/mucoepidermal
What is the incidence of anal carcinoma?	Rare (1% of colon cancers incidence)
What is anal Bowen's disease?	Squamous carcinoma in situ
How is it treated?	With local wide excision
What is Paget's disease of the anus?	Adenocarcinoma in situ of the anus
How is it treated?	With local wide excision
What are the risk factors for anal cancer?	Any chronic inflammatory process: fistula, abscess, infections (e.g., condyloma), Crohn's disease Also, incidence is higher in homosexual men, renal transplant patients, Herpes patients, and patients who smoke
What is the most common symptom of anal carcinoma?	Anal bleeding
What are the other signs/symptoms of anal carcinoma?	Pain, mass, mucous per rectum, pruritus

What percentage of patients with anal cancer are asymptomatic?	Approximately 25%
To what locations do anal cancers metastasize?	Lymph nodes, liver, bone, lung
Are most patients with anal cancer diagnosed early or late?	Late (diagnosis is often missed)
What is the workup of a patient with suspected anal carcinoma?	History Physical exam: digital rectal exam, proctoscopic exam, and colonoscopy Biopsy of mass Abdominal/pelvic CT scan, with or without pelvic MRI or transanal U/S CXR LFTs
What are the epidermal cancers?	Squamous cell carcinoma, cloacogenic carcinoma, mucoepidermal carcinoma
How is an anal canal epidermal carcinoma treated?	Nigro protocol: 1. Chemotherapy 2. Radiation 3. Postradiation therapy scar biopsy
How is a small (< 2 cm) anal margin epidermal cancer treated?	Usually by surgical excision with 1 cm margins
What is the treatment of anal basal cell carcinoma?	Local excision
What is the treatment of anal melanoma?	Wide excision or APR (especially if tumor is large)
What percentage of patients have an amelanotic anal tumor?	Approximately one-third, thus making diagnosis difficult
What is the prognosis of anal melanoma?	Less than 5% five-year survival rate

FISTULA IN ANO

What is it?	Anal fistula from the rectum to the perianal skin
What are the causes?	Usually due to anal crypt/gland (at dentate line) infection with extension/ abscess formation
What are the signs/ symptoms?	Perianal drainage, perirectal abscess, recurrent perirectal abscess, "diaper rash" due to drainage (i.e., excoriation), itching
What disease should be considered with fistula in ano?	Crohn's disease (also consider ulcerative colitis, pilonidal abscess)
How is the diagnosis made?	Exam, proctoscope
What is Goodsall's rule?	Fistulas originating **anterior** to a transverse line through the anus will course **straight** ahead and exit anteriorly, whereas those exiting **posteriorly** have a **curved** tract.
How can Goodsall's rule be remembered?	Think of a dog with a straight nose (anterior) and a curved tail (posterior)
What is the management of anorectal fistulas?	1. Define the pathoanatomy 2. Marsupialization of fistula tract (i.e., fillet tract open) 3. Wound care—routine Sitz baths and dressing changes, stool softeners 4. Seton placement, if fistula is through the sphincter muscle
What is a Sitz bath?	Sitting in a warm bath (usually done after bowel movement and TID)
What percentage of patients with a perirectal abscess develop a fistula in ano?	Approximately 50%

PERIRECTAL ABSCESS

What is it?	Abscess formation around the anus/ rectum
What are the signs/ symptoms?	Rectal pain, drainage of pus, fever, perianal mass
How is the diagnosis made?	Physical/digital exam reveals perianal/ rectal submucosal mass/fluctuance
What is the cause?	Crypt abscess in dentate line with spread
What is the treatment?	As with all abscesses (except simple liver amebic abscess), **drainage**, with or without antibiotics against colonic flora (antibiotics are absolutely indicated with diabetes, artificial or prosthetic heart valve, spreading infection, or immunocompromised patients), Sitz bath, anal hygiene, stool softeners
What percentage of patients develop a fistula in ano in the subsequent 6 months after surgery?	Approximately 50%

ANAL FISSURE

What is it?	Tear or fissure in the anal epithelium
What is the most common site?	Posterior midline (comparatively low blood flow)
What is the cause?	Hard stool passage (constipation), hyperactive sphincter, disease process (e.g., Crohn's disease)
What are the signs/ symptoms?	Pain in the anus, painful (can be excruciating) bowel movement, rectal bleeding, blood on toilet tissue after bowel movement, sentinel tag, tear in the anal skin, extremely painful rectal exam, sentinel pile, hypertrophic papilla

What is a sentinel pile?	Thickened mucosa/skin at the distal end of an anal fissure that looks like a small hemorrhoid
What is the conservative treatment?	Sitz baths, stool softeners, high fiber diet, excellent anal hygiene
What disease processes must be considered with a chronic anal fissure?	Crohn's disease, anal cancer, sexually transmitted disease, ulcerative colitis, AIDS
What are the indications for surgery?	Chronic fissure refractory to conservative treatment
What are the surgical options?	Lateral internal sphincterotomy (i.e., cut the integral sphincter to release it from spasm) Anal dilatation (3–4 fingers)

PERIANAL WARTS

What are they?	Warts around the anus/perineum
What is the cause?	Condyloma acuminatum (human papilloma virus)
What is the major risk?	Squamous cell carcinoma
What is the treatment if warts are small?	Topical podophyllin
What is the treatment if warts are large?	Surgical resection or laser ablation

HEMORRHOIDS

What are they?	Engorgement of the venous plexi of the rectum and/or anus, with protrusion of the mucosa and/or anal margin
What are the signs/ symptoms?	Anal mass/prolapse, bleeding, itching, pain
Which type, internal or external, is painful?	External, below the dentate line

If a patient has excruciating anal pain and history of hemorrhoids, what is the likely diagnosis?
Thrombosed external hemorrhoid

What are the causes of hemorrhoids?
Constipation/straining, portal hypertension, pregnancy

What is an internal hemorrhoid?
Hemorrhoid above the (proximal) dentate line

What is an external hemorrhoid?
Hemorrhoid below the dentate line

What are the three "hemorrhoid quadrants"?
1. Left lateral
2. Right posterior
3. Right anterior

Classification By Degrees

Define the following terms for internal hemorrhoids:

First degree hemorrhoid
Hemorrhoid that does not prolapse

Second degree hemorrhoid
Prolapses with defecation, but returns on its own

Third degree hemorrhoid
Prolapses with defecation or any type of Valsalva maneuver and requires active manual reduction (eat fiber!)

Fourth degree hemorrhoid
Prolapsed hemorrhoid that cannot be reduced

What is the treatment?
High-fiber diet, anal hygiene, topical steroids, Sitz baths
Rubber band ligation (in most cases anesthetic is not necessary for internal hemorrhoids)
Surgical resection for large refractory hemorrhoids

What are the dreaded complications of hemorrhoidectomy?
Exsanguination (bleeding may pool proximally in lumen of colon without any signs of external bleeding)
Pelvic infection (may be extensive and potentially fatal)
Incontinence (injury to sphincter complex)
Anal stricture

What condition is a contraindication for hemorrhoidectomy?	Crohn's disease
What must be ruled out with lower GI bleeding believed to be caused by hemorrhoids?	Colon cancer (colonoscopy or proctoscopy followed up with a barium enema)

43

Lower GI Bleeding

What is the definition of lower GI bleeding?

Bleeding distal to the ligament of Treitz; vast majority occurs in the colon

What are the symptoms?

Hematochezia (bright red blood per rectum [BRBPR]), with or without abdominal pain, melena, anorexia, fatigue, syncope, shortness of breath, shock

What are the signs?

BRBPR, positive hemoccult, abdominal tenderness, hypovolemic shock, orthostasis

What are the causes?

Diverticulosis (usually **right**-sided in severe hemorrhage), vascular ectasia, colon cancer, hemorrhoids, trauma, hereditary hemorrhagic telangiectasia, intussusception, volvulus, ischemic colitis, IBD (especially ulcerative colitis), anticoagulation, rectal cancer, Meckel's diverticulum (with ectopic gastric mucosa), colonic ulcer, chemotherapy, irradiation injury, infarcted bowel, strangulated hernia, anal fissure

What are the most common causes of massive lower GI bleeding?

1. **Diverticulosis**
2. Vascular ectasia

What lab tests should be performed?

CBC, Chem-7, PT/PTT, type and cross

What is the initial treatment?

IVFs: lactated Ringer's; packed red blood cells, as needed (through at least a 16 G peripheral IV X 2); Foley catheter, to follow urine output

What diagnostic tests should be performed for all lower GI bleeds?

History, physical exam, NGT aspiration (to rule out UGI bleeding; bile or blood must be seen; otherwise, perform EGD), anoscopy/proctoscopic exam

What must be ruled out in patients with lower GI bleeding?

Upper GI bleeding! Remember, NGT aspiration is not 100% accurate (even if you get bile without blood)
If there is any question, perform EGD

What would an algorithm for diagnosing and treating lower GI bleeding look like?

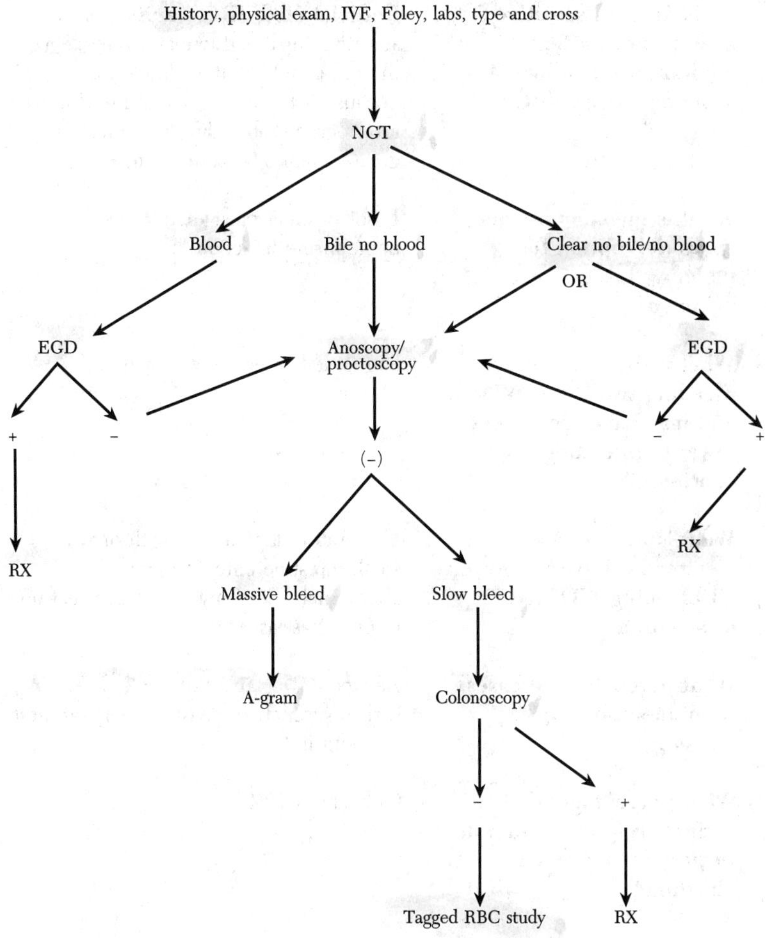

What is the diagnostic test of choice for localizing a slow to moderate lower GI bleeding source?

Colonoscopy

What test is performed to localize bleeding if there is too much active bleeding to see the source with a colonoscope?

A-gram

What is more sensitive for a slow, intermittent amount of blood loss: A-gram or tagged RBC study?

Radiolabeled RBC scan is more sensitive for blood loss at a rate of 0.1 ml/min or intermittent blood loss because it has a longer half life (for arteriography, bleeding rate must be greater than 0.5–1.0 ml/min)

What is the colonoscopic treatment option for bleeding vascular ectasia or polyp?

Laser or electrocoagulation; local epinephrine injection

What is the treatment if bleeding site is KNOWN and massive or recurrent lower GI bleeding continues?

Segmental resection of the bowel

What is the surgical treatment of massive lower GI bleeding WITHOUT localization?

Exploratory laparotomy with or without small intestine enteroscopy and abdominal colectomy (i.e., leave rectum in place) as last resort

What percentage of cases spontaneously stop bleeding?

Between **80% and 90% stop bleeding** with resuscitative measures only (at least temporarily)

What percentage of patients require emergent surgery for lower GI bleeding?

Only about 10%

44

Inflammatory Bowel Disease (IBD): Crohn's Disease and Ulcerative Colitis

What is it?	Inflammatory disease of the GI tract
What are the two inflammatory bowel diseases?	Crohn's Disease and Ulcerative Colitis
What is another name for Crohn's disease?	"Regional enteritis"
What is the cause of IBD?	**No one knows,** but probably an autoimmune process with environmental factors playing a part
What is the differential diagnosis?	Crohn's versus ulcerative colitis, infectious colitis (e.g., C. difficile, amebiasis, shigellosis), ischemic colitis, irritable bowel syndrome, diverticulitis, Zollinger-Ellison (Z-E) syndrome, colon cancer, carcinoid, ischemic bowel
What are the extraintestinal manifestations seen in both types of IBD?	Ankylosing spondylitis, aphthous (oral) ulcers, iritis, pyoderma gangrenosum, erythema nodosum, clubbing of fingers, sclerosing cholangitis, arthritis, kidney disease (nephrotic syndrome, amyloid deposits)
How can these manifestations be remembered?	Think of the acronym "A PIE SACK": **A:** Aphthous ulcers **P:** Pyoderma gangrenosum **I:** Iritis **E:** Erythema nodosum

S: Sclerosing cholangitis
A: Arthritis, ankylosis spondylitis
C: Clubbing of fingers
K: Kidney (amyloid deposits, nephrotic syndrome)

COMPARISON OF CROHN'S DISEASE AND ULCERATIVE COLITIS

Incidence

Crohn's disease?

High in the Jewish population, low in the African-American population
Female > male
Bimodal distribution: peak incidence at 25 to 40 years; second bimodal distribution peak at 50 to 65 years

Ulcerative colitis?

High in the Jewish population, low in the African-American population
Seen in families
Male > female
Bimodal distribution (i.e., two peaks in incidence) at ages 20 to 35 and 50 to 65 years of age

Initial symptoms

Crohn's disease?

Abdominal pain, fever, diarrhea, weight loss, anal disease

Ulcerative colitis?

Bloody diarrhea, fever, weight loss

Anatomic distribution

Crohn's disease?

Classically said to involve **"mouth to anus"**
Small bowel alone—20%
Small bowel **and** colon—40%
Colon alone— ≈ 30%

Ulcerative colitis?

Colon alone (can have "backwash ileitis")

Route of spread

Crohn's disease?

Small bowel and/or colon **with "skip areas"** of normal bowel; hence, the name "regional enteritis"

Ulcerative colitis?

Almost always involves the rectum and spreads proximally always in a continuous route without "skip areas"

What is "backwash" ileitis?

Mild inflammation of the terminal ileum in ulcerative colitis, thought to be "backwash" of inflammatory mediators from the colon into the terminal ileum.

Bowel wall involvement

Crohn's disease?

Full thickness (transmural involvement)

Ulcerative colitis?

Mucosa/submucosa only

Anal involvement

Crohn's disease?

Common (fistulae, abscess, fissures, ulcers)

Ulcerative colitis?

Uncommon

Rectal involvement

Crohn's disease?

Rare

Ulcerative colitis?

100%

Mucosal findings

Crohn's disease (6)?

1. Aphthoid ulcers
2. **Granulomas**
3. Linear ulcers
4. Transverse fissures
5. Swollen mucosa
6. Full-thickness wall involvement

Ulcerative colitis (5)?

1. Granular, flat mucosa
2. Ulcers
3. **Crypt abscess**
4. Dilated mucosal vessels
5. **Pseudopolyps**

Diagnostic tests

Crohn's disease?

Colonoscopy with biopsy, barium enema, UGI with small bowel follow through, stool cultures

Ulcerative colitis?

Colonoscopy, barium enema, UGI with small bowel follow through (to look for Crohn's disease), stool cultures

Complications

Crohn's disease?

Anal fistula/abscess, **fistula,** stricture, perforation, **abscesses,** toxic megacolon, colovesical fistula, enterovaginal fistula, hemorrhage, **obstruction,** cancer

Ulcerative colitis?

Cancer, toxic megacolon, colonic perforation, hemorrhage, strictures, obstruction, complications of surgery

Why are fistulae and abscesses more often Crohn's disease versus ulcerative colitis?

Crohn's disease involves the entire bowel wall (transmural), whereas ulcerative colitis only involves the mucosa/submucosa.

Cancer risk

Crohn's disease?

High risk in areas surgically bypassed from the fecal stream; overall increased risk, but much less than that of ulcerative colitis

Ulcerative colitis?

Approximately 2% risk of developing colon cancer at 10 years and then increases approximately 2% per year; thus, an incidence of about 20% after 20 years of the disease

Incidence of toxic megacolon

Crohn's disease?

Approximately 5%

Ulcerative colitis?

Approximately 10%

Indications for surgery

Crohn's disease?

Obstruction, massive bleeding, fistula, perforation, suspicion of cancer, abscess refractory to medical treatment, toxic megacolon (refractory to medial treatment)

Ulcerative colitis?

Toxic megacolon (refractory to medical treatment); cancer prophylaxis; massive bleeding; failure of child to mature because of disease and steroids, perforation, suspicion of or documented cancer, acute severe symptoms refractory to medical treatment, inability to wean off of chronic steroids, obstruction

What are the common surgical options for ulcerative colitis?

1. Total proctocolectomy, distal rectal mucosectomy, and ileoanal pull through
2. Total proctocolectomy and Brooke ileostomy

What is "toxic megacolon"?

Toxic patient: sepsis, febrile, abdominal pain
Megacolon: acutely and massively distended colon

What is the medical treatment of IBD?

Sulfasalazine, mesalamine (5-aminosalicylic acid)
Steroids, metronidazole (Flagyl)

What is the active metabolite of sulfasalazine?

5′-aminosalicylate (5′-ASA), which is released in the colon

Which disease has "cobblestoning" more often on endoscopic exam?

Crohn's disease (think: **C**rohn's = **C**obblestoning)

Which disease has pseudopolyps on colonoscopic exam?

Ulcerative colitis; pseudopolyps are polyps of hypertrophied mucosa surrounded by mucosal atrophy

Which disease has a "lead pipe" appearance on barium enema?

Chronic ulcerative colitis

Rectal bleeding/bloody diarrhea is a hallmark of which disease?

Ulcerative colitis (rare in Crohn's disease)

What is the most common indication for surgery in patients with Crohn's disease?	Small bowel obstruction (SBO)
What are the intraoperative findings of Crohn's disease?	Mesenteric **"fat creeping"** onto the antimesenteric border of the small bowel Shortened (and thick) mesentery Thick bowel wall Fistula(e) Abscess(es)
What is the operation for a short chronic stricture of the small bowel in Crohn's disease?	Stricturoplasty; basically a Heineke-Mikulicz pyloroplasty on the strictured segment (i.e., opened longitudinally and sewn closed in a transverse direction)
Should the appendix be removed during a laparotomy for abdominal pain if Crohn's disease is discovered?	Yes, if the cecum is not involved with active Crohn's disease
What is the medical treatment of choice for perianal Crohn's disease?	PO metronidazole (Flagyl)
What are the treatment options for long-term remission of IBD?	6-Mercaptopurine (6-MP), azathioprine, mesalamine
What is pouchitis?	Inflammation of the pouch of an ileoanal pull through; treat with metronidazole (Flagyl)

45 Liver

ANATOMY

What is the name of the liver capsule?
Glisson's capsule

What is the bare area?
The posterior section of the liver against the diaphragm without peritoneal covering

What is Cantlie's line?
A line drawn between the gallbladder to just left of the inferior vena cava that transects the liver into the right and left lobes

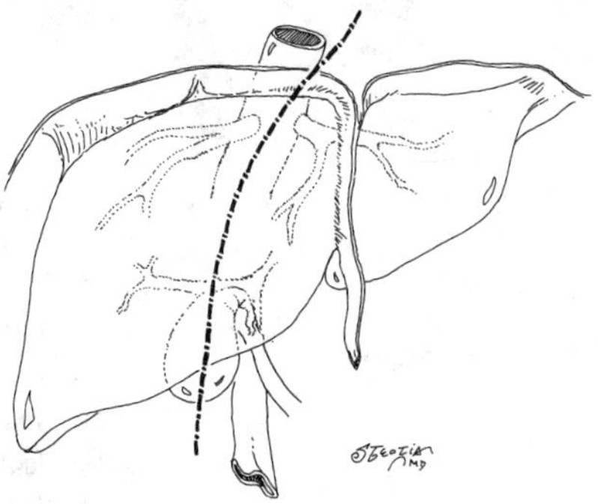

Which ligament goes from the anterior abdominal wall to the liver?
Falciform ligament (contains the ligament teres, which is the obliterated umbilical vein)

What is the coronary ligament?
The peritoneal reflection on top of the liver that crowns (coronary) the liver and attaches it to the diaphragm

What are the triangular ligaments of the liver?
The right and left lateral extents of the coronary ligament, which form triangles

What is the origin of the hepatic arterial supply?
From the proper hepatic artery off of the celiac trunk (celiac trunk to common hepatic artery to proper hepatic artery)

Identify the arterial branches of the celiac trunk.

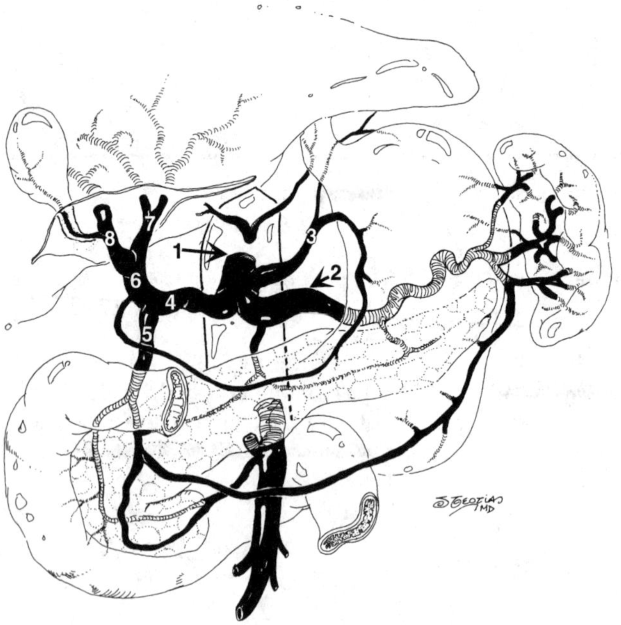

1. Celiac trunk
2. Splenic artery
3. Left gastric artery
4. Common hepatic artery
5. Gastroduodenal artery
6. Proper hepatic artery
7. Left hepatic artery
8. Right hepatic artery

What is the venous supply?

Portal vein (formed from the splenic vein and the superior mesenteric vein)

What is the hepatic venous drainage?

Via the hepatic veins, which drain into the IVC (three veins: left, middle, and right)

What sources provide oxygen to the liver?

Portal vein blood—50%
Hepatic artery blood—50%

From what sources does the liver receive blood?

Portal system—75%
Hepatic artery system—25%

What is the maximum amount of liver that can be resected while retaining adequate liver function?

More than 80%; if given adequate recovery time, the original mass can be **regenerated.**

What are the signs/symptoms of liver disease?

Hepatomegaly, splenomegaly, icterus, pruritus (from bile salts in skin), blanching spider telangiectasia, gynecomastia, testicular atrophy, caput medusae, dark urine, clay-colored stools, bradycardia, edema, ascites, fever, fetor hepaticus (sweet musty smell), hemorrhoids, variceal bleeding, anemia, body hair loss, liver tenderness, palmar erythema

Which liver enzymes are made by hepatocytes?

AST and ALT

What is the source of alkaline phosphatase?

Ductal epithelium (thus, elevated with ductal obstruction)

What is Child's class?

A classification system that estimates hepatic reserve in patients with hepatic failure

What comprises the Child's classification?

Lab: bilirubin, albumin
Clinical: nutrition, encephalopathy, ascites

How can the criteria comprising the Child's classification be remembered?

Acronym: "A BEAN":
A: Ascites

B: Bilirubin
E: Encephalopathy
A: Albumin
N: Nutrition

Define Child's classification

	Bili	ALB	Nutrit	Enceph	Ascites
A?	< 2	> 3.5	excellent	none	none
B?	2–3	3.–3.5	good	minimal	easily controlled
C?	> 3	< 3	poor	severe	poorly controlled

Think, as in a letter grading system, A is better than B, B is better than C

	A	B	C
A	>3.5	3–3.5	<3.
B	<2	2–3	>3
E	NONE	Minimal	Severe
A	NONE	easily Controlled	poorly Controlled
N	Excellent	good	poor

What is the operative mortality for a portocaval shunt in the following Child's classes:	
A?	Less than 5%
B?	Less than 15%
C?	Approximately 33%

TUMORS OF THE LIVER

What is the most common liver tumor?	**Metastatic disease** outnumbers primary tumors 20:1. Primary site is usually the GI tract.
What is the most common primary malignant liver tumor?	Hepatocellular carcinoma (hepatoma)
What is the most common primary benign liver tumor?	Hemangioma
What lab tests comprise the workup for liver metastasis?	LFTs (SGOT and alkaline phosphatase are most useful), CEA for suspected primary colon cancer
What are the associated imaging studies?	CT, ultrasound, A-gram
What is a right hepatic lobectomy?	Removal of the right lobe of the liver (i.e., all tissue to the right of Cantlie's line is removed)
What is a left hepatic lobectomy?	Removal of the left lobe of the liver (i.e., removal of all the liver tissue to the left of Cantlie's line)
What is a right trisegmentectomy?	Removal of all the liver tissue to the right of the falciform ligament
What are the three common types of primary benign liver tumors?	1. Hemangioma 2. Hepatocellular adenoma 3. Focal nodular hyperplasia

What are the four common types of primary malignant liver tumors?

1. Hepatocellular carcinoma (hepatoma)
2. Cholangiocarcinoma (when intrahepatic)
3. Angiosarcoma (associated with vinyl chloride, arsenic, or thorotrast contrast exposure)
4. Hepatoblastoma (most common in infants and children)

What is a "hepatoma"?

Hepatocellular carcinoma, NOT a Hepatic Adenoma

What are the other benign liver masses?

Benign liver cyst, bile duct hamartomas, bile duct adenoma

HEPATOCELLULAR ADENOMA

What is it?

Benign liver tumor

Describe the histology.

Normal hepatocytes without bile ducts

What are the associated risk factors?

Women, birth control pills (think: **ABC** = **A**denoma **B**irth **C**ontrol), anabolic steroids (e.g., misguided athletes), glycogen storage disease

What is the female:male ratio?

9 to 1 F > M

What is the average age of occurrence?

Between 30 and 35 years

What are the signs/symptoms?

Right upper quadrant pain/mass,right upper quadrant fullness, bleeding (rare)

What are the possible complications?

Rupture with bleeding, necrosis, pain, risk of hepatocellular carcinoma

How is the diagnosis made?

CT, U/S, +/- biopsy

What is the treatment?

Surgical resection, discontinuation of birth control pills/steroids, avoidance of pregnancy

FOCAL NODULAR HYPERPLASIA

What is it?

Benign liver tumor

Describe the histology.	Normal hepatocytes and **bile ducts (adenoma has no bile ducts)**
What is the average age of occurrence?	Approximately 40 years
What are the associated risk factors?	Women
Are the tumors associated with birth control pills?	No clear association
How is the diagnosis made?	Nuclear technetium 99 study, U/S, CT, A-gram, biopsy
What is the classic CT finding?	Liver mass with "central scar'
What are the possible complications?	Pain (no risk of cancer, very rarely hemorrhage)
What is the treatment?	Resection, if patient is symptomatic; otherwise, follow if diagnosis is confirmed
What study helps to differentiate focal nodular hyperplasia and hepatic adenoma?	Nuclear technetium 99 study (focal nodular hyperplasia will show up on the study and adenoma usually will not)

HEPATIC HEMANGIOMA

What is it?	Benign vascular tumor of the liver
What is its claim to fame?	Most common primary benign liver tumor
What are the signs/ symptoms?	Right upper quadrant pain/mass, bruits, shock with bleeding, congestive heart failure
What are the possible complications?	Hemorrhage, congestive heart failure, coagulopathy, obstructive jaundice, gastric outlet obstruction
How is the diagnosis made?	CT with IV contrast, ultrasound, tagged red blood scan, MRI

Should biopsy be performed?	No (chance of hemorrhage with biopsy)
What is the treatment?	**Observation** Resection, if the patient is symptomatic (or if easy removal is possible)

HEPATOCELLULAR CARCINOMA

What is the incidence?	Most common primary malignant liver tumor (accounts for more than 75% of all primary malignant tumors)
What are the geographic high-risk areas?	Africa and Asia
What are the associated risk factors?	**Hepatitis B virus, cirrhosis, aflatoxin** (fungi toxin of *Aspergillus flavus)* Other risk factors: α-1-antitrypsin deficiency, hemochromatosis, schistosomiasis, androgens, BCP, glycogen storage disease (type I)
What percentage of patients with cirrhosis will develop hepatocellular carcinoma?	Approximately 10%
What are the signs/ symptoms?	Dull right upper quadrant pain, hepatomegaly, (classic presentation: **painful hepatomegaly**) abdominal mass, weight loss, paraneoplastic syndromes, signs of portal hypertension, ascites, jaundice, fever, anemia, splenomegaly
How is the diagnosis made?	Ultrasound, CT, angiography, tumor marker elevation
What is the tumor marker?	Elevated α-fetoprotein
What is the most common site of metastasis?	Lungs
What is the treatment of hepatocellular carcinoma?	Surgical resection, if possible (e.g., lobectomy) (Liver transplant, percutaneous ethanol tumor injection, liquid nitrogen cryotherapy, and intra-arterial chemotherapy are other options)

What is the prognosis under the following conditions:

Unresectable? Almost none survive a year

Resectable? Approximately 25% are alive at 5 years

Which subtype has the best prognosis? Fibrolamellar hepatoma (young adults)

LIVER ABSCESSES

What is it? Abscess (collection of pus) in the liver parenchyma

What are the types of liver abscess? Pyogenic (bacterial), parasitic (amebic), fungal

What is the most common location of abscess in the liver? Right lobe > left lobe

What are the sources?
Direct spread from biliary tract infection
or
Portal spread from GI infection (e.g., appendicitis, diverticulitis)
Systemic source (bacteremia)
Liver trauma (e.g., liver gunshot wound)
Cryptogenic (unknown source)

What are the two most common types? **Bacterial** (most common in the United States) and amebic (most common worldwide)

Define pyogenic. Caused by bacteria

BACTERIAL

What are the three most common organisms? *E. coli, Klebsiella, and Proteus* (also: *Bacteroides,* anaerobic streptococci, mixed infection)

What are the most common sources/causes of bacterial liver abscesses? Cholangitis, diverticulitis, liver cancer, liver metastasis

What are the signs/ symptoms?	**Fever, chills,** leukocytosis, **right upper quadrant pain,** increased LFTs, jaundice, sepsis, weight loss
What is the treatment?	IV antibiotics (triple antibiotics with metronidazole), percutaneous drainage with CT or U/S guidance
What are the indications for operative drainage?	Surgical drainage of multiple/loculated abscesses or if multiple percutaneous attempts have failed

AMEBIC

What is the etiology?	*Entamoeba histolytica* (typically reaches liver via portal vein from intestinal amebiasis)
How does it spread?	Fecal–oral transmission
What are the risk factors?	Patients from countries below the US–Mexican border, institutionalized patients, homosexual men, alcoholic patients
What are the signs/ symptoms?	Right upper quadrant pain, fever, hepatomegaly, diarrhea Note: chills are much less common with amebic abscesses versus pyogenic abscesses.
Which lobe is most commonly involved?	The right lobe of the liver ("**anchovy paste pus**" present in the abscess)
How is the diagnosis made?	Lab tests, ultrasound, CT
What lab tests should be performed?	Indirect hemagglutination titers for *Entamoeba* antibodies elevated in more than 95% of cases, elevated LFTs
What is the treatment?	Metronidazole IV; surgical drainage if refractory to metronidazole, if bacterial co-infection is present, peritoneal rupture

What are the possible complications of large left lobe liver amebic abscess?

Erosion into the pericardial sac (potentially fatal!)

HYDATID LIVER CYSTS

What is it?

Usually a right lobe cyst filled with Echinococcus *granulosus* (think granule = cyst) parasite or *Echinococcus multilocularis*

What are the risk factors?

Travel, exposure to dogs, sheep, cattle (carriers)

What are the signs/ symptoms?

Right upper quadrant abdominal pain, jaundice, right upper quadrant mass

How is the diagnosis made?

Indirect hemagglutination antibody test (serologic testing), Casoni skin test, ultrasound, CT, radiographic imaging

What are the findings on AXR?

Possible calcified outline of cyst

What are the major risks?

Erosion into the pleural cavity, pericardial sac, or biliary tree
Rupture into the peritoneal cavity causing **fatal anaphylaxis**

What is the risk of surgical removal of echinococcal (hydatid) cysts?

Rupture or leakage of cyst contents into the abdomen may cause a fatal **anaphylactic** reaction

When should percutaneous drainage be performed?

Never; may cause leaking into the peritoneal cavity and anaphylaxis

What is the treatment?

Mebendazole, followed by surgical resection; large cysts can be drained and then injected with toxic irrigant (scoliocide) into the cyst unless aspirate is bilious (which means there is a biliary connection) followed by cyst removal

Which toxic irrigations are used?

Hypertonic saline, ethanol

HEMOBILIA

What is it?	Blood draining via the common bile duct into the duodenum
What are the signs/ symptoms of hemobilia?	Triad: 1. Right upper quadrant pain 2. Guaiac positive/upper GI bleeding 3. Jaundice
What are the causes?	Trauma, percutaneous transhepatic cholangiography (PTC), tumors, etc.
How is the diagnosis made?	EGD (blood out of the ampulla of Vater), A-gram
What is the treatment?	A-Gram with embolization of the bleeding vessel

MISCELLANEOUS

What vitamin should every patient with liver failure and a coagulopathy receive?	Vitamin K (remember: 2, 7, 9, 10 are liver clotting factors)
Define the Pringle maneuver.	**Compression of the hepatoduodenal ligament** and its contents (i.e., hepatic artery and portal vein) to control bleeding from the liver, usually from trauma
What is the hepatorenal syndrome?	Renal failure of unknown cause in patients with liver failure (kidneys work fine when transplanted into a patient with a normal liver!)

46

Portal Hypertension

Define the anatomy of the portal venous system.

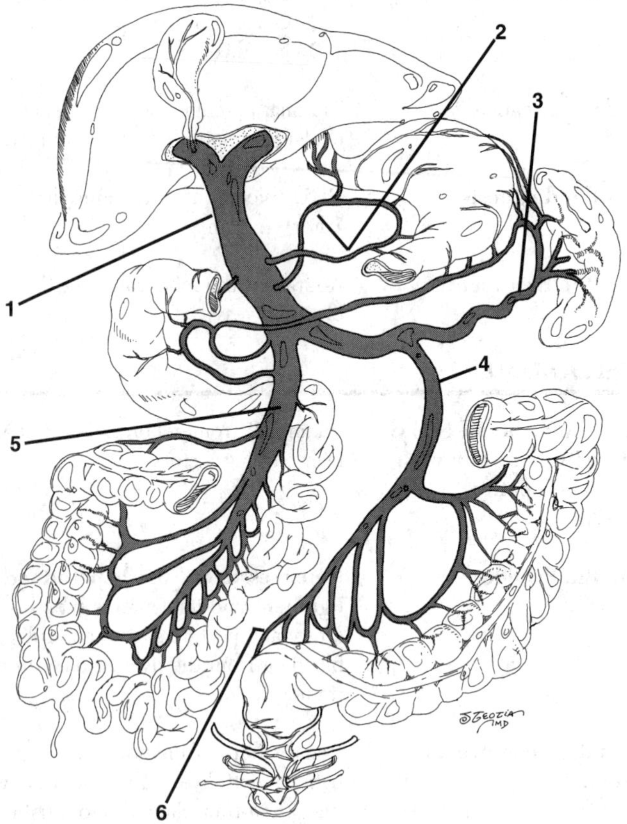

1. Portal vein
2. Coronary vein
3. Splenic vein
4. IMV (inferior mesenteric vein)
5. SMV (superior mesenteric vein)
6. Superior hemorrhoidal vein

Describe drainage of blood from the superior hemorrhoidal vein.

To the IMV, the splenic vein, and then the portal vein

Where does blood drain to from the IMV?	Into the splenic vein
Where does the portal vein begin?	At the confluence of the splenic vein and the SMV
What are the (6) potential routes of portal-systemic collateral blood flow (as seen with portal hypertension)?	1. Umbilical vein 2. Coronary vein to esophageal venous plexi 3. Retroperitoneal veins (veins of Retzius) 4. Diaphragm veins (veins of Sappey) 5. Superior hemorrhoidal vein to middle and inferior hemorrhoidal veins and then to the iliac vein 6. Splenic veins to the short gastric veins
What is the pathophysiology of portal hypertension?	Elevated portal pressure due to resistance to portal flow
What level of portal pressure is normal?	About 6 mm Hg **(< 10 mm Hg)**
What is the etiology?	**Prehepatic**—Thrombosis of portal vein **Hepatic—Cirrhosis** (distortion of normal parenchyma by regenerating hepatic nodules), hepatocellular carcinoma, etc. **Post-hepatic**—Budd Chiari syndrome: thrombosis of hepatic veins
What is the most common cause of portal hypertension in the United States?	Cirrhosis (> 90% of cases)
What percentage of patients with alcoholism develop cirrhosis?	Surprisingly, less than 1 in 5
What percentage of patients with cirrhosis develop esophageal varices?	Approximately 40%

What percentage of patients with cirrhosis develop portal hypertension?

Approximately two-thirds

What is the most common physical finding in patients with portal hypertension?

Splenomegaly

What are the associated CLINICAL findings in portal hypertension (4)?

1. Caput medusa (periumbilical veins engorgement)
2. Hemorrhoids
3. Splenomegaly
4. Esophageal varices

What other physical findings are associated with cirrhosis and portal hypertension?

Spider angioma, palmer erythema, ascites, truncal obesity and peripheral wasting, encephalopathy, liver flap, jaundice

What is the name of the periumbilical bruit seen with caput medusa?

Cruveilhier-Baumgarten bruit

How is portal pressure measured?

Indirect hepatic vein wedge pressure

What constitutes the portal-systemic collateral circulation in portal hypertension in the following conditions:

Esophageal varices?

Coronary vein backing up into the azygous system

Caput medusa?

Umbilical vein (via falciform ligament) draining into the epigastric veins

Retroperitoneal varices?

Small mesenteric veins (veins of Retzius) draining retroperitoneally into lumbar veins

Hemorrhoids?

Superior hemorrhoidal vein (which normally drains into the inferior mesenteric vein) backing up into the middle and inferior hemorrhoidal veins

What is the etiology?	**Cirrhosis (90%),** schistosomiasis, hepatitis, Budd-Chiari syndrome, hemochromatosis, Wilson's disease, portal vein thrombosis, tumors, splenic vein thrombosis
What is the most common cause of portal hypertension outside of North America?	Schistosomiasis
What is Budd-Chiari syndrome?	Thrombosis of the hepatic veins
What is the most feared complication of portal hypertension?	Bleeding from esophageal varices (up to 50% mortality!)
What are esophageal varices?	Engorgement of the esophageal venous plexi secondary to increased collateral blood flow from the portal system due to portal hypertension
What is the "rule of two-thirds" of portal hypertension?	**Two-thirds** of patients with cirrhosis will develop portal hypertension **Two-thirds** of patients with portal hypertension will develop esophageal varices **Two-thirds** of patients with esophageal varices will bleed from the varices
In patients with cirrhosis and known varices suffering upper GI bleeding, how often is that bleeding due to the varices?	Only about 50% of the time
What are the signs/ symptoms?	Hematemesis, melena, hematochezia
What is the mortality of an acute esophageal variceal bleed?	Approximately 50%

What is the initial treatment of variceal bleeding?

As with all upper GI bleeding: large bore IVS x 2, IV fluid, Foley catheter, NG tube, type and cross blood, send labs, correct coags (vitamin K, FFP)

What is the diagnostic test of choice?

EGD (upper GI endoscopy)
Remember, bleeding is due to varices only half the time; must rule out ulcers, etc.

If bleeding is due to esophageal varices, what is the initial treatment?

Emergent endoscopic sclerotherapy: a sclerosing substance is injected into the esophageal varices under direct endoscopic vision

What is the next step if the patient continues to bleed after the initial treatment?

IV vasopressin (and nitroglycerin, to avoid MI) Somatostatin is another choice to achieve vasoconstriction of the mesenteric vessels. If bleeding continues, consider balloon (**Sengstaken-Blakemore tube**) tamponade of the varices.

What is the next therapy after the bleeding is controlled?

Repeat endoscopic sclerotherapy

What are the options if sclerotherapy and conservative methods fail to stop the variceal bleeding or bleeding recurs?

Repeat sclerotherapy and treat conservatively
TIPS
Surgical shunt
Liver transplantation

What is the preferred shunt in the following cases:

If patient is a liver transplant candidate or very poor operative candidate?

TIPS procedure

Nonalcoholic patient who is not a transplant candidate?

Warren selective shunt (distal splenorenal shunt)

If the patient is an alcoholic and a good operative candidate, but not a liver transplant candidate?	Partial shunt: portocaval synthetic H-graft
What is a TIPS procedure?	**T**ransjugular **I**ntrahepatic **P**ortacaval **S**hunt (angiographic procedure!); a small tube is placed intrahepatically between the hepatic vein and a branch of the portal vein by the angiographic radiologist
What is a Warren shunt?	Distal splenorenal shunt—elective shunt procedure associated with low incidence of encephalopathy in nonalcoholic patients postoperatively because only the splenic flow is diverted to decompress the varices Not appropriate for long-term treatment in alcoholic patients: splenorenal vein anastomosis and **ligation of the coronary vein**

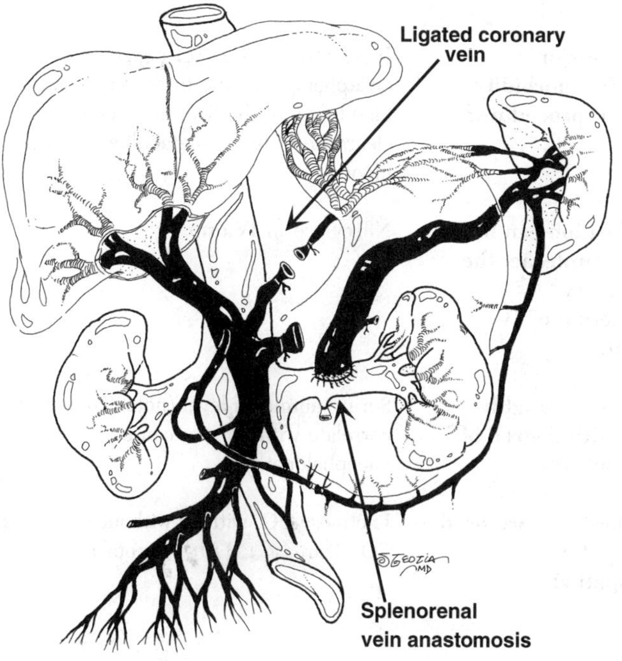

Define the following shunts:

End-to-side portocaval shunt?

"Total shunt"—portal vein (end) to IVC (side)

Side-to-side portocaval shunt?

Side of portal vein anastomosed to side of IVC—partially preserves portal flow ("partial shunt")

Synthetic portocaval H-graft?

"Partial shunt"—synthetic tube graft from the portal vein to the IVC (good option for acholic patients; associated with lower incidence of encephalopathy and easier transplantation later)

Synthetic mesocaval H-graft?

Synthetic graft from the SMV to the IVC

What does the acronym TIPS stand for?

Transjugular **I**ntrahepatic **P**ortal caval **S**hunt (angiographic procedure)

What is the most common perioperative cause of death following shunt procedure?

Hepatic failure, secondary to decreased blood flow (accounts for two-thirds of deaths)

What is the major postoperative morbidity after a shunt procedure?

Increased incidence of hepatic encephalopathy due to decreased portal blood flow to the liver and decreased clearance of toxins/metabolites from the blood

What medication can be infused to counteract the coronary artery vasoconstriction of IV vasopressin?

Nitroglycerin IV drip

What lab value roughly correlates with degree of encephalopathy?

Serum ammonia level (note: Thought to correlate with but not cause encephalopathy)

What medications are used to treat hepatic encephalopathy?

Lactulose PO, with or without neomycin PO; decrease PO protein intake

47 Biliary Tract

ANATOMY

Name structures 1 through 8 (below) of the biliary tract.

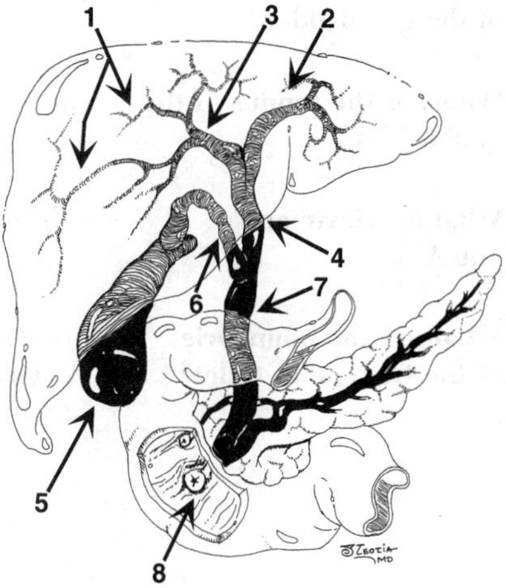

1. Intrahepatic ducts
2. Left hepatic duct
3. Right hepatic duct
4. Common hepatic duct
5. Gallbladder
6. Cystic duct
7. Common bile duct
8. Ampulla of Vater

Which is the proximal and which is the distal bile duct?

Proximal is close to the liver. (Bile and the liver is analogous to blood and the heart; they both flow distally.)

What is the name of the node in Calot's triangle?

Calot's node

What are the small ducts that drain bile directly into the gallbladder from the liver?

Ducts of Luschka

Which artery is susceptible to injury during cholecystectomy?
Right hepatic artery, because of its proximity to the cystic artery and Calot's triangle

What is the name of the valves of the gallbladder?
Spiral valves of Heister

Where is the infundibulum of the gallbladder?
Near the cystic duct

Where is the fundus of the gallbladder?
At the end of the gallbladder

What is "Hartmann's pouch"?
The gallbladder infundibulum

What are the boundaries of the triangle of Calot?
1. Cystic duct
2. Common hepatic duct
3. Inferior border of the liver

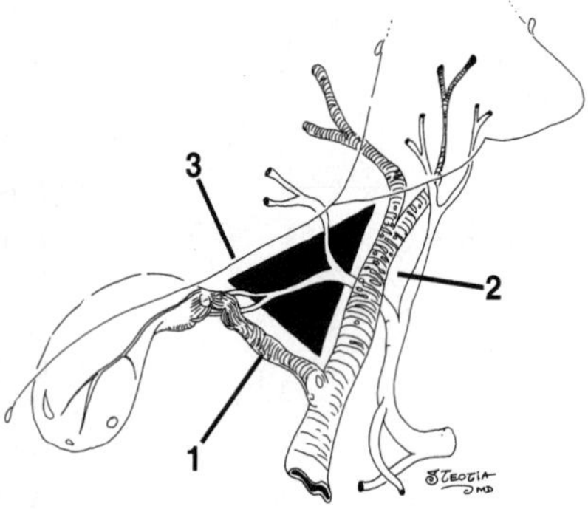

What is found in the triangle of Calot?
The cystic artery (and possibly the right hepatic artery)

PHYSIOLOGY

What is the source of alkaline phosphatase?
Bile duct epithelium. Expect alkaline phosphatase to be elevated in bile duct obstruction

What is in bile?
Cholesterol, lecithin (phospholipid), bile acids, and bilirubin

What does bile do?
Emulsify fats

What is the enterohepatic circulation?
Circulation of bile acids from liver to gut and back to the liver

Where are most of the bile acids absorbed?
In the terminal ileum

What stimulates gallbladder emptying?
Cholecystokinin and vagal input

What is the source of cholecystokinin?
Duodenal mucosal cells

What stimulates the release of cholecystokinin?
Fat, protein, amino acids, and HCl

What inhibits its release?
Trypsin and chymotrypsin

What are its actions?
Gallbladder emptying
Opening of ampulla of Vater
Slowing of gastric emptying
Pancreas acinar cell growth and release of exocrine products

PATHOPHYSIOLOGY

At what level of serum total bilirubin does one start to get jaundiced?
Greater than 2.5

Classically, what is thought to be the anatomic location where one first finds evidence of jaundice?
Under the tongue

With good renal function, how high can the serum total bilirubin go?
Very rarely, over 20

What are the signs and symptoms of obstructive jaundice?
Jaundice
Dark urine
Clay-colored stools (acholic stools)
Pruritus (itching)
Loss of appetite
Nausea

What causes the itching in obstructive jaundice?
Bile salts in the dermis (not bilirubin!)

Define the following conditions:

Cholelithiasis — Gallstones in gallbladder

Choledocholithiasis — Gallstone in common bile duct

Cholecystitis — Inflammation of gallbladder

Cholangitis — Infection of biliary tract

Cholangiocarcinoma — Adenocarcinoma of bile ducts

Klatskin's tumor — Cholangiocarcinoma of bile duct at the **junction** of the right and left hepatic ducts

Biliary colic — Pain due to gallstones, usually from a stone at cystic duct. The pain is located in the right upper quadrant, epigastrium, or right subscapular region of the back. It usually lasts minutes to hours but eventually goes away. It is often postprandial, especially after fatty foods

DIAGNOSTIC STUDIES

Define the following diagnostic studies:

ERCP — **E**ndoscopic **R**etrograde **C**holangio**P**ancreatography

PTC — **P**ercutaneous **T**ranshepatic **C**holangiogram

IOC — **I**ntra**O**perative **C**holangiogram (done laparoscopically or open to rule out choledocholithiasis)

Name the types of biliary tract radiographic evaluations.

- Abdominal films (about 10%–15% of all stones and 50% of pigmented stones are radiopaque)
- Ultrasound (may show stones, sludge, thickened walls, fluid)
- Endoscopic retrograde cholangiopancreatography (ERCP)
- Percutaneous transhepatic cholangiography (PTC)
- HIDA/PRIDA scan (radioisotope evaluation can show cystic duct obstruction)

What is the initial diagnostic study of choice for evaluation of the biliary tract/cholelithiasis?	Ultrasound!

BILIARY SURGERY

What is a cholecystectomy?	Removal of the gallbladder done laparoscopically or through standard Kocher incision
What is the Kocher incision?	Right subcostal incision
What is a sphincterotomy?	Cut through sphincter of Oddi to allow passage of gallstones from the common bile duct; most often done at ERCP; also known as papillotomy

OBSTRUCTIVE JAUNDICE

What is it?	Jaundice (hyperbilirubinemia greater than 2.5) due to obstruction of bile flow to the duodenum
What is the differential diagnosis of proximal bile duct obstruction?	Cholangiocarcinoma Lymphadenopathy Metastatic tumor Gallbladder carcinoma Sclerosing cholangitis Gallstones Tumor embolus Parasites Postsurgical stricture Hepatoma Benign bile duct tumor
What is the differential diagnosis of distal bile duct obstruction?	Choledocholithiasis **(gallstones)** Pancreatic carcinoma Pancreatitis Ampullary carcinoma Lymphadenopathy Pseudocyst Postsurgical stricture Ampulla of Vater dysfunction Lymphoma Benign bile duct tumor Parasites

What is the initial study of choice for obstructive jaundice?
Ultrasound

What lab results are associated with obstructive jaundice?
Elevated alkaline phosphatase, elevated bilirubin with or without elevated LFTs

CHOLELITHIASIS

What is it?
The formation of gallstones

What is the incidence?
About 10% of U.S. population will develop gallstones

What are the risk factors?
The "four Fs": **female**, **fat**, **forty**, **fertile** (multiparity); also:
Oral contraceptives
Bile stasis
Chronic hemolysis (pigment stones)
Cirrhosis
Infection
Native American heritage
Rapid weight loss
Obesity
Inflammatory bowel disease (IBD)
Ileal resection
Total parenteral nutrition (TPN)
Vagotomy
Advanced age
Hyperlipidemia
Somatostatin therapy

What are the types of stones?
Cholesterol stones (75% of all stones) and pigment stones (25% of all stones)

What are the types of pigmented stones?
Black stones (contain calcium bilirubinate) and brown stones (associated with biliary tract infection)

What are the causes of black-pigmented stones?
Cirrhosis, hemolysis

What is the pathogenesis of cholesterol stones?
Secretion of bile **supersaturated** with cholesterol (relatively decreased amounts of lecithin and bile salts); then, cholesterol precipitates out and forms solid crystals, then gallstones

Is hypercholesterolemia a risk factor for gallstone formation?	No (but hyperlipidemia is)
What are the signs and symptoms?	Signs and symptoms of biliary colic: right upper quadrant pain, usually postprandially (i.e., after eating a fatty meal) Referred right subscapular pain Epigastric pain Nausea Vomiting (Signs and symptoms usually last for hours; therefore, colic is a misnomer!)
What percentage of patients with gallstones are asymptomatic?	Eighty percent of patients with cholelithiasis are asymptomatic!
What is thought to cause biliary colic?	Gallbladder contraction against a stone temporarily at the gallbladder/cystic duct junction; a stone in the cystic duct; or a stone passing through the cystic duct
What is Boas's sign?	The referred right subscapular pain of biliary colic
What are the complications of gallstones?	Acute cholecystitis Choledocholithiasis Gallstone pancreatitis Gallstone ileus
How is cholelithiasis diagnosed?	History Physical examination **Ultrasound** Laboratory tests
How often does ultrasound detect cholelithiasis?	More than 98% of the time!
How often does ultrasound detect choledocholithiasis?	About 33% of the time . . . not a very good study for choledocholithiasis!
How are symptomatic or complicated cases of cholelithiasis treated?	By cholecystectomy (most by laparoscopic cholecystectomy – "lap chole")

What are the possible complications of a "lap chole"?

Common bile duct injury
Right hepatic duct/artery injury
Cystic duct leak
Biloma (collection of bile)

What are the indications for cholecystectomy in the asymptomatic patient?

Sickle cell disease
Calcified gallbladder (porcelain gallbladder)
The patient is a child
+/- Large gallstone (larger than 2–3 cm)

Define IOC.

Intra**O**perative **C**holangiogram (dye in bile duct by way of the cystic duct with fluoro/x-ray)

When are the indications for an IOC?

Should be performed if there is any evidence of choledocholithiasis:

1. Jaundice
2. Hyperbilirubinemia
3. Gallstone pancreatitis
4. Elevated alkaline phosphatase
5. Choledocholithiasis on ultrasound
6. To define anatomy

What is choledocholithiasis?

Gallstones in the bile ducts

What is the management of choledocholithiasis?

Operative stone removal by common bile duct exploration by means of open or laparoscopic methods (if open exploration, leave T-tube in common bile duct); or ERCP with basket retrieval and papillotomy (cut sphincter of Oddi)

What medication may dissolve a cholesterol gallstone?

Chenodeoxycholic acid, ursodeoxycholic acid (Actigall®)

ACUTE CHOLECYSTITIS

What is the pathogenesis of acute cholecystitis?

Obstruction of cystic duct leads to inflammation of the gallbladder; about 95% of cases are due to calculi, and about 5% to acalculus obstruction

What are the risk factors?

Gallstones

What are the signs and symptoms?	**Unrelenting** right upper quadrant pain or tenderness Fever Nausea/vomiting **Painful** palpable gallbladder in 33% Positive Murphy's sign Right subscapular pain (referred) Epigastric discomfort (referred)
What is Murphy's sign?	Acute pain and inspiratory arrest elicited by palpation of the right upper quadrant during inspiration
What are the complications of acute cholecystitis?	Abscess Perforation Choledocholithiasis Cholecystenteric fistula formation Gallstone ileus
What lab results are associated with acute cholecystitis?	Increased WBC ± slight elevation in alkaline phosphatase, LFTs ± slight elevation in amylase, T. Bili
What is the diagnostic test of choice for acute cholecystitis?	Ultrasound
What are the signs of acute cholecystitis on ultrasound?	Thickened gallbladder wall (thicker than 3 mm) Pericholecystic fluid Distended gallbladder Gallstones present/cystic duct stone Sonographic Murphy's sign (pain on placement of ultrasound probe over gallbladder)
What is the treatment of acute cholelithiasis?	IVFs; antibiotics, with or without NG tube decompression; and **cholecystectomy, open or laparoscopically, early**

ACUTE ACALCULUS CHOLECYSTITIS

What is it?	Acute cholecystitis without evidence of stones

What is the pathogenesis? It is believed to be due to sludge and gallbladder disuse and **biliary stasis,** perhaps secondary to absence of cholecystokinin stimulation (decreased contraction of gallbladder).

What are the risk factors?
Prolonged fasting
TPN
Trauma
Multiple transfusions
Dehydration
Often occurs in prolonged postop or ICU setting

What is the diagnostic test of choice? **Ultrasound.** Sludge and inflammation will be present with acute acalculus cholecystitis

What is the management of acute acalculus cholecystitis? Cholecystectomy, or cholecystostomy tube if the patient is unstable (placed percutaneously by radiology or open surgery)

CHOLANGITIS

What is it? Bacterial infection of the biliary tract due to obstruction (either partial or complete); potentially life-threatening

What are the common causes of obstruction?
Choledocholithiasis
Stricture (usually postop)
Neoplasm (usually ampullary carcinoma)
Extrinsic compression (pancreatic pseudocyst/pancreatitis)
Instrumentation of the bile ducts (e.g., PTC/ERCP)
Biliary stent

What is the most common cause of cholangitis? Gallstones in common bile duct (choledocholithiasis)

What are the signs and symptoms?
Charcot's triad: fever/chills, right upper quadrant pain, and jaundice
Reynold's pentad: Charcot's triad plus altered mental status and shock

What lab results are associated with cholangitis?

Increased WBC, bilirubin, and alkaline phosphatase; ± blood cultures

Which organisms are most commonly isolated with cholangitis?

Gram-negative organisms (*E. coli, Klebsiella, Pseudomonas, Enterobacter, Proteus, Serratia*) are the most common.
Enterococci are the most common gram-positive bacteria.
Less commonly, anaerobes (*B. fragilis* most frequently)
Even less commonly, fungus (*Candida*)

What are the diagnostic tests of choice?

Ultrasound followed by a contrast study (i.e., PTC or ERCP) after patient has "cooled off" with IV antibiotics

What is suppurative cholangitis?

Severe infection with sepsis—"pus under pressure"

What is the management of cholangitis?

Nonsuppurative: IVF and antibiotics, with definitive treatment later
Suppurative: IVF, antibiotics, and decompression; decompression can be obtained by ERCP with papillotomy, PTC with catheter drainage, or laparotomy with T-tube placement if refractory to ERCP/PTC

SCLEROSING CHOLANGITIS

What is it?

Multiple inflammatory fibrous thickenings of bile duct walls resulting in biliary strictures

What is its natural history?

Progressive obstruction possibly leading to cirrhosis and liver failure; 10% of patients will develop cholangiocarcinoma

What is the etiology?

Unknown, but probably autoimmune

What are the risk factors?

Inflammatory bowel disease (about 60%); pancreatitis (20%); diabetes (10%)

What are the signs and symptoms of sclerosing cholangitis?

The same as the signs of obstructive jaundice:
Jaundice
Itching (pruritus)
Dark urine
Clay-colored stools
Loss of energy
Weight loss
(Many patients are asymptomatic.)

What are the complications?

Cirrhosis
Cholangiocarcinoma (10%)
Cholangitis
Obstructive jaundice

How is it diagnosed?

Elevated alkaline phosphatase, and PTC or ERCP revealing "beads on a string" appearance on contrast study

What are the management options?

Hepatoenteric anastomosis (if primarily extrahepatic ducts are involved) and removal of extrahepatic bile ducts because of the risk of cholangiocarcinoma
Transplant (if primarily intrahepatic disease or cirrhosis)
Endoscopic balloon dilations

What percentage of patients with IBD develop sclerosing cholangitis?

Less than 5%

GALLSTONE ILEUS

What is it?

Small bowel obstruction due to a large gallstone (larger than 2.5 cm) that has eroded through the gallbladder and into the duodenum/small bowel (i.e., a gallstone creates a cholecystenteric fistula and lodges in the ileocecal valve, causing obstruction). A large gallstone may also gain access to the GI tract after an endoscopic sphincterotomy (papillotomy transection of the sphincter of Oddi)

What is the classic site of obstruction?	The ileocecal valve (but may cause obstruction in the duodenum, sigmoid colon)
What is the population at risk?	Gallstone ileus is most commonly seen in **women over 70 years.**
What are the signs and symptoms?	Symptoms of small bowel obstruction: distention, vomiting, hypovolemia, right upper quadrant pain
What is the differential diagnosis?	Other causes of small bowel obstruction (A, B, C: adhesions, bulge/hernia, cancer)
Gallstone ileus causes what percentage of small bowel obstruction?	Less than 1%
What are the diagnostic tests of choice?	**Abdominal x-ray:** occasionally reveals radiopaque gallstone in the bowel; **40% of patients show air in the biliary tract,** small bowel distention, and air fluid levels secondary to ileus UGI: used if diagnosis is in question; will show cholecystenteric fistula and the obstruction **Abdominal CT:** reveals air in biliary tract, small bowel obstruction +/- gallstone in intestine
What is the management?	Surgery: enterotomy with removal of the stone ± cholecystectomy/closure of fistula.

CARCINOMA OF THE GALLBLADDER

What is it?	Malignant neoplasm arising in the gallbladder; very low incidence, vast majority are **adenocarcinoma (90%)**
What are the risk factors?	**Gallstones** (approximately 100% of cases, especially large gallstones), cholecystenteric fistula, **porcelain gallbladder** (approximately 50% will have gallbladder cancer)

What is the incidence?	**About 1% of all patients with cholelithiasis over a lifetime!**
What are the symptoms?	Biliary colic, weight loss, anorexia; many patients are asymptomatic until late; may present as acute cholecystitis
What are the signs?	Jaundice (from invasion of the common duct or compression by involved pericholedochal lymph nodes), right upper quadrant mass, palpable gallbladder (advanced disease)
What are the diagnostic tests of choice?	Ultrasound, abdominal CT, ERCP
What is the route of spread?	Contiguous spread to the liver is most common.
What is the management under the following conditions?	
Confined to mucosa	Cholecystectomy
Confined to muscularis/ serosa	Radical cholecystectomy: cholecystectomy and wedge resection of overlying liver, and lymph node dissection
What is the main complication of laparoscopic cholecystectomy for gallbladder cancer?	Trocar site tumor implants (so if known preoperatively, perform open cholecystectomy)

CHOLANGIOCARCINOMA

What is it?	Malignancy of the extrahepatic or intrahepatic ducts – **primary bile duct cancer**
What is the histology?	Almost all are adenocarcinomas
What is the average age of the patient?	About 65 years

What are the signs and symptoms?

The signs and symptoms of biliary obstruction: jaundice, **pruritus, dark urine, clay-colored stools**

What are the risk factors?

Choledochal cysts
Ulcerative colitis
Thorotrast contrast dye (used in 1950s)
Sclerosing cholangitis
Liver flukes (clonorchiasis)
Toxin exposures (e.g., agent orange?)

What is a Klatskin tumor?

Tumor that involves the junction of the right and left hepatic ducts

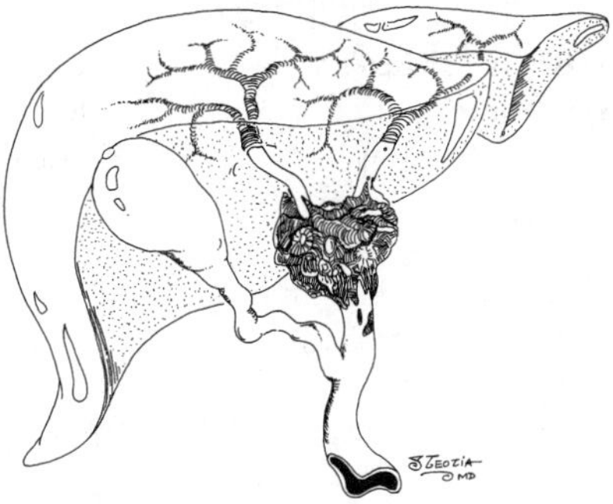

What are the diagnostic tests of choice?

Ultrasound, CT, ERCP/PTC with biopsy/brushings for cytology

What is the management of proximal bile duct cholangiocarcinoma?

Resection with Roux-en-Y hepaticojejunostomy (anastomose bile ducts to jejunum)

What is the management of distal common bile duct cholangiocarcinoma?

Whipple procedure

MISCELLANEOUS CONDITIONS

What is a porcelain gallbladder?

Calcified gallbladder seen on abdominal x-ray; due to chronic cholelithiasis/cholecystitis with calcified scar tissue in gallbladder wall; **cholecystectomy** required because of the strong association of **gallbladder carcinoma** with this condition

What is hydrops of the gallbladder?	Complete obstruction of the cystic duct by a gallstone, with filling of the gallbladder with fluid (not bile) from the gallbladder mucosa
What is Gilbert syndrome?	Inborn error in liver bilirubin uptake and glucuronyl transferase resulting in hyperbilirubinemia
What is Courvoisier's gallbladder?	A palpable, **nontender** gallbladder (unlike acute cholecystitis) associated with cancer of the head of the pancreas; able to distend because it has not been "scarred down" by gallstones
What is Mirizzi's syndrome?	Common hepatic duct obstruction due to extrinsic obstruction from a gallstone impacted in the cystic duct

48 Pancreas

Identify the regions of the pancreas.

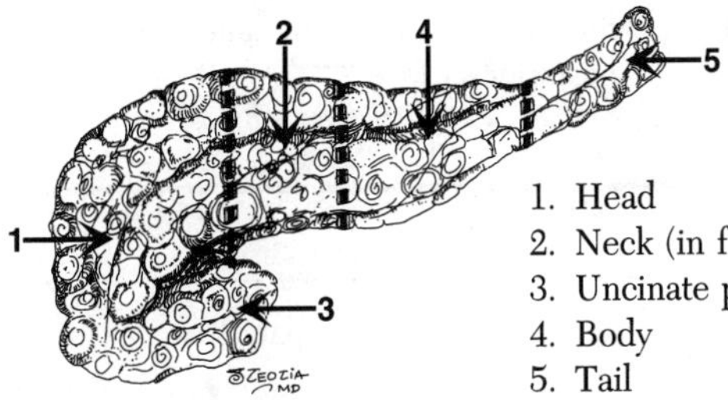

1. Head
2. Neck (in front of the SMV)
3. Uncinate process
4. Body
5. Tail

What structure is the tail of the pancreas said to "tickle"?

The spleen

Name the two pancreatic ducts.

1. Wirsung duct
2. Santorini duct

Which duct is the main duct?

Duct of Wirsung is the major duct (think: **S**antorini = **S**mall duct)

How is blood supplied to the head of the pancreas?

Celiac trunk → gastroduodenal →
- Anterior superior pancreaticoduodenal artery
- Posterior superior pancreaticoduodenal artery

Superior mesenteric artery →
- Anterior inferior pancreaticoduodenal artery
- Posterior inferior pancreaticoduodenal artery

Splenic artery →
- Dorsal pancreatic artery

Why must the duodenum be removed if the head of the pancreas is removed?

They share the same blood supply (gastroduodenal artery)

What is the endocrine function of the pancreas?

Islets of Langerhans
α-cells: glucagon
β-cells: insulin

What is the exocrine function of the pancreas?

Digestive enzymes: amylase, lipase, trypsin, chymotrypsin, carboxypeptidase

What maneuver is used to mobilize the duodenum and pancreas and evaluate the entire pancreas?

Kocher maneuver: incise the lateral attachments of the duodenum and then lift the pancreas to examine the posterior surface

PANCREATITIS

ACUTE PANCREATITIS

What is it?

Inflammation of the pancreas

What are the most common etiologies in the United States?

1. **Alcohol abuse (50%)**
2. **Gallstones (30%)**
3. Idiopathic (10%)

Other causes:
- Hypercalcemia
- Trauma
- Hyperlipidemia
- Iatrogenic (ERCP)
- Cardiopulmonary bypass (decreased blood flow)
- Familial
- Drugs (e.g., thiazide diuretics, steroids, valproic acid)

What are the symptoms?

Epigastric pain (frequently radiates to another quadrant or back); nausea and vomiting

What are the signs of pancreatitis?

Epigastric tenderness
Diffuse abdominal tenderness
Decreased bowel sounds (adynamic ileus)
± Fever
Dehydration/shock

What is the differential diagnosis?

Gastritis/PUD
Perforated viscus
Acute cholecystitis
Small bowel obstruction
Mesenteric ischemia/infarction
Ruptured AAA
Biliary colic
Inferior myocardial infarction/pneumonia

What is the differential diagnosis of increased amylase?

Pancreatitis, salivary tumor/inflammation
Liver disease
Renal failure
Small bowel obstruction
Ovarian tumor
Ectopic pregnancy
Macroamylasemia, pancreatic tumor/abscess/pseudocyst, pancreatic ascites, diabetic ketoacidosis, ruptured AAA, afferent loop syndrome, pneumonia, mesenteric ischemia, renal tx

What lab tests should be ordered?

CBC
LFT
Amylase/lipase
Type and cross
ABG
Ca^{2+}
Chem 10
Coags
Serum lipids

What are the associated diagnostic findings?

Lab—High amylase, high lipase, high WBC
Abdominal X-ray—Sentinel loop, colon cutoff, possibly gallstones (only 10% visible on X-ray)
U/S—Pseudocyst, phlegmon, abscess, cholelithiasis
CT—Pseudocyst, phlegmon, abscess, pancreatic necrosis

What is the most common sign of pancreatitis on AXR?

Sentinel loop(s)

What is the treatment?

NPO
NG tube
IVF
TPN
H_2 blocker
Analgesia (Demerol, not morphine—less sphincter of Oddi spasm)
Correction of coags/electrolytes
"Tincture of time"

What are the possible complications?

Pseudocyst
Abscess/infection

Pancreatic necrosis
Splenic/mesenteric/portal vessel rupture or thrombosis
Pancreatic ascites/pancreatic pleural effusion
Diabetes
ARDS/sepsis/MOF
Coagulopathy/DIC
Encephalopathy
Severe hypocalcemia

What is the prognosis?
Based on Ranson's criteria

What is Ranson's criteria for the following stages:

At presentation?
1. Age > 55
2. WBC > 16,000
3. Glc > 200
4. AST > 250
5. LDH > 350

During the initial 48 hours?
1. Base deficit > 4
2. BUN increase > 5 mg/dl
3. Fluid sequestration > 6 L
4. Serum Ca^{2+} < 8
5. Hct decrease > 10%
6. Po_2 (ABG) < 60 mm Hg

Amylase value is NOT one of Ranson's criteria!

What is the mortality per positive criteria:

0 to 2?
Less than 5%

3 to 4?
Approximately 15%

5 to 6?
Approximately 40%

7 to 8?
Approximately 100%

How can the admission Ranson criteria be remembered?
GA LAW ("Georgia law")
G—Glucose
A—Age > 55

L—LDH > 350
A—AST > 250
W—WBC > 16,000
"Don't mess with the pancreas and don't mess with the Georgia law."

How can Ranson's criteria at less than 48 hours be remembered?	**C HOBBS** ("Calvin and Hobbs") **C**—Calcium < 8 mg/dl **H**—Hct drop of > 10% **O**—O_2 < 60 (Pao_2) **B**—Base deficit > 4 **B**—Bun > 5 increase **S**—Sequestration > 6 L
How can the AST versus LDH values in Ranson's criteria be remembered?	Alphabetically: A before L and 250 before 350 Therefore, AST > 250 and LDH > 350
What is the etiology of hypocalcemia with pancreatitis?	Fat saponification; fat necrosis binds to calcium
What complication is associated with splenic vein thrombosis?	Gastric varices
Can TPN with lipids be given to a patient with pancreatitis?	Yes, if the patient does not suffer from hyperlipidemia
What is the least common cause of acute pancreatitis (and possibly the most commonly asked cause on rounds!)	Scorpion bite (not the US type; found on Pacific islands)

GALLSTONE PANCREATITIS

What is it?	Acute pancreatitis due to a gallstone in or passing through the ampulla of Vater (the exact mechanism is unknown)
How is the diagnosis made?	Acute pancreatitis and cholelithiasis and/ or choledocholithiasis and no other cause of pancreatitis (e.g., no history of alcohol abuse)
What radiologic tests should be performed?	U/S to look for gallstones CT to look at the pancreas, if symptoms are severe

What is the treatment?
Conservative measures and early interval cholecystectomy (laparoscopic cholecystectomy or open cholecystectomy) and intraoperatic cholangiogram (IOC) 3 to 5 days (after pancreatic inflammation resolves)

Why should early interval cholecystectomy be performed on patients with gallstone pancreatitis?
Pancreatitis will recur in approximately 33% of patients within 8 weeks (so always perform early interval cholecystectomy and IOC in 3–5 days)

HEMORRHAGIC PANCREATITIS

What is it?
Bleeding into the parenchyma and retroperitoneal structures with extensive pancreatic necrosis

What are the signs?
Abdominal pain, shock/ARDS, Cullen's sign, Grey Turner's sign, Fox's sign

Define the following terms:

Cullen's sign
Bluish discoloration of the periumbilical area due to retroperitoneal hemorrhage tracking around to the anterior abdominal wall through fascial planes

Grey Turner's sign
Ecchymosis or discoloration of the flank in patients with retroperitoneal hemorrhage due to dissecting blood from the retroperitoneum (think: Grey Turner = turn side to side = flank [side] hematoma)

Fox's sign
Ecchymosis of the inguinal ligament due to blood tracking from the retroperitoneum and collecting at the inguinal ligament

What are the significant lab values?
Increased amylase/lipase
Decreased Hct
Decreased calcium levels

What radiologic test should be performed?
CT scan with IV contrast

PANCREATIC ABSCESS

What is it?	Infected peripancreatic purulent fluid collection
What are the signs/ symptoms?	Fever, unresolving pancreatitis, epigastric mass
What radiographic tests should be performed?	Abdominal CT with needle aspiration→send for Gram stain/culture
What are the associated lab findings?	Positive Gram stain and culture of bacteria
Which organisms are found in pancreatic abscesses?	Gram negative (most common): *E. coli, Pseudomonas, Klebsiella* Gram positive: *Staphylococcus aureus* *Candida*
What is the treatment?	Antibiotics and percutaneous drain placement, or operative debridement and placement of drains

PANCREATIC NECROSIS

What is it?	Dead pancreatic tissue, usually following acute pancreatitis
How is the diagnosis made?	Abdominal CT with IV contrast; dead pancreatic tissue does not take up IV contrast and is not enhanced on CT scan
What is the treatment?	Surgical debridement and drain placement IF there is infected necrosis or patient is severely ill and refractory to medical management

CHRONIC PANCREATITIS

What is it?	Chronic inflammation of the pancreas; causes destruction of the parenchyma, fibrosis, and calcification, resulting in loss of endocrine and exocrine tissue
What are the subtypes?	1. Chronic calcific pancreatitis 2. Chronic obstructive pancreatitis (5%)

What are the causes?

Alcohol abuse (most common; 70% of cases)
Idiopathic (15%)
Hypercalcemia (hyperparathyroidism)
Hyperlipidemia
Familial (found in families without any other risk factors)
Trauma
Iatrogenic
Gallstones

What are the symptoms?

Epigastric and/or back pain, weight loss, steatorrhea

What are the signs of pancreatic exocrine insufficiency?

Steatorrhea (fat malabsorption due to lipase insufficiency—stools float in water)

What are the signs of pancreatic endocrine insufficiency?

Diabetes (glucose intolerance)

What are the common pain patterns?

Unrelenting pain
Recurrent pain

What are the associated signs?

IDDM (up to one-third)
Steatorrhea (up to one-fourth)

What is the differential diagnosis?

PUD, biliary tract disease, AAA, pancreatic cancer, angina

What percentage of patients with chronic pancreatitis have or will develop pancreatic cancer?

Approximately 2%

Lab tests?

Amylase/lipase
72-hour fecal fat analysis
Glc tolerance test (IDDM)

Why may amylase/lipase be normal in a patient with chronic pancreatitis?

Because of extensive pancreatic tissue loss ("burned-out pancreas")

What radiographic tests should be performed?

CT—Has greatest sensitivity for gland enlargement/atrophy, calcifications, masses, pseudocysts
KUB—Calcification in the pancreas
ERCP—Ductal irregularities with dilation and stenosis (Chain of Lakes), pseudocysts

What is the medical treatment?

Discontinuation of alcohol use—can stop attacks, though parenchymal damage continues secondary to ductal obstruction and fibrosis
Insulin for IDDM
Pancreatic enzyme replacement
Narcotics for pain (watch for addiction)

What is the surgical treatment?

Peustow—longitudinal pancreaticojejunostomy (pancreatic duct **must be dilated**)
DuVal—distal pancreaticojejunostomy
Near-total pancreatectomy

What is the indication for surgical treatment of chronic pancreatitis?

Severe, prolonged/refractory pain

What are the possible complications of chronic pancreatitis?

IDDM (glucose intolerance)
Steatorrhea
Malnutrition
Biliary obstruction
Splenic vein thrombosis
Gastric varices
Pancreatic pseudocyst/abscess
Narcotic addiction
Pancreatic ascites/pleural effusion
Splenic artery aneurysm

PANCREATIC ASCITES/PLEURAL EFFUSION

What is it?

Fluid collections (chest = pleural effusion and peritoneal cavity = ascites) from fluid draining from a pancreatic duct disruption

What are the associated risk factors?

Occurs with acute or chronic pancreatitis, trauma, pancreatic surgery

What diagnostic tests should be performed?

Paracentesis/thoracentesis
Amylase—level of fluid
ERCP—to locate disrupted duct, if fluid continues to accumulate

What is the initial treatment?

Nonoperative; peritoneal drains (for ascites), chest tube (for pleural effusion), supportive NPO/TPN/octreotide

What is the surgical treatment?

If unresolved after medical treatment, distal pancreatectomy (body/tail fistula), or Roux-en-Y pancreaticojejunostomy

PANCREATIC PSEUDOCYST

What is it?

Encapsulated collection of pancreatic fluid ("pseudo" = wall formed by inflammatory fibrosis, NOT epithelial cell lining)

What is the incidence?

Approximately 1 in 10 after alcoholic pancreatitis

What are the associated risk factors?

Acute pancreatitis < chronic pancreatitis due to alcohol

What is the most common cause of pancreatic pseudocyst in the United States?

Chronic alcoholic pancreatitis

What are the symptoms?

Epigastric pain
Emesis
Mild fever
Weight loss
Should be suspected when a patient with acute pancreatitis fails to resolve pain

What are the signs?

Palpable epigastric mass; tender epigastrium, ileus

What lab tests should be performed?

Amylase/lipase
Bilirubin
CBC

What are the diagnostic findings?	Lab—High amylase, leukocytosis, high bilirubin (if there is obstruction) U/S—Fluid-filled mass CT—Fluid-filled mass, good for showing multiple cysts ERCP—Radiopaque contrast material fills cyst if there is a communicating pseudocyst (i.e., pancreatic duct communicates with pseudocyst)
What is the differential diagnosis of a pseudocyst?	Cystadenocarcinoma, cystadenoma
What are the possible complications of a pancreatic pseudocyst?	Infection, bleeding into the cyst, fistula, pancreatic ascites, gastric outlet obstruction
What is the treatment?	Drainage of the cyst or observation
What is the waiting period before a pseudocyst should be drained?	It takes 6 weeks for pseudocyst walls to "mature" or become firm enough to hold sutures and most will resolve in this period of time if they are going to.
What percentage of pseudocysts resolve spontaneously?	Approximately 50%
What size pseudocyst should be drained?	Controversial, but most experts say those larger than 5 cm as: Pseudocysts larger than 5 cm have a small chance of resolving and have a higher chance of complications (e.g., bleeding, infection). Many experts advocate close follow-up only for pancreatic pseudocysts less than 5 cm.
What are the treatment options for pancreatic pseudocyst?	Percutaneous/aspiration/drain Operative drainage
What are the surgical options for the following conditions:	
Pseudocyst adherent to the stomach?	Cystogastrostomy (drain into the stomach)

Pseudocyst adherent to the duodenum?	Cystoduodenostomy (drain into the duodenum)
Pseudocyst not adherent to the stomach or duodenum?	Roux-en-Y cystojejunostomy (drain into the Roux limb of the jejunum)
Pseudocyst in the tail of the pancreas?	Resection of the pancreatic tail with the pseudocyst
What is the other endoscopic option for drainage of a pseudocyst?	Controversial and evolving: **endoscopic** cystogastrostomy
What must be done during a surgical drainage procedure for a pancreatic pseudocyst?	**Biopsy** of the cyst wall to rule out a cystic carcinoma (e.g., cystadenocarcinoma)
What is the most common cause of death due to pancreatic pseudocyst?	Massive hemorrhage into the pseudocyst

PANCREATIC CARCINOMA

What is it?	Adenocarcinoma of the pancreas arising from duct cells
What are the associated risk factors?	**Smoking,** diabetes mellitus, heavy alcohol use, exposure to the chemicals benzidine and β-naphthylamine may be associated
What is the male : female ratio?	3 : 2
What is the African-American : white ratio?	2 : 1
What is the average age?	Greater than 60 years
What are the different types?	Over 90% are duct cell adenocarcinomas; other types include cystadenocarcinoma and acinar cell carcinoma

What percentage arise in the pancreatic head?
Two-thirds arise in the **head** of the pancreas; **one-third** arise in the **body and tail**

What are the signs/ symptoms of tumors based on location:

Head of the pancreas?
Painless jaundice (80%) due to obstruction of the common bile duct, weight loss, and abdominal pain; weakness, **pruritus** due to bile salts in the skin, anorexia, palpable, nontender distended gallbladder **(Courvoisier's sign)**, acholic stools (clay-colored), and dark urine

Body or tail?
Weight loss and pain (90%); migratory thrombophlebitis (10%); jaundice (< 10%); nausea and vomiting; fatigue

What is the classic presentation of pancreatic cancer in the head of the pancreas?
Painless jaundice

What are the associated lab findings?
Increased direct bilirubin and alkaline phosphatase (as a result of biliary obstruction)
± increased LFTs
Elevated pancreatic tumor markers

Which tumor markers are associated with pancreatic cancer?
CEA and CA 19-9

Diagnostic studies?
Abdominal CT, U/S, cholangiography (PTC or ERCP with possible biopsy/ brushings), selective angiography (for staging and defining arterial and venous involvement and anatomy)

What is the treatment based on location:

Head of the pancreas?
Whipple procedure (pancreaticoduodenectomy)

Body or tail?
Distal resection

What factors signify inoperability?

Vascular encasement (portal vein, SMV, SMA)
Liver metastasis
Peritoneal implants
Distant lymph node metastasis (periaortic/celiac nodes)

Define the Whipple procedure (pancreaticoduodenectomy).

Cholecystectomy
± Truncal vagotomy
± Antrectomy
Pancreaticoduodenectomy—removal of the head of the pancreas and duodenum
Choledochojejunostomy—anastomosis of the common bile duct to the jejunum
Pancreaticojejunostomy—anastomosis of the distal pancreas remnant to the jejunum
Gastrojejunostomy—anastomosis of the stomach to the jejunum

What is the complication rate after a Whipple procedure?

Approximately 25%

What mortality rate is associated with a Whipple procedure?

Approximately 5%

What is the "pylorus-preserving Whipple"?

No antrectomy; anastomose duodenum to jejunum

What are the possible post-Whipple complications?

Delayed gastric emptying (if antrectomy is performed); anastomotic leak (from the bile duct or pancreatic anastomosis); wound infection; pancreatic fistula; postgastrectomy syndromes

Why must the duodenum be removed if the head of the pancreas is resected?

They share the same blood supply

What is the postoperative adjuvant therapy?

Chemotherapy (5-FU) and x-ray therapy

What is the palliative treatment if the tumor is inoperable and biliary obstruction is present?

PTC or ERCP and placement of stent across obstruction

What is the prognosis?

Dismal; 90% of patients die within 1 year of diagnosis; overall survival rate is 5% to 15% at 5 years after resection/obstruction

MISCELLANEOUS

What is an annular pancreas?

Pancreas encircling the duodenum; if obstruction is present, bypass, **do not resect**

What is pancreatic divisum?

Failure of the two pancreatic ducts to fuse; the normally small duct (**s**mall = **S**antorini) of Santorini acts as the main duct in pancreatic divisum (think: the two pancreatic ducts are **D**ivided = **D**ivisum)

What is heterotopic pancreatic tissue?

Heterotopic pancreatic tissue usually found in the stomach, intestine, duodenum

What is a Puestow procedure?

Longitudinal filleting of the pancreas with a side-to-side anastomosis with the small bowel

What medication decreases output from a pancreatic fistula?

Somatostatin (GI-inhibitory hormone)

Which has a longer half life: amylase or lipase?

Lipase; therefore, amylase may be normal and lipase will remain elevated longer

What is the WDHA syndrome?

A pancreatic **VIP**oma (**V**asoactive **I**ntestinal **P**olypeptide tumor)

Also known as Verner-Morrison syndrome

Tumor secretes VIP, which causes:

- **W: Water**
- **D: Diarrhea**
- **H: Hypokalemia**
- **A: Achlorhydria** (no gastric acid secretion, or decreased secretion)

What is the Whipple triad of pancreatic insulinoma?

1. Hypoglycemia (Glc < 50)
2. Symptoms of hypoglycemia: mental status changes/vasomotor instability
3. Relief of symptoms with administration of glucose

What is the most common islet cell tumor?

Insulinoma

What pancreatic tumor is associated with gallstone formation?

Somatostatinoma (inhibits gallbladder contraction)

What is the triad found with pancreatic somatostatinoma tumor?

1. Gallstones
2. Diabetes
3. Steatorrhea

What are the two classic findings with pancreatic glucagonoma tumors?

1. Diabetes
2. Dermatitis/rash (necrotizing migratory erythema)

What is Zollinger-Ellison syndrome?

Pancreatic gastrinoma and peptic ulcer disease due to gastrin-induced excessive gastric acid production

49 The Breast

ANATOMY OF THE BREAST AND AXILLA

Name the boundaries of the axilla for dissection:

Superior boundary
Axillary vein

Posterior boundary
Long thoracic nerve

Lateral boundary
Latissimus dorsi muscle

Medial boundary
Lateral to, deep to, or medial to pectoral minor muscle, depending on level of nodes taken.

What four nerves must the surgeon be aware of during an axillary dissection?

1. **Long thoracic nerve**
2. **Thoracodorsal nerve**
3. Medial pectoral nerve
4. Lateral pectoral nerve

Describe the location of these nerves and the muscle each innervates.

Long thoracic nerve
Courses along lateral chest wall in midaxillary line on serratus anterior muscle; innervates serratus anterior muscle

Thoracodorsal nerve
Courses lateral to long thoracic nerve on latissimus dorsi muscle; innervates latissimus dorsi muscle

Medial pectoral nerve
Runs **lateral** to or through the pectoral minor muscle, actually lateral to the lateral pectoral nerve; innervates the pectoral minor and pectoral major muscles; also known as the medial thoracic nerve

Lateral pectoral nerve — Runs **medial** to the lateral pectoral nerve through the pectoral minor muscle (names describe orientation from the brachial plexus!); innervates the pectoral major; also known as the lateral thoracic nerve

Identify the nerves in the axilla on the illustration below.

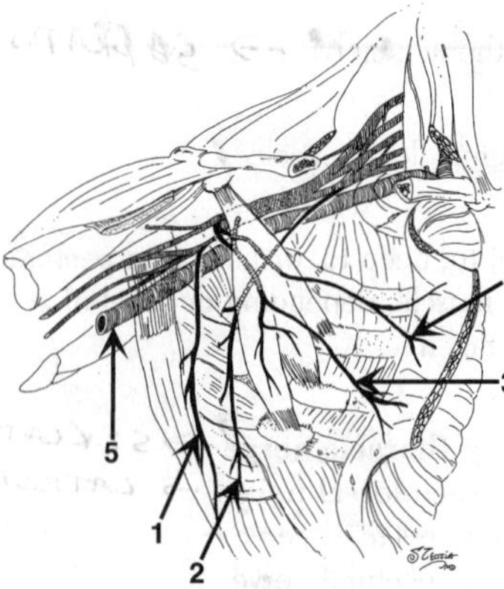

1. Thoracodorsal nerve
2. Long thoracic nerve
3. Medial pectoral nerve
4. Lateral pectoral nerve
5. Axillary vein

What is the deformity if you cut the long thoracic nerve in this area? — "Winged scapula"

What is the name of the CUTANEOUS nerve that crosses the axilla in a transverse fashion? (Many surgeons try to preserve this nerve.) — Intercostobrachial nerve

What is the name of the large vein that marks the upper limit of the axilla? — Axillary vein

What arteries supply blood to the breast? — Internal mammary artery (via perforators)
Intercostal arteries
Axillary artery (via the lateral thoracic and thoracoacromial arteries)

What veins drain blood from the breast?

Axillary vein (main route of drainage)
Internal mammary vein
Intercostal veins

What is the lymphatic drainage of the breast?

Lateral: axillary lymph nodes
Medial: parasternal nodes that run with internal mammary artery

What are the levels of axillary lymph nodes?

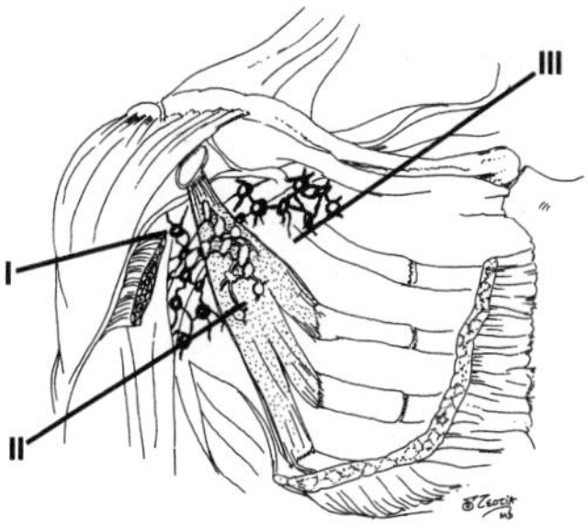

Level I (low): lateral to pectoral minor
Level II (middle): deep to pectoral minor
Level III (high): medial to pectoral minor
In breast cancer, a higher level of involvement has a worse prognosis, but the level of involvement is not as important as the number of positive nodes. (**think:** Levels I, II, III are in the same superior–inferior anatomic order as the LeFort facial fractures and the trauma neck zones; *I dare you to forget!*)

What are Rotter's nodes?

Nodes between the pectoralis major and the pectoralis minor muscles; not usually removed unless there is clinical evidence of metastasis

What are the suspensory breast ligaments called?

Cooper's ligaments

What is the mammary "milk line"?

The embryological line from shoulder to thigh where "supernumerary" breast nipples can be found

What is the "tail of Spence"?

The "tail" of breast tissue that tapers into the axilla

Which hormone is mainly responsible for breast milk production?

Prolactin

BREAST CANCER

What is the incidence of breast cancer?

One in ten American women will develop breast cancer.

What percentage of all breast cancers occur in women younger than 30 years?

Approximately 2%

What percentage of all breast cancers occur in women older than 70 years?

33%

What is the most common motivation for medicolegal cases involving the breast?

Failure to diagnose a breast carcinoma

What are the risk factors for breast cancer?

Age (risk increases with age)
Family history (especially first degree and especially if premenopausal)
Nulliparity or late first pregnancy
Cancer in ipsilateral/contralateral breast
Early menarche, late menopause (To remember **early** menarche and **late** menopause: Consider that the woman with early menarche and late menopause will have more menstrual cycles, and thus the breast will have to go through a greater number of cyclic changes.)
DCIS
LCIS
Hyperplasia
Atypia
Previous negative breast biopsy
Radiation exposure

Is "run of the mill" fibrocystic disease a risk factor for breast cancer?

No

What are the possible symptoms of breast cancer?

No symptoms
Mass in the breast
Pain (**most are painless**)
Nipple discharge
Local edema
Nipple retraction
Dimple
Nipple rash

Why does skin retraction occur?

Tumor involvement of Cooper's ligaments and subsequent traction on ligaments, causing skin to be pulled inward

What are the signs of breast cancer?

Mass
- 1 cm is usually the smallest lesion that can be palpated on examination

Dimple
Nipple rash
Edema
Axillary/supraclavicular nodes

What is the most common site of breast cancer?

Approximately one-half of cancers develop in the upper outer quadrants

What are the major types of invasive carcinoma?

Invasive ductal carcinoma (90%)
Invasive lobular carcinoma (10%)
Inflammatory carcinoma

What is the most common type of breast cancer?

Infiltrating ductal carcinoma

What is the differential diagnosis?

Fibrocystic disease of the breast
Fibroadenoma
Intraductal papilloma
Duct ectasia
Fat necrosis
Abscess
Radial scar
Adenitis

Describe the appearance of the edema of the dermis in inflammatory carcinoma of the breast.

Peau d'orange (orange peel)

What are the screening recommendations for breast cancer?

Breast exam recommendations:
- Self-examination of breasts monthly
- Age 20 to 40: breast exam every 2 to 3 years by a physician
- Over 40 years: Annual breast exam by physician

Mammograms: Recommendations are controversial! . . . but most experts say:
- Baseline mammogram between 35 and 40 years
- Mammogram every year or every other year for ages 40 to 50
- Mammogram yearly after age 50

When is the best time for breast self exams?

One week after menstrual period

Why is mammography a more useful diagnostic tool in older women than in younger women?

Breast tissue undergoes fatty replacement with age, making masses more visible. Younger women have more fibrous tissue, which makes mammograms harder to interpret.

What are the radiographic tests for breast cancer?

Mammography and breast ultrasound

What is the test of choice to evaluate a breast mass in a woman younger than 30 years?

Breast ultrasound

What are the methods for obtaining tissue for pathologic examination?

Fine needle aspiration (FNA), core biopsy (larger needle core sample), and open biopsy. Open biopsy can be incisional (cutting a **piece** of the mass) or excisional (cutting out the **entire** mass).

What are the indications for biopsy?

- Persistent mass after aspiration
- Solid mass
- Blood in cyst aspirate
- Suspicious lesion by mammography
- Bloody nipple discharge
- Ulcer or dermatitis of nipple
- Patient's concern of persistent breast abnormality

What is the process for performing a biopsy when a nonpalpable mass is seen on mammogram?

Needle localization by radiologist, followed by biopsy. Removed breast tissue must be checked by mammogram to ensure all of suspicious lesion has been excised or mammogram-guided core biopsy.

What is obtained first, the mammogram or the biopsy?

The mammogram is obtained first; otherwise tissue extraction (core or open) may alter the mammographic findings. (Fine needle aspiration may be done prior to the mammogram because the fine needle will not affect the mammographic findings.)

What would be suspicious mammographic findings?

Mass, microcalcifications, stellate/spiculated mass

What is the "workup" for a breast mass?

1. Physical exam
2. Mammogram or breast ultrasound
3. Fine needle aspiration, core biopsy, or open biopsy

How do you proceed if the mass appears to be a cyst?

Aspirate it with a needle.

Is the fluid from a breast cyst sent for cytology?

Not routinely; bloody fluid should be sent for cytology

When do you proceed to open biopsy for a breast cyst?

1. In the case of a second cyst recurrence
2. Bloody fluid in the cyst
3. Palpable mass after aspiration

What is the preoperative staging workup in a patient with breast cancer?

Bilateral mammogram (Cancer in one breast is a risk factor for cancer in the contralateral breast!)
Chest x-ray (to check for lung metastasis)
LFTs (to check for liver metastasis)
Serum calcium level, alkaline phosphatase (If these tests indicate bone metastasis, proceed to bone scan.)
Other tests, depending on signs/symptoms (e.g., head CT if patient has focal neurologic deficit, to look for brain metastasis)

What hormone receptors must be checked for in the biopsy specimen?

Estrogen and progesterone receptors. This is **key for determining adjuvant treatment.** This information must be obtained on all specimens (including fine needle aspirates).

What staging system is used for breast cancer?

TMN: tumor/metastases/nodes (AJCC)

Describe the staging (simplified).

Stage I

Tumor ≤ 2 cm in diameter without metastases, **no nodes**

Stage IIA

Tumor ≤ 2 cm in diameter with mobile axillary nodes or
Tumor 2 to 5 cm in diameter, no nodes

Stage IIB

Tumor 2 to 5 cm in diameter with mobile axillary nodes or
Tumor larger than 5 cm **with no nodes**

Stage IIIA

Tumor larger than 5 cm with mobile axillary nodes or
Any size tumor with **fixed** axillary nodes, no metastases

Stage IIIB

Peau d'orange (skin edema) or
Chest wall invasion/fixation or
Inflammatory cancer or
Breast skin ulceration or
Breast skin satellite metastases or
Any tumor and + ipsilateral **internal mammary** lymph nodes

Stage IV

Distant Metastases (including ipsilateral supraclavicular nodes)

Sites of metastases?

Lymph nodes (most common)
Lung/pleura
Liver
Bones
Brain

What are the major treatments of breast cancer?

Modified radical mastectomy
Lumpectomy and radiation
(Both treatments either with or without postop chemotherapy/Tamoxifen)

What breast carcinomas are candidates for lumpectomy and radiation?

Stage I and stage II (tumors < 5 cm)

What is the treatment of inflammatory carcinoma of the breast?

Chemotherapy first! Then often followed by radiation and/or mastectomy

What is a lumpectomy and radiation?

Lumpectomy (segmental mastectomy: removal of a **part** of the breast); axillary node dissection; and course of radiation therapy **after** operation, over a period of several weeks

What is the major absolute contraindication to lumpectomy and radiation?

Pregnancy

What are other contraindications to lumpectomy and radiation?

Previous radiation to the chest
Positive margins
Collagen vascular disease
Extensive DCIS (often seen as diffuse microcalcification)
Relative contraindications:
Lesion that cannot be seen on the mammograms (i.e., early recurrence will be missed on follow-up mammograms)
Very small breast (no cosmetic advantage)

What is a modified radical mastectomy?

Removal of the breast, axillary nodes (level II, I), and nipple–areolar complex
Pectoralis major and minor muscles are **not** removed (Auchincloss modification).
Drains are placed to drain lymph fluid.

What are the potential complications after a modified radical mastectomy?

Ipsilateral arm lymphedema, infection, and injury to nerves

During an axillary dissection, should the patient be paralyzed?

NO, because the nerves (long thoracic/thoracodorsal) are stimulated with resultant muscle contraction to help identify them

How can the long thoracic and thoracodorsal nerves be identified during an axillary dissection?	The nerves can be stimulated with a forcep, which results in contraction of the latissimus dorsi (thoracodorsal nerve) or anterior serratus (long thoracic nerve)
When do you remove the drains after an axillary dissection?	When there is less than 30 to 40 cc of drainage per day
How does tamoxifen work?	It binds estrogen receptors.
Give the common adjuvant therapy for the following breast cancer patients. (These are rough guidelines; check for current guidelines, as they are always changing):	
Premenopausal, node +, ER –	Chemotherapy
Premenopausal, node +, ER+	Chemotherapy ± Tamoxifen
Premenopausal, tumor less than 1 cm, node –, ER +/–	Close follow-up only ± Tamoxifen
Postmenopausal, node +, ER +	Tamoxifen
Postmenopausal, node +, ER –	Chemotherapy
Postmenopausal, tumor less than 1 cm, node –	Close follow-up only ± Tamoxifen (**Note:** ER = estrogen receptor)

DCIS

What does DCIS stand for?	**D**uctal **C**arcinoma **I**n **S**itu
What is DCIS also known as?	Intraductal carcinoma
Describe DCIS.	Cancer cells in the duct without invasion (in situ: cells do not penetrate the basement membrane)

What are the signs and symptoms of DCIS?	Usually none; usually nonpalpable
What are the mammographic findings?	Microcalcifications
How is the diagnosis made?	Core or open biopsy
What is the most aggressive histologic type?	Comedo
What is the risk of lymph node metastasis with DCIS?	Less than 2% (usually when microinvasion is seen)
What is the major risk with DCIS?	Subsequent development of infiltrating ductal carcinoma in the same breast
What is the treatment for DCIS in the following cases:	
Tumor less than 5 mm	Remove with clear margins and close follow up
Tumor 5 mm to 2 cm	Lumpectomy with 1 cm margins and radiation
Tumor larger than 2 cm	Lumpectomy with 1-cm margins and radiation, **or** total (simple) mastectomy (**no** axillary dissection)
What is a simple mastectomy?	Removal of the breast and nipple without removal of the axillary nodes. (Always remove nodes with invasive cancer)
When must a simple mastectomy be performed for DCIS?	Diffuse breast involvement (e.g., diffuse microcalcifications)
What is the role of axillary node dissection with DCIS?	No role in true DCIS (i.e., without microinvasion)

LCIS

What is LCIS?

Lobular **C**arcinoma **I**n **S**itu (carcinoma cells in the lobules of the breast without invasion)

What are the signs and symptoms?

There are none.

What are the mammographic findings?

There are none.

How is the diagnosis made?

LCIS is found **incidentally** on biopsy.

What is the major risk with LCIS?

Carcinoma of **either** breast

Which breast is most at risk for developing an invasive carcinoma?

Equal risk in both breasts! (Think of LCIS as a **risk marker** for future development of cancer in either breast.)

What percentage of women with LCIS develop an invasive breast carcinoma?

About 30% in the 20 years after diagnosis of LCIS!

What type of invasive breast cancer do patients with LCIS develop?

Most commonly, **infiltrating ductal carcinoma, with equal distribution** in the contralateral and ipsilateral breasts (Note: counterintuitive!)

What is the treatment of LCIS?

None – close follow-up (or bilateral simple mastectomy in high-risk patients)

What is the major difference in the subsequent development of invasive breast cancer with DCIS and LCIS?

LCIS cancer develops in *either* breast; DCIS cancer develops in the ipsilateral breast.

What is the most common cause of a bloody nipple discharge in a young woman?

Intraductal papilloma

What is the most common breast tumor in patients younger than 30 years of age?

Fibroadenoma

What is Paget's disease of the breast?

Scaling rash/dermatitis of the nipple caused by invasion of skin by cells from a ductal carcinoma

What are the common options for breast reconstruction after a mastectomy?

Saline implant
Transverse **R**ectus **A**bdominis **M**yocutaneous (TRAM) flap: bring rectus muscle up and create a new breast

MALE BREAST CANCER

What is the incidence of breast cancer in men?

Less than 1% of all cases of breast cancer (1/150)

What is the average age at diagnosis?

65 years of age

What are the risk factors?

Increased estrogen
Radiation
Gynecomastia due to increased estrogen
Estrogen therapy
Klinefelter's syndrome (XXY)

What type of breast cancer do men develop?

Nearly 100% of cases are ductal carcinoma. (Men do not usually have breast lobules.)

What are the signs and symptoms of breast cancer in men?

Breast mass (most are painless), breast skin changes (ulcers, retraction), and nipple discharge (usually blood or a blood-tinged discharge)

How is breast cancer in men diagnosed?

Biopsy and mammogram

What is the treatment?

One of the more aggressive surgical approaches (radical mastectomy or modified radical mastectomy) is used because of early involvement of the pectoralis major and the skin. **Radical mastectomy:** removal of skin, nipple, **pectoral muscles,** and axillary nodes, +/– skin graft). **Modified radical**

mastectomy: removal of involved underlying pectoralis major muscle. Most patients then receive tamoxifen or chemotherapy, or both

BENIGN BREAST DISEASE

What is the most common cause of green, straw-colored, or brown nipple discharge?

Fibrocystic disease

What is the most common cause of a bloody nipple discharge in a young woman?

Intraductal papilloma

What is the most common cause of breast mass after breast trauma?

Fat necrosis

What is Mondor's disease?

Thrombophlebitis of superficial breast veins

CYSTOSARCOMA PHYLLODES

What is it?

Mesenchymal tumor arising from breast lobular tissue. Most are benign. "Sarcoma" is a misnomer, as the vast majority are benign.

What is the usual age of the patient with this tumor?

Older than 30 years. She is usually older than the patient with fibroadenoma.

What are the signs and symptoms?

Mobile, smooth breast mass that looks like a fibroadenoma on mammogram/ultrasound

How is it diagnosed?

Through biopsy or excision

What is the treatment?

If benign, wide local excision; if malignant, simple total mastectomy

What is the role of axillary dissection with cystosarcoma phyllodes tumor?

None, as the malignant form rarely spreads to nodes (most common site of metastasis is the lung)

FIBROADENOMA

What is it?	Benign tumor of the breast consisting of collagen arranged in "swirls"
What is the clinical presentation of a fibroadenoma?	Young women less than 30 years of age with a solid, mobile, **well-circumscribed** round breast mass
How is fibroadenoma diagnosed?	Negative needle aspiration looking for fluid; ultrasound; core biopsy
What is the treatment?	Surgical resection for large or growing lesions; small fibroadenomas can be observed closely
What is this disease's claim to fame?	It is the most common breast tumor in women younger than 30 years of age.

FIBROCYSTIC DISEASE

What is it?	A common benign breast condition consisting of fibrous (rubbery) and cystic changes in the breast
What are the signs and symptoms?	Pain or tenderness of the breast that varies with the menstrual cycle; cysts; and fibrous ("nodular") fullness
How is it diagnosed?	Through breast exam, history, and aspirated cysts (usually straw-colored or green fluid)
What is the treatment for symptomatic fibrocystic disease?	**Stop caffeine** Stop tobacco Pain medications (NSAIDs) Vitamin E, evening primrose oil, danazol, OCP
What is done if the patient has a breast cyst?	Needle drainage. If aspirate is bloody or a palpable mass remains after aspiration, an open biopsy is performed. If the aspirate is straw colored or green, the patient is followed closely; then, if there is recurrence, a second aspiration is performed. A re-recurrence requires open biopsy.

MASTITIS

What is it?	Superficial infection of the breast (cellulitis)
In what circumstance does it most often occur?	Breast-feeding
What bacteria are most commonly the cause?	*Staphylococcus aureus*
How is mastitis treated?	Stop breast-feeding and use a breast pump instead; application of heat; administration of antibiotics
Why must the patient with mastitis have close follow-up?	To make sure that she does not have inflammatory breast cancer!

BREAST ABSCESS

What are the causes?	Mammary ductal ectasia (stenosis of breast duct) and mastitis
What is the treatment of breast abscess?	Antibiotics Needle or open drainage with cultures taken Resection of involved ducts if recurrent Breast pump if breast feeding

MALE GYNECOMASTIA

What is it?	Enlargement of the male breast
What are the causes?	**Medications** Illicit drugs (marijuana) Liver failure Increased estrogen Decreased testosterone
What is the major differential diagnosis?	Male breast cancer
What is the treatment?	Stop or change medications; correct underlying cause if there is a hormonal imbalance; perform subcutaneous mastectomy (i.e., leave nipple) if refractory to conservative measures and time, and if patient wishes removal

50 Endocrine

ADRENAL GLAND

NORMAL ADRENAL PHYSIOLOGY

What is CRH?	**Corticotropin-Releasing Hormone:** released from the anterior hypothalamus and causes release of ACTH from the anterior pituitary
What is ACTH?	**AdrenoCorticoTropic Hormone:** released normally by the anterior pituitary, which in turn causes release of cortisol by the adrenal gland
What feeds back to inhibit ACTH secretion?	Cortisol

CUSHING'S SYNDROME

What is Cushing's syndrome?	Excessive **cortisol** production
What is the most common cause of Cushing's syndrome?	Iatrogenic (i.e., prescribed prednisone)
What is the second most common cause of Cushing's syndrome?	Cushing's disease (most common noniatrogenic cause)
What is Cushing's disease?	Cushing's syndrome caused by excess production of ACTH by the anterior **pituitary**
What is an ectopic ACTH source?	A tumor not found in the pituitary that secretes ACTH, which in turn causes a release of cortisol by the adrenal without the normal negative feedback loop

What are the signs/ symptoms of Cushing's syndrome?

Truncal obesity, hirsutism, "moon" facies, acne, "buffalo hump," purple striae, hypertension, diabetes, weakness, depression, easy bruisability, myopathy

How can cortisol levels be indirectly measured over a short duration?

By measuring urine cortisol or the breakdown product of cortisol, 17-hydroxycorticosteroid (**17-OHCS**), in the urine

What is a direct test of serum cortisol?

Serum cortisol level (highest in the morning and lowest at night in healthy patients)

Can ACTH levels be checked directly?

Yes (but many hospitals do not offer direct testing)

What initial tests should be performed in Cushing's syndrome?

Electrolytes
Serum cortisol
Urine free cortisol, urine 17-OHCS
Low-dose dexamethasone suppression test

What is the low-dose dexamethasone suppression test?

Dexamethasone is a synthetic cortisol that results in negative feedback on ACTH secretion and subsequent cortisol secretion in healthy patients. Patients with Cushing's syndrome do not suppress their cortisol secretion.

What test should be performed if a patient fails to suppress with the low-dose dexamethasone test?

High-dose dexamethasone suppression test

What is the high-dose dexamethasone suppression test?

Dexamethasone is a **cortisol analog** that suppresses pituitary secretion of ACTH by the cortisol negative feedback. The decreased ACTH results in decreased cortisol, as measured by serum cortisol and/or decreased urine 17-OHCS.

What findings on HIGH-dose dexamethasone test are associated with the following conditions:

Healthy patient?

Decreased urinary 17-OHCS/ serum cortisol level less than half the previous baseline levels

Cushing's disease (pituitary cause)?	**Decreased** urinary 17-OHCS/serum cortisol to about half the previous baseline levels
Ectopic ACTH-producing tumor?	**No effect** in more than 70% of cases (no response to cortisol; autonomous ACTH production)
Adrenal tumor?	**No effect** (autonomous cortisol production)
What is the corticotropin-releasing hormone (CRH) stimulation test?	CRH is administered via an IV, causing an increase in ACTH
What findings on CRH-stimulation test are associated with the following conditions:	
Healthy patients?	**Mild increase** in ACTH/cortisol
Cushing's disease (pituitary cause)?	**Great increase** in ACTH/cortisol
Ectopic ACTH-producing tumor?	**No effect** (ACTH is already high)
Adrenal tumor?	**No effect** (cortisol production does not respond to ACTH)
Summarize the "Cushing's syndrome" lab values found in the majority of patients with the following conditions:	
Healthy patients	Normal cortisol, normal ACTH, suppression with low-dose dexamethasone, suppression with high-dose dexamethasone (< 1/2), mild increase with CRH test
Cushing's disease (pituitary ACTH hypersecretion)	High cortisol, high ACTH, no suppression with low-dose dexamethasone, suppression with high-dose dexamethasone, great increase in cortisol with CRH test

Adrenal tumor	High cortisol, low ACTH, no suppression with low-dose dexamethasone, no suppression with high-dose dexamethasone, no change after CRH test
Ectopic ACTH-producing tumor	High cortisol, high ACTH, no suppression with low-dose dexamethasone test, no suppression with high-dose dexamethasone test, no change with CRH test
What is the most common site of ectopic ACTH-producing tumor?	More than two-thirds are oat cell tumors of the lung
How are the following tumors treated:	
Adrenal adenoma?	Adrenalectomy (almost always **unilateral**)
Adrenal carcinoma?	Surgical excision (only one-third of cases are operable)
Ectopic ACTH-producing tumor?	Surgical excision, if feasible
What is mitotane?	Medication that selectively **kills the cells that produce cortisol** (kills zona fasciculata and zona reticularis); used in inoperable cases of adrenal carcinoma (think: **MIT**otane = un**MIT**igated murder of cortisol-producing cells)
What medication must be given to a patient who is undergoing surgical correction of Cushing's syndrome?	Cortisol (usually hydrocortisone until PO is resumed)
What medication can be given to a patient with SEVERE cortisol excess?	Metyrapone (inhibits cortisol production by inhibiting the enzyme 11b-hydroxylase)

What is Nelson's syndrome?	Pituitary hypersecretion of some or all of the anterior pituitary hormones occurring in approximately 20% of all Cushing patients after adrenalectomy This condition can lead to hyperpigmentation, headache, exophthalmos, ↑ sex hormones, and pituitary enlargement, which can cause visual field deficits/blindness (think of it as an acute loss of the abnormal massive negative cortisol feedback) Think: **N**elson = **N**uclear reaction in the pituitary

ADRENAL INCIDENTALOMA

What is an incidentaloma?	A tumor found in the adrenal gland **incidentally** on a CT scan performed for an unrelated reason
What is the risk factor for carcinoma?	Solid tumor more than 5 cm in diameter
What is the treatment?	Controversial for smaller/medium-sized tumors; but almost all surgeons would agree that resection is indicated for solid incidentalomas more than 5 cm in diameter
What are the indications for removal of adrenal incidentaloma less than 5 cm?	MRI T2 signal greater than 2 Hormonally active Enlarging cystic lesion
What tumor must be ruled out prior to biopsy or surgery for any adrenal mass?	Pheochromocytoma

PHEOCHROMOCYTOMA

What is it?	Tumor of the adrenal medulla and sympathetic ganglion (from chromaffin cell lines) that produces **catecholamines** (norepinephrine > epinephrine)

What is the incidence?	It is the cause of hypertension in approximately 1/500 hypertensive patients (≈ 10% of the US population has hypertension)
Which age group is most likely to be affected?	Any age (children and adults); average age is 40 to 60 years
What are the associated risk factors?	MEN-II, family history, neuroectodermal dysplasia (e.g., neurofibromatosis)
What are the signs/ symptoms?	"Classic" triad: 1. **Palpitations** 2. **Headache** 3. **Episodic diaphoresis** Also, hypertension (50%), pallor → flushing, anxiety, weight loss, tachycardia, hyperglycemia
How can the pheochromocytoma SYMPTOMS triad be remembered?	Think of the first three letters in the word **PHE**ochromocytoma: **P**alpitations **H**eadache **E**pisodic diaphoresis
What is the most common sign of pheochromocytoma?	Hypertension
What is the differential diagnosis?	Renovascular hypertension, menopause, migraine headache, carcinoid syndrome, preeclampsia, neuroblastoma, anxiety disorder with panic attacks, hyperthyroidism, insulinoma
What diagnostic tests should be performed?	Urine screen: vanillylmandelic acid (**VMA**), **metanephrine,** and **normetanephrine** (all breakdown products of the catechols) Urine/serum **epinephrine/ norepinephrine** levels
What are the other common lab findings?	Hyperglycemia (epinephrine increases glucose, norepinephrine decreases insulin) Polycythemia (due to intravascular volume depletion)

What are the most common sites of pheochromocytoma?

Adrenal (approximately 90%)
Organ of Zuckerkandl
Thorax (mediastinum)
Bladder
Scrotum

What are the tumor localization tests?

CT, MRI, ^{131}**I-MIBG**

What does ^{131}I-MIBG stand for?

MetaIodoBenzylGuanidine

How does the ^{131}I-MIBG scan work?

^{131}I-MIBG is a norepinephrine analog that collects in adrenergic vesicles and, thus, in pheochromocytomas

What is the scan for imaging adrenal cortical pheochromocytoma?

NP-59 (a cholesterol analog)

What is the localizing option if a tumor is not seen on CT, MRI, I-MIBG?

IVC venous sampling for catecholamines (gradient will help localize the tumor)

What is the tumor site if epinephrine is elevated?

It must be adrenal or near the adrenal gland (e.g., organs of Zuckerkandl), because nonadrenal tumors lack the capability to methylate norepinephrine to epinephrine

What percentage of patients have malignant tumors?

Approximately 10%

Can histology be used to determine malignancy?

No; only distant metastasis or invasion can determine malignancy

What is the classic pheochromocytoma "rule of 10's"?

10% malignant
10% bilateral
10% in children
10% multiple tumors
10% extraadrenal

What is the preoperative/ medical treatment?
Increase intravascular volume with **α**-blockade (e.g., phenoxybenzamine or prazosin) to allow reduction in catecholamine-induced vasoconstriction and resulting volume depletion
Treatment should be started as soon as diagnosis is made

What is the surgical treatment?
Tumor resection with early ligation of venous drainage (lower possibility of catecholamine release/crisis by tying off drainage)

What are the possible perioperative complications?
Anesthetic challenge: hypertensive crisis with manipulation (treat with nitroprusside), hypotension with total removal of the tumor, cardiac arrhythmias

In the patient with pheochromocytoma, what must be ruled out?
MEN type II; almost all cases are bilateral

What is the most likely tumor site in a patient with palpitations, headache, and diaphoresis with urination?
Bladder pheochromocytoma

What risk is associated with angiography to localize a pheochromocytoma?
May precipitate a hypertensive crisis

What are the organs of Zuckerkandl?
Embryonic chromaffin cells around the abdominal aorta (near the inferior mesenteric artery) that normally atrophy during childhood but are a major site of extraadrenal pheochromocytoma

CONN'S SYNDROME

What is it?
Hyper**aldosteronism** (primary)

What are the common sources?

Adrenal adenoma or adrenal hyperplasia; aldosterone is abnormally secreted by an adrenal adenoma (two-thirds) > hyperplasia > carcinoma

What are the signs/ symptoms?

Hypertension, headache, fatigue, nocturia/polydipsia

What are the two classic clues of Conn's syndrome?

1. Hypertension
2. Hypokalemia

What are the associated lab findings?

Increased serum sodium, decreased serum potassium (makes sense: aldosterone results in sodium/H_2O retention with loss of K^+), increase in urinary aldosterone, **normal or low renin** serum levels, high urine potassium

What is secondary hyperaldosteronism?

Hyperaldosteronism due to abnormally high **renin** levels (renin causes an increase in angiotensin/aldosterone)

What diagnostic tests should be performed?

CT, Adrenal **venous sampling** for aldosterone levels, iodocholesterol scanning, arteriography/venography (retrograde), Captopril test, saline infusion

What are the saline infusion and Captopril tests?

1. Saline infusion: will decrease aldosterone levels in normal patients but not in Conn's syndrome
2. Captopril test: will decrease aldosterone levels in normal patients but not in patients with Conn's syndrome

What is the preoperative treatment?

Spironolactone

What is spironolactone?

An antialdosterone medication (works at the kidney tubule)

What is the treatment of the following conditions:

Adenoma?

Surgical resection (adrenalectomy)

Unilateral hyperplasia?	Unilateral adrenalectomy
Bilateral hyperplasia?	Spironolactone (no surgery)
What are the renin levels in patients with PRIMARY hyperaldosteronism?	Normal or low (key point!)

INSULINOMA

What is it?	Insulin-producing tumor arising from β cells
What is the incidence?	Number one islet cell neoplasm; half of β cell tumors of the pancreas produce insulin
What are the associated risks?	Associated with MEN-I syndrome (ppp = pituitary, pancreas, parathyroid tumors)
What are the signs and symptoms?	**Sympathetic nervous system symptoms due to hypoglycemia:** Palpitations, diaphoresis, tremulousness, irritability, weakness
What are the neurologic symptoms?	Personality changes, confusion, obtundation, seizures, coma
What is Whipple's triad?	1. Hypoglycemic symptoms produced by fasting 2. Blood Glc < 50 mg/dl during symptomatic attack 3. Relief of symptoms by administration of glucose
What is the differential diagnosis?	Reactive hypoglycemia Functional hypoglycemia with gastrectomy Adrenal insufficiency Hypopituitarism Hepatic insufficiency Munchausen syndrome (insulin self-injections) Nonislet cell tumor causing hypoglycemia (hemangiopericytoma, fibrosarcoma, leiomyosarcoma, hepatoma, adrenocortical carcinoma)

	Surreptitious administration of insulin by others (the Sonny von Bulow case comes to mind!)
What lab tests should be performed?	Glucose and insulin levels during fast; proinsulin levels (if self-injection of insulin is a concern, as insulin injections have **no** proinsulin)
What diagnostic tests should be performed?	Fasting hypoglycemia in the presence of inappropriately high levels of insulin **72-hour fast,** then check glucose and insulin levels q 6 hr (monitor very closely because the patient can develop hypoglycemic crisis)
Localizing tests?	CT A-gram Endoscopic ultrasound Venous catheterization (to sample blood along portal and splenic veins to measure insulin and localize tumor) Intraoperative ultrasound
What is the medical treatment?	Diazoxide, to suppress insulin release
What is the surgical treatment?	Surgical resection
What is the prognosis?	Approximately 80% of patients have a benign solitary adenoma that is cured by surgical resection

GLUCAGONOMA

What is it?	Glucagon-producing tumor
Where is it located?	Pancreas (usually in the tail)
What are the symptoms?	**Necrotizing migratory erythema** (usually below the waist), glossitis, stomatitis, diabetes
What are the associated lab findings?	Hyperglycemia, low amino acid levels, high glucagon levels

What stimulation test is used for glucagonoma?	Tolbutamide stimulation test: IV tolbutamide results in elevated glucagon levels
What test is used for localization?	CT
What is the medical treatment of necrotizing migratory erythema?	Somatostatin, IV amino acids
What is the treatment?	Surgical resection

ZOLLINGER-ELLISON SYNDROME

What is it?	**Gastrinoma:** Non-β islet cell tumor of the pancreas (or other locale) that produces gastrin, causing gastric hypersecretion of HCl acid resulting in GI **ulcers**
What is the incidence?	1/1000 in patients with peptic ulcer disease, but nearly 2% in patients with **recurrent ulcers**
What is the associated syndrome?	MEN-I syndrome
What percentage of patients with pheochromocytoma have this syndrome?	Approximately 25%
What percentage of patients with MEN-I will have a gastrinoma?	Approximately 50%
What are the signs/ symptoms?	Peptic ulcers, diarrhea, weight loss, abdominal pain
What causes the diarrhea?	Massive acid hypersecretion and destruction of digestive enzymes
What are the signs?	**PUD:** epigastric pain, hematemesis, melena, hematochezia, GE reflux, diarrhea, **recurrent ulcers**

What are the possible complications?

GI hemorrhage
GI Perforation
Gastric outlet obstruction/stricture
Metastatic disease

What is the differential diagnosis of increased gastrin?

Postvagotomy
Gastric outlet obstruction
Antral G-cell hyperplasia/hyperfunction
Pernicious anemia
Atrophic gastritis
Short gut syndrome
Renal failure
H_2 blocker, omeprazole (remember: a gastric pH < 2 inhibits gastrin in normal patients)

Which patients should have a gastrin level checked?

Those with recurrent ulcers, ulcers in an unusual position (e.g., jejunum), ulcer refractory to medical management, or prior to any operation for an ulcer

What lab tests should be performed?

Fasting gastrin level
Postsecretin challenge gastrin level
Calcium (screen for MEN-I)
Chem 7

What are the associated gastrin levels?

NL fasting = 100 pg/ml
ZES fasting = 200-1000 pg/ml
Basal acid secretion; (ZES > 15 mEq/hr, nl < 10mEq/hr)

What is the secretin stimulation test?

IV secretin is administered and the gastrin level is determined. Patients with Zollinger-Ellison syndrome have a paradoxic increase in gastrin

Lab results with secretin challenge:

NL—Decreased gastrin
Zollinger-Ellison syndrome—Increased gastrin (increased by > 200 pg/ml)

What tests are used to evaluate ulcers?

EGD and/or UGI

What tests are used to localize the tumor?

Abdominal CT, MRE **octreotide scan,** selective angiography, selective venous sampling for gastrin

What is the most common site?
Pancreas

What is the most common NONpancreatic site?
Duodenum

What are some other sites?
Stomach, lymph nodes, liver, kidney, ovary

Define the "gastrinoma triangle."
A triangle drawn from the following points:
1. Cystic duct
2. Junction of the second and third portions of the duodenum
3. Neck of the pancreas (90% of gastrinomas are in this triangle)

What is the next step if the tumor cannot be localized?
Exploratory surgery (if the tumor is not in pancreas, open the duodenum and look), proximal gastric vagotomy if not found

What is the medical treatment?
H_2 blockers, omeprazole, somatostatin

What is the surgical treatment?
If the tumor is in the head of pancreas, remove (enucleation); if the tumor is in the body/tail of the pancreas, perform distal pancreatic resection; if the tumor is in the duodenum, remove locally

What percentage have malignant tumors?
Two-thirds

What is the most common site of metastasis?
Liver

What is the treatment of patients with liver metastasis?
Excise, if technically feasible

What is the surgical option if gastrinoma is in the duodenum/head of the pancreas and is too large or has too many lymph node metastases for local resection?
Whipple procedure

What is the treatment of widely metastatic or incurable gastrinoma?	Debulking surgery Chemotherapy: 5-FU, streptozotocin, doxorubicin
What is the prognosis with the following procedures:	
Complete excision?	90% 10-year survival
Incomplete excision?	25% 10-year survival

MULTIPLE ENDOCRINE NEOPLASIA

What is it also known as?	MEN syndrome
What is it?	Inherited condition of propensity to develop multiple endocrine tumors
How is it inherited?	Autosomal dominant (but with a significant degree of variation in penetrance)
Which patients should be screened for MEN?	All family members of patients diagnosed with MEN

MEN TYPE I

What is the common eponym?	Wermer's syndrome (think: Wermer = Winner = # 1 = type **1**)
What are the most common tumors and their incidences?	**PPP:** **P**arathyroid hyperplasia (≈ 90%) **P**ancreatic islet cell tumors (≈ 2/3) Gastrinoma: Zollinger-Ellison syndrome (50%) Insulinoma (20%) **P**ituitary tumors (≈ 66%)
How can tumors for MEN-I be remembered?	Think: type 1 = primary, primary, primary = **PPP** = parathyroid, pancreas, pituitary
How can the P's associated with MEN-I be remembered?	All the P's are followed by a vowel: PA, PA, PI
What percentage of patients with MEN-I have parathyroid hyperplasia?	Approximately 90%

What percentage of patients with MEN-I have a gastrinoma?

Approximately 50%

What other tumors (in addition to PPP) are associated with MEN- I?

Adrenal (30%) and thyroid (15%) adenomas

MEN TYPE IIA

What is the common eponym?

Sipple's syndrome (think: Sipple = Second = # 2 = type **2**)

What are the most common tumors and their incidences?

MPH:
Medullary thyroid carcinoma (100%)
  Calcitonin secreted
Pheochromocytoma (> 33%)
  Catecholamine excess
Hyperparathyroidism (about 50%)
  Hypercalcemia

How can the tumors involved with MEN-II be remembered?

Think: type 2 = 2 MPH or 2 **M**iles **P**er **H**our = **MPH** = **M**edullary, **P**heochromocytoma, **H**yperparathyroid

How can the P of MPH be remembered?

Followed by the consonant "H"—PHEOCHROMOCYTOMA (remember, the P's of MEN-I are followed by vowels)

What percentage of patients with MEN-IIA have medullary carcinoma of the thyroid?

100%

MEN TYPE IIB

What are the most common abnormalities, their incidences, and symptoms?

MMMP:
Mucosal neuromas (100%)—in the nasopharynx, oropharynx, larynx, and conjunctiva
Medullary thyroid carcinoma (≈ 85%)—more aggressive than in MEN-IIa
Marfanoid body habitus (long/lanky)
Pheochromocytoma (≈ 50%) and found bilaterally**

How can the features of MEN-IIB be remembered?	MMMP (think: **3M P**lastics)
What are the physical findings/signs of MEN-IIB?	Mucosal neuromas (e.g., mouth, eyes) Marfanoid body habitus Pes cavus/planum (large arch of foot/ flatfooted) Constipation
What is the most common GI complaint of patients with MEN-IIB?	**Constipation** due to ganglioneuromatosis of GI tract
What percentage of pheochromocytomas in MEN-IIA/B are bilateral?	Approximately 70% (but found bilaterally in only 10% of **all** patients diagnosed with pheochromocytoma)
What is the major difference between MEN-IIA and MEN-IIB?	MEN-IIa = parathyroid hyperplasia MEN-IIb = **no** parathyroid hyperplasia (and neuromas, marfanoid habitus, pes cavus [extensive arch of foot], etc.)
What type of parathyroid disease is associated with MEN-I and MEN-IIA?	**Hyperplasia** (treat with removal of all parathyroid tissue with autotransplant of some of the parathyroid tissue to the forearm)
What percentage of patients with Zollinger-Ellison syndrome have MEN-I?	Approximately 25%

51 Thyroid Gland

THYROID DISEASE

ANATOMY

Identify the following structures:

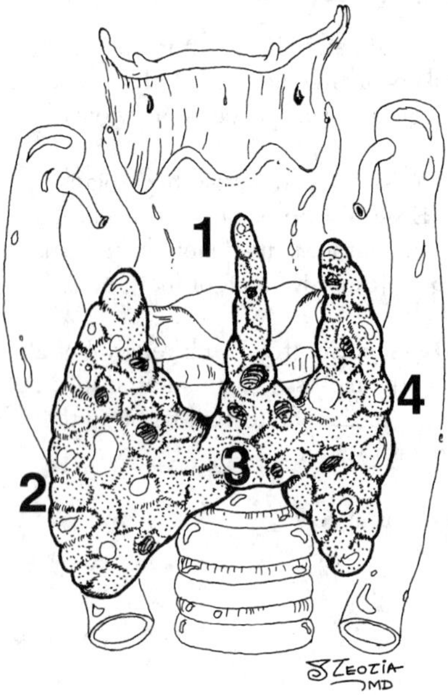

1. Pyramidal lobe
2. Right lobe
3. Isthmus
4. Left lobe

Define the arterial blood supply to the thyroid.

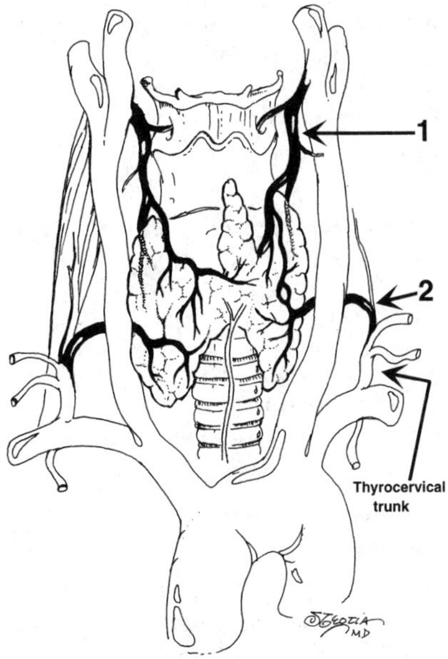

Two arteries:

1. Superior thyroid artery (first branch of the external carotid artery)
2. Inferior thyroid artery (branch of the thyrocervical trunk)

(IMA artery rare)

What is the venous drainage of the thyroid?

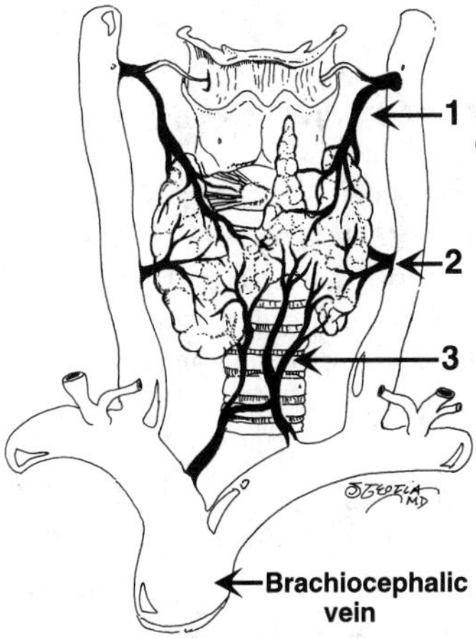

Three veins:

1. Superior thyroid vein
2. **Middle** thyroid vein
3. Inferior thyroid vein

Name the thyroid lobe appendage coursing toward the hyoid bone from around the thyroid isthmus?	Pyramidal lobe
What percentage of patients have a pyramidal lobe?	Approximately 50%
Name the lymph node group around the pyramidal thyroid lobe?	Delphian lymph node group
What is the thyroid isthmus?	Midline border between the left and right thyroid lobes
Which ligament connects the thyroid to the trachea?	Ligament of Berry
What is the IMA (not I.M.A.) artery?	A small inferior artery to the thyroid from the aorta or innominate artery
What percentage of patients have an IMA artery?	Approximately 3%
Name the most posterior extension of the lateral thyroid lobes?	Tubercle of Zuckerkandl
Which paired nerves must be carefully identified during a thyroidectomy?	The **recurrent laryngeal nerves**, which are found in the tracheoesophageal grooves and dive behind the cricothyroid muscle; damage to these nerves paralyzes laryngeal abductors and causes hoarseness if unilateral and airway obstruction if bilateral.
What other nerve is at risk during a thyroidectomy and what are the symptoms?	**Superior laryngeal nerve**—if damaged, the patient will have a deeper and quieter voice (opera singers are unable to hit the high pitches)

What is the name of the famous opera singer whose superior laryngeal nerve was injured during a thyroidectomy?

Gallicurci; his career was ended

THYROID PHYSIOLOGY

What is TRH?

Thyrotropin-**r**eleasing **H**ormone released from the hypothalamus

What is TSH?

Thyroid-**s**timulating **H**ormone released by the anterior pituitary; causes release of thyroid hormone from the thyroid

What are the thyroid hormones?

T3 and T4

What is the most active form of thyroid hormone?

T3

What is a negative feedback loop?

T3 and T4 feed back negatively on the anterior pituitary (causing decreased release of TSH in response to TRH)

What is the most common site of conversion of T4 to T3?

Peripheral (e.g., liver, pituitary gland)

THYROID NODULE

What is the differential diagnosis of a thyroid nodule?

Adenomatous goiter
Adenoma
Hyperfunctioning adenoma
Cyst
Thyroiditis
Carcinoma/lymphoma
Parathyroid carcinoma

Name 3 types of nonthyroidal neck masses.

1. Inflammatory lesions (e.g., abscess, lymphadenitis)
2. Congenital lesions (i.e., thyroglossal duct [midline], branchial cleft cyst [lateral])
3. Malignant lesions: lymphoma, metastases, squamous cell carcinoma

What studies can be used to evaluate a thyroid nodule?

Ultrasound—solid or cystic nodule
Fine needle aspirate (FNA) → cytology
Radioiodide
^{123}I or ^{99m}Tc scan—hot or cold nodule
Thyroid panel (T3/T4)
Thyroid antibody
TSH

What is meant by a hot versus a cold nodule?

Nodule uptake of IV ^{131}I or ^{99m}T
Hot—Increased ^{123}I or ^{99m}T uptake = functioning/hyperfunctioning nodule
Cold—Decreased ^{123}I or ^{99m}T uptakc = nonfunctioning nodule

What is the test of choice for DIAGNOSIS of a thyroid nodule?

FNA

What is the percentage of false negative results for FNA and thyroid nodules?

Approximately 5%

What is the role of thyroid suppression of a thyroid nodule?

Diagnostic and therapeutic; administration of thyroid hormone suppresses TSH secretion and up to half of the benign thyroid nodule will disappear!

In evaluating thyroid nodules, what history, labs, symptoms, and signs suggest carcinoma?

History of radiation therapy to the neck
History of rapid development
Vocal cord paralysis (recurrent laryngeal nerve paralysis)
Cervical adenopathy
Invasion outside the thyroid
Hard fixed mass in the thyroid
Elevated serum calcitonin

MALIGNANT THYROID NODULES

What percentage of cold thyroid nodules are malignant?

Approximately 25% in adults

What are the risk factors for a malignant nodule?

History of neck irradiation, young > old, cold nodule, solitary nodule > multiple nodules

What percentage of multinodular masses are malignant?

Approximately 1%

What percentage of cystic masses larger than 4 cm in diameter are malignant?

Almost none; diagnosis is confirmed by ultrasound or needle aspiration (many patients will need surgical resection because masses will come back even after multiple aspirations)

What are the pros and cons of fine needle aspiration?

Pros—Safe, cost-effective diagnosis of papillary, medullary, and anaplastic carcinomas

Cons—false negative results; FNA cannot accurately distinguish between benign and malignant follicular tumors or Hürthle cell tumors

What is the treatment of a patient with a history of radiation exposure, thyroid nodule, and negative FNA?

Most experts would remove the nodule surgically (due to the high risk of radiation)

THYROID CARCINOMA

Name the FIVE main types of thyroid carcinoma and their relative percentages.

1. Papillary carcinoma: 80% (**P**opular = **P**apillary)
2. Follicular carcinoma: 10%
3. Medullary carcinoma: 5%
4. Hürthle cell carcinoma: 4%
5. Anaplastic/undifferentiated carcinoma: 1% to 2%

What are the signs and symptoms?

Mass/nodule, lymphadenopathy; most are **euthyroid,** (rarely hyperfunctioning)

What comprises the work up?

Thyroid function test: T4, T3, TSH
FNA
CXR
± Radioisotope scan
Thyroid ultrasound

PAPILLARY ADENOCARCINOMA

With what condition is it associated?

Gardner's syndrome and neck irradiation

What are the associated histologic findings?

Psammoma bodies (remember, **p** = **p**sammoma = **p**apillary, which constitute 80% of thyroid tumors; therefore, **p**apillary = **p**opular)

Describe the route and rate of spread.

Most spread via lymphatics (cervical adenopathy); spread occurs slowly

^{131}I uptake?

Good uptake

What is the 10-year survival rate?

Approximately 95%

What is the treatment?

1. Thyroid lobectomy and isthmectomy
2. Near-total thyroidectomy
3. Total thyroidectomy (usually used if diffuse/bilateral)

What postoperative medication should be administered?

Thyroid hormone replacement, to suppress TSH

What is the advantage of total thyroidectomy?

Postoperative ^{131}I scan can locate residual tumor and distant metastasis that can be treated with ablative doses of ^{131}I (disadvantage is increased risk to recurrent laryngeal nerve and parathyroid glands)

What are the "P's" of papillary thyroid cancer?

Papillary cancer:
Popular (most common type)
Psammoma bodies
Palpable lymph nodes (spreads most commonly by lymphatics, seen in up to one-third of patients)
Positive ^{131}I uptake
Positive prognosis
Postoperative ^{131}I scan to diagnose/treat metastases

FOLLICULAR ADENOCARCINOMA

What percentage of thyroid cancers does it comprise?

Approximately 10%

Describe the nodule consistency.
Rubbery, encapsulated

What is the route of spread?
Hematogenous, more aggressive than papillary adenocarcinoma

What is the male: female ratio?
1:3

^{131}I uptake?
Good uptake

What is the 10-year survival rate?
Approximately 90%

Can the diagnosis be made by FNA?
No; tissue structure is needed for a diagnosis of cancer

What histologic findings define malignancy in follicular cancer?
Capsular or blood vessel invasion

What is the most common site of distant metastasis?
Bone

What is the treatment?
1. Near total thyroidectomy or lobectomy/isthmectomy for small tumors
2. Total thyroidectomy for large or diffuse tumors
3. Postoperative ^{131}I scan for diagnosis/treatment of metastasis if total thyroidectomy is performed

What are the "F's" of follicular cancer?
Follicular cancer:
Far-away metastasis (spreads hematogenously)
Female (3 to 1 ratio)
FNA, NOT (cancer CANNOT be diagnosed by FNA)
Favorable prognosis

MEDULLARY CARCINOMA

What percentage of all thyroid cancers does it comprise?
Approximately **5%**

With what other conditions is it associated?
Multiple endocrine neoplasia type II; autosomal dominant genetic transmission

Histology?
Amyloid (a**M**yloid = **M**edullary)

What does it secrete?
Calcitonin

What is the appropriate stimulation test?
Pentagastrin

Describe the route and rate of spread.
Lymphatic and hematogenous distant metastasis

How is the diagnosis made?
FNA

^{131}I uptake?
Poor uptake

What is the prognosis?
Ten-year survival rate is 50%; however, the cure rate is 95% when occult tumors are found in MEN family members who are being screened for elevated calcitonin.
If detected when clinically palpable, the cure rate is less than 20%

What is the treatment?
Total thyroidectomy and median lymph node dissection
Modified neck dissection, if lateral cervical nodes are positive

What are the "M's" of medullary carcinoma?
Medullary cancer:
MEN
a**M**yloid
Median lymph node dissection
Modified neck dissection if lateral nodes are positive

HÜRTHLE CELL THYROID CANCER

What is it?
Thyroid cancer of Hürthle cells

What percentage of thyroid cancers does it comprise?
Approximately 4%

What is the cell of origin?
Follicular cells

^{131}I uptake?	No uptake
How is the diagnosis made?	FNA can identify cells, but malignancy can only be determined by tissue histology (like follicular cancer)
What is the route of metastasis?	Lymphatic > hematogenous
What is the treatment of the following disorders:	
Hürthle cell adenoma?	**Lobectomy** and isthmectomy
Hürthle cell carcinoma?	**Total thyroidectomy** and modified radical neck dissection, if lateral nodes are positive
What is the role of postoperative ^{131}I?	No role

ANAPLASTIC CARCINOMA

What is it also known as?	Undifferentiated carcinoma
What is it?	An undifferentiated cancer arising in approximately 75% of previously differentiated thyroid cancers (most commonly, follicular carcinoma)
What percentage of all thyroid cancers does it comprise?	Approximately 1% to 2%
What is the gender preference?	Women > men
What are the associated histologic findings?	Giant cells, spindle cells
^{131}I uptake?	Very poor uptake
How is the diagnosis made?	FNA (large tumor)
What is the major differential diagnosis?	Thyroid lymphoma (much better prognosis!)

What is the treatment of the following disorders:

Small tumors? Total thyroidectomy ± external beam x-ray therapy

Airway compromise? Debulking surgery and tracheostomy

What is the prognosis? Dismal, because most patients are at stage IV at presentation (distant metastasis); survival past 2 years is rare

What laboratory value must be followed postoperatively after a thyroidectomy? **Calcium** decreased secondary to parathyroid damage; during lobectomy, the parathyroids must be spared and their blood supply protected; if blood supply is compromised intraoperatively, they can be autografted into the sternocleomastoid muscle or forearm

What is the differential diagnosis of postoperative dyspnea after a thyroidectomy?

Neck hematoma (remove sutures and clot at the **bedside**)

Bilateral recurrent laryngeal nerve damage

What is a "lateral aberrant rest" of the thyroid? A misnomer; it is **papillary** cancer of a lymph node from metastasis

BENIGN THYROID DISEASE

What is Graves' disease? Diffuse goiter with hyperthyroidism, exophthalmos, and pretibial myxedema

What is the etiology of Graves' disease? Caused by circulating **antibodies** that stimulate TSH receptors on follicular cells of the thyroid and cause deregulated production of thyroid hormones (i.e., hyperthyroidism)

What is the female: male ratio with Graves' disease? 6:1

What specific physical finding is associated with Graves'? Exophthalmus

How is the diagnosis made? Increased TFT's; global uptake of radioiodine

Name three main treatment modalities of Graves' disease.

1. **Medical Blockade:** iodide, propranolol, propylthiouracil (PTU), methimazole, Lugol's solution (potassium iodide)
2. **Radioiodide ablation:** most popular therapy
3. **Surgical resection:** (near-total thyroidectomy) used if there is also a suspicious nodule, if patient is noncompliant or refractory to medicines, pregnant or planning pregnancy within a year, a child, or if patient refuses radioiodide

What is the major complication of radioiodide or surgery for Graves' disease?

Hypothyroidism

What does PTU stand for?

Propylthiouracil

How does PTU work?

1. Inhibits incorporation of iodine into T4/T3 (by blocking peroxidase oxidation of iodide to iodine)
2. Inhibits peripheral conversion of T4 to T3

How does methimazole work?

Inhibits incorporation of iodine into T4/T3 **only** (by blocking peroxidase oxidation of iodide to iodine)

TOXIC MULTINODULAR GOITER

What is it?

Multiple thyroid nodules that produce thyroid hormone, resulting in hyperthyroidism (or a "toxic" thyroid state)

What are the associated physical findings?

Multiple thyroid nodules

What is the treatment?

1. Thyroidectomy
2. Subtotal thyroidectomy removing all nodules
3. ^{131}I (used rarely) in poor operative candidates

THYROIDITIS

What are the features of acute thyroiditis?	Painful, swollen thyroid; fever; overlying skin erythema
What is the cause of ACUTE thyroiditis?	Bacteria (usually *Streptococcus, Staphylococcus*); usually caused by a thyroglossal fistula or anatomic variant
What is the treatment of ACUTE thyroiditis?	Antibiotics, drainage of abscess, needle aspiration for culture; most patients need definitive surgery later to remove the fistula
What are the features of subacute thyroiditis?	Glandular swelling, tenderness, often follows upper respiratory infection, elevated ESR
What is the cause of subacute thyroiditis?	Viral infection
What is the treatment of subacute thyroiditis?	Supportive: NSAIDS, ± steroids
What is DeQuervain's thyroiditis?	Just another name for subacute thyroiditis caused by a virus (think: DeQuer**VAIN**: **VIRUS**)
How can the differences between etiologies of ACUTE and SUBACUTE thyroiditis be remembered?	Alphabetically: **A** before **S, B** before **V** (i.e., **A**cute before **S**ubacute and **B**acterial before **V**iral and thus: **A**cute = **B**acterial and **S**ubacute = **V**iral)
What are the two types of chronic thyroiditis?	1. Hashimoto's thyroiditis 2. Riedel's thyroiditis
What are the features of Hashimoto's (chronic) thyroiditis?	Firm and rubbery gland, 95% in women, lymphocyte invasion
What is the claim to fame of Hashimoto's disease?	Most common cause of hypothyroidism in the United States
What is the etiology of Hashimoto's disease?	Autoimmune (think: HashimOTO = AUTO and thus; Hashimoto = autoimmune)

What lab tests should be performed to diagnose Hashimoto's disease?

Antithyroglobulin and microsomal antibodies

What is Riedel's thyroiditis?

Benign inflammatory thyroid enlargement **with fibrosis** of thyroid
Patients present with painless, large thyroid
Fibrosis may involve surrounding tissues

52 Parathyroid

ANATOMY

How many parathyroids are there?	Usually **four** (two superior and two inferior)
What percentage of patients have five parathyroid glands?	Approximately 5%
What is the usual position of the inferior parathyroid glands?	Posterior and lateral behind the thyroid and below the inferior thyroid artery
What is the most common site of an "extra" gland?	Thymus gland
What percentage of patients have a parathyroid gland in the mediastinum?	Approximately 1%
If only three parathyroid glands are found at surgery, where can the fourth one be hiding?	Thyroid gland Thymus/mediastinum Carotid sheath Tracheoesophageal groove Behind the esophagus
What is the embryologic origin of the following structures:	
Superior parathyroid glands?	Fourth pharyngeal pouch
Inferior parathyroid glands?	Third pharyngeal pouch (counterintuitive)
What supplies blood to the parathyroid glands?	Inferior thyroid artery

What percentage of patients have all four parathyroid glands supplied by the inferior thyroid arteries exclusively?

Approximately 80%

PHYSIOLOGY

What cell type produces PTH?

Chief cells

What are the major actions of parathyroid hormone (PTH)?

Increases blood **calcium** levels (takes from bone breakdown, GI absorption, increased reabsorption from kidney, excretion of phosphate by kidney)

HYPERPARATHYROIDISM (↑PTH)

Define primary ↑PTH.

Increased secretion of PTH by parathyroid gland(s); marked by elevated calcium, low phosphorus

Define secondary ↑PTH.

Increase in serum PTH due to **renal failure or decreased GI calcium absorption;** calcium levels are normal or **low**

Define tertiary ↑PTH

Persistent ↑PTH after correction of secondary hyperparathyroidism; calcium levels are elevated (e.g., renal transplant in patients with secondary hyperparathyroidism due to **refractory hyperplasia** caused by second degree ↑PTH; after serum Ca^{2+} is corrected following renal transplant, Ca^{2+} fails to regulate/inhibit PTH secretion)

What are the methods of imaging the parathyroids?

Surgical operation (**"photon scan"**) is most common
Ultrasound
Sestamibi scan
^{201}TI(technetium)–thallium subtraction scan
CT/MRI
A-gram (rare)
Venous sampling for PTH (rare)

What are the indications for a localizing preoperative study?

Reoperation for recurrent hyperparathyroidism

PRIMARY HYPERPARATHYROIDISM

What is the most common cause of primary hyperparathyroidism?

Adenoma (> 85%)

What are the etiologies of primary ↑PTH and percentages?

Adenoma (~ 85%)
Hyperplasia (~ 10%)
Carcinoma (~ 1%)

What is the incidence of primary ↑PTH in the United States?

Approximately 1/4000

What are the risk factors for primary ↑PTH (2)

Family history, MEN I and IIa, irradiation

What are the signs/ symptoms of primary ↑PTH hypercalcemia?

"Stones, bones, groans, and psychiatric overtones":
- **Stones:** kidney stones
- **Bones:** Bone pain, pathologic fractures, subperiosteal resorption
- **Groans:** Muscle pain and weakness, pancreatitis, gout, constipation
- **Psychiatric overtones:** Depression, anorexia, anxiety
- **Other symptoms:** Polydipsia, weight loss, HTN (10%), polyuria, lethargy

What is the "33 to 1" rule?

Patients with first degree hyperparathyroidism have a ratio of serum [Cl^-<] to phosphate ≥ 33

What plain x-ray findings are associated with hyperparathyroidism?

Subperiosteal bone resorption (usually in hand digits; said to be "pathognomonic" for hyperparathyroidism!)

How is primary ↑PTH diagnosed?

Labs—**elevated parathyroid hormone** (hypercalcemia, ↑phosphorus, ↑chloride); urine calcium should be checked for familial hypocalciuric hypercalcemia

What is familial hypocalciuric hypercalcemia?

Familial inheritance (autosomal dominant) of a condition of **asymptomatic** hypercalcemia and low urine calcium, with or without elevated parathyroid hormone; in contrast, hypercalcemia due to hyperparathyroid results in high levels of calcium in the urine
(Surgery to remove parathyroid glands is not indicated for this diagnosis.)

How many of the glands are USUALLY affected by the following conditions:

Hyperplasia?

Four

Adenoma?

One

Carcinoma?

One

What percentage of adenomas are not single, but are found in more than one gland?

Approximately 5%

What is the differential diagnosis of hypercalcemia?

"CHIMPANZEES":
↑**C**alcium
Hyperparathyroidism (1°/2°/3°)
Hyperthyroidism, **H**ypocalciuric **H**ypercalcemia (familial)
Immobility/iatrogenic (thiazide diuretics)
Metastasis/milk alkali syndrome (rare)
Paget's disease (bone)
Addison's disease/acromegaly
Neoplasm (colon, lung, breast, prostate, multiple myeloma)
Zollinger-Ellison syndrome
Excessive vitamin D
Excessive vitamin A
Sarcoid

What is the initial medical treatment of hypercalcemia (1° ↑PTH)?

Medical—IV fluids, furosemide, **NOT** thiazide diuretics

What is the definitive treatment of hyperparathyroidism in the following cases:

Primary hyperparathyroidism due to HYPERPLASIA?

Neck exploration removing all parathyroid glands and leaving at least 30 mg of parathyroid tissue placed in the forearm muscles (nondominant arm, of course!)

Primary hyperparathyroidism due to parathyroid ADENOMA?

Surgically remove adenoma (send for frozen section) and biopsy all abnormally enlarged parathyroid glands (some experts biopsy all glands)

Primary hyperparathyroidism due to parathyroid CARCINOMA?

Remove carcinoma, ipsilateral thyroid lobe, and all enlarged lymph nodes

Secondary hyperparathyroidism?

Correct calcium and phosphate, perform renal transplantation (no role for parathyroid surgery)

Tertiary hyperparathyroidism?

Correct calcium and phosphate, perform renal transplantation, surgical operation to remove all parathyroid glands and reimplant 30 to 40 mg in the forearm if **REFRACTORY** to medical management

Why place 30 to 40 mg of sliced parathyroid gland in the forearm?

To retain parathyroid function; if hyperparathyroidism recurs, it is easy to remove some of the parathyroid gland from the easily accessible forearm

What must be ruled out in the patient with 1° ↑PTH due to hyperplasia?

MEN type I and MEN type IIa

What carcinomas are commonly associated with hypercalcemia?	**Breast cancer metastases,** prostate cancer, kidney cancer, lung cancer
What is the most likely diagnosis if a patient has a PALPABLE neck mass, hypercalcemia, and elevated parathyroid hormone?	Parathyroid carcinoma (vast majority of other causes of primary hyperparathyroidism have nonpalpable parathyroids)

PARATHYROID CARCINOMA

What is it?	Primary carcinoma of the parathyroid gland
What is the number of glands usually affected?	One
What are the signs/ symptoms?	Hypercalcemia, elevated PTH, **PALPABLE** parathyroid gland (50%), pain in neck, recurrent laryngeal nerve paralysis (change in voice), hypercalcemic crisis (usually associated with calcium levels > 13)
What is the common tumor marker?	Human chorionic gonadotrophin
What is the treatment?	Surgical resection with ipsilateral thyroid lobectomy, ipsilateral lymph node resection
What percentage of all cases of primary hyperparathyroidism are caused by parathyroid carcinoma?	Approximately 1%
What are the possible postoperative complications after a parathyroidectomy?	Recurrent nerve injury (unilateral: voice change; bilateral: airway obstruction), neck hematoma (open at bedside if breathing is compromised), hypocalcemia, superior laryngeal nerve injury

What is "hungry bone syndrome"?

Severe hypocalcemia seen after surgical correction of hyperparathyroidism, as the chronically calcium-deprived bone aggressively absorbs calcium (most patients have a preoperative elevated alkaline phosphate level)

What are the signs/ symptoms of postoperative hypocalcemia?

Perioral tingling, paresthesia, positive Chvostek's sign, positive Trousseau's sign, positive tetany

53

Spleen and Splenectomy

Which arteries supply the spleen?	The splenic artery, a branch of the celiac trunk, and the short gastric arteries that arise from the gastroepiploic arteries
What is the venous drainage of the spleen?	The **portal** vein, via the splenic vein and the left gastroepiploic vein
What is said to "tickle" the spleen?	The tail of the pancreas
What percentage of people have an accessory spleen?	Approximately 1 in 5
What percentage of the total body platelets are stored in the spleen?	One-third
What are the functions of the spleen?	Filters abnormal RBCs, stores platelets, produces tuftsin and properdin (opsins), produces antibodies (especially IGM), is the site of phagocytosis (the human spleen does NOT store RBCs like the canine!)
What is the spleen's claim to fame?	The **spleen** is the **most common** intra-abdominal organ injured in **blunt trauma (although this assertion has been challenged by new studies that conclude that the liver is the most common)**
What is "delayed splenic rupture"?	A subcapsular hematoma may rupture at a later time after blunt trauma causing "delayed splenic rupture." Rupture most often occurs about 2 weeks after the injury and presents with shock/abdominal pain.

What are the signs/symptoms of ruptured/injured spleen?

Hemoperitoneum and Kehr's sign (referred pain to the tip of the left shoulder), left upper quadrant abdominal pain, and a left upper quadrant mass (Ballance's sign)

How is a spleen injury diagnosed?

Abdominal **CT, if the patient is stable;** DPL →exploratory laparotomy, if the patient is unstable

What is the treatment?

1. Nonoperative in a stable patient with an **isolated** splenic injury without hilar involvement, complete rupture, or if the patient can be stabilized
2. If patient is unstable, DPL → laparotomy with splenorrhaphy or splenectomy

What is a splenorrhaphy?

Splenic salvage operation with wrapping vicral mesh, aid of topical hemostatic agents, partial splenectomy, (VAST majority of pediatric patients undergo nonoperative treatment for blunt spleen injury)

What are the other indications for splenectomy?

Control/staging of disease/hypersplenism
Gaucher's disease
Splenic vein thrombosis
Sickle cell disease
Thrombocytopenia associated with drug abuse
Spherocytosis
Lymphomas (especially Hodgkin's disease)
Idiopathic thrombocytopenic purpura (ITP)
Thrombotic thrombocytopenic purpura (TTP)
Splenic tumors
Splenic trauma
Felty's syndrome
Lymphoproliferative disorders (i.e., NHL, CLL)
Hairy cell leukemia
Thalassemia major

Is G6PD deficiency an indication for splenectomy?	**NO**
What are the possible postsplenectomy complications?	Thrombocytosis (treat with **ASA** if platelet count is $\leq$ 1 million), subphrenic abscess, gastric dilation, and **overwhelming postsplenectomy sepsis** (**OPSS**)
What causes OPSS?	Increased susceptibility to fulminant bacteremia, meningitis, or pneumonia because of loss of splenic function
What is the incidence of OPSS in adults?	Very rare; less than 1% (more common in young children)
What is the typical presentation of OPSS?	Fever, lethargy, common cold, sore throat, URI followed by confusion, shock, and coma with death ensuing within 24 hours in up to 50% of patients
What are the common organisms associated with OPSS?	**Encapsulated:** *Streptococcus pneumoniae* accounts for more than 50% of cases Meningococcus *H. influenzae* *E. coli*
What is the most common bacteria in OPSS?	Streptococcus
What is the preventive treatment of OPSS?	**Vaccinations** for **pneumococcus,** *H. influenza,* and meningococcus Prophylactic penicillin for all minor infections/illnesses and immediate medical care if febrile illness develops
What is the best time to give immunizations to splenectomy patients?	**Preoperatively,** if at all possible
Why is an NG tube necessary after splenectomy?	To prevent gastric distention, which can blow out suture ties used to control the short gastric vessels resulting in postoperative bleeding

What lab tests are abnormal after splenectomy?

WBC count increases by 50% over the baseline; marked **thrombocytosis** occurs; RBC smear is abnormal

What are the findings on postsplenectomy RBC smear?

Peripheral smear will show Pappenheimer bodies and Howell-Jolly bodies

When and how should thrombocytopenia be treated?

When platelet count is more than 1 million (according to most experts)
Treat with **aspirin**

What is the most common cause of splenic vein thrombosis?

Pancreatitis

What opsonins are produced by the spleen?

Properdin, tuftsin (think: "PROfessionally TUF spleen")

What is the most common cause of ISOLATED GASTRIC varices?

Splenic vein thrombosis (usually due to pancreatitis)

What is the treatment of gastric varices due to splenic vein thrombosis?

Splenectomy

Which patients develop hyposplenism?

Patients with ulcerative colitis

What vaccinations should every patient with a splenectomy receive?

Pneumococcus
Meningococcus
Haemophilus influenzae type B

Define hypersplenism.

Hyperfunctioning spleen
Documented loss of blood elements (WBC, Hct, platelets)
Large spleen (splenomegaly)
Hyperactive bone marrow (trying to keep up with the loss of blood elements)

Define splenomegaly.

Enlarged spleen

What is ITP?

Autoimmune (antiplatelet antibodies in > 80% of patients) platelet destruction leading to troublesome bleeding and purpura

What is the most common cause of failure to correct thrombocytopenia after splenectomy for ITP?	Missed accessory spleen
What are the "I's" of ITP?	**I**mmune etiology (thought to be an autoimmune phenomenon) **I**mmunosuppressive treatment (initially treated with steroids) **I**mprovement with splenectomy (75% of patients have improved platelet counts after splenectomy)
What is the treatment of choice for TTP?	Plasmapheresis (splenectomy reserved as a last resort)
What is the most common physical finding of portal hypertension?	Splenomegaly

54 Surgically Correctable HTN

What is it?

Hypertension caused by conditions that are amenable to surgical correction

What percentage of patients with HTN have a surgically correctable cause?

Approximately 7%

What are the diseases that cause HTN and are surgically correctable?

Renal artery stenosis
Pheochromocytoma
Unilateral renal parenchymal disease
Cushing's syndrome
Conn's syndrome (primary hyperaldosteronism)
Hyperparathyroidism/hyperthyroidism
Coarctation of the aorta
Cancer
Neuroblastoma
Increased intracranial pressure

What is the formula for pressure?

Pressure = flow × resistance or P = F × R (think: **P**ower **F**o**R**ward); thus, an increase in flow and/or resistance results in an increase in pressure

NEUROBLASTOMA

What is it?

Embryonal tumor of neural crest origin; seen in children

What causes HTN in neuroblastoma?

Increased catecholamines

PHEOCHROMOCYTOMA

What is it?

Tumor of the adrenal medulla and other similar tissues (e.g., sympathetic ganglion) that produces catecholamines (epinephrine, norepinephrine, dopamine)

What causes HTN in pheochromocytoma?	Increased catecholamines

RENAL ARTERY STENOSIS

What is it?	Stenosis of the renal artery, resulting in decreased perfusion of the juxtaglomerular apparatus and subsequent activation of the aldosterone–renin–angiotensin system
What are the signs/ symptoms?	Most patients are asymptomatic, but may have headache, **diastolic HTN,** flank bruits (present in 50% of cases), and decreased renal function Note: Approximately 7% of patients with essential HTN also have flank bruits
What causes HTN in renal artery stenosis?	Increased renin→angiotensin/ aldosterone
Which antihypertensive is contraindicated in patients with renal artery stenosis?	Ace inhibitors

COARCTATION OF THE AORTA

What is it?	Congenital abnormality consisting of narrowing of thoracic aorta with or without intraluminal "shelf" (infolding of the media), usually found near the ductus/ligamentum arteriosum
What causes HTN in coarctation?	Increase in resistance to flow to the distal body and, thus, increased flow to the upper body

HYPERPARATHYROIDISM (↑PTH)

Define ↑PTH.	Increased secretion of PTH
What percentage of patients with hyperparathyroidism have HTN?	Approximately 10%

What causes HTN in hyperparathyroidism?

Hypercalcemia

CONN'S SYNDROME

What is it?

Hyperaldosteronism; aldosterone is abnormally secreted by an adrenal adenoma/carcinoma/hyperplasia or by an ovarian tumor

What are the two classic signs of Conn's syndrome?

HTN and hypokalemia

What causes HTN in Conn's syndrome?

Hypervolemia

CUSHING'S SYNDROME

What is it?

Excessive cortisol production

What percentage of patients with Cushing's syndrome have hypertension?

More than 75%!

What causes HTN in Cushing's syndrome?

Hypervolemia

INCREASED INTRACRANIAL PRESSURE

What causes HTN in increased ICP?

The Cushing's response (reflex), consisting of **HTN** and **bradycardia**

CANCER

What causes HTN in cancer?

Paraneoplastic syndromes

RENAL PARENCHYMAL DISEASE

What causes HTN in renal parenchymal disease?

Hypervolemia
Increased renin (which increases angiotensin [vasoconstriction] and aldosterone [hypervolemia])

55

Soft Tissue Sarcomas and Lymphomas

SOFT TISSUE SARCOMAS

What is it?	Soft tissue tumors; derived from mesoderm
How common are they?	Comprise 1% of malignant tumors
What are the risk factors?	Usually none; possibly radiation, AIDS (Kaposi's)
Name the following types of malignant sarcoma:	
Fat	Liposarcoma
Smooth muscle	Leiomyosarcoma
Histiocyte	Malignant fibrous histiocytoma
Striated muscle	Rhabdomyosarcoma
Vascular endothelium	Angiosarcoma
Fibroblast	Fibrosarcoma
Lymph vessel	Lymphangiosarcoma
Peripheral nerve	Malignant neurilemmoma or schwannoma
AIDS	Kaposi's sarcoma
What are the signs/ symptoms?	Soft tissue mass, pain from compression of adjacent structures, often noticed after minor trauma to area of mass
How do most sarcomas metastasize?	Hematogenously (i.e., via blood)

What is the most common location and route of metastasis?
Lungs via hematogenous route

What tests should be done in the preoperative workup?
CXR, ± chest CT, LFTs

What are the three most common malignant sarcomas in adults?
Fibrous histiocytoma (25%), liposarcoma (20%), leiomyosarcoma (15%)

What are the two most common in children?
Rhabdomyosarcoma (about 50%)
Fibrosarcoma (20%)

What is the most common type to metastasize to the lymph nodes?
Malignant fibrous histiocytoma

What is the most common sarcoma of the retroperitoneum?
Liposarcoma

How do sarcomas locally invade?
Usually along anatomic planes such as fascia, vessels, etc.

How is the diagnosis made?
Imaging workup—MRI is superior to CT at distinguishing the tumor from adjacent structures
Mass less than 3 cm: excisional biopsy
Mass more than 3 cm: incisional biopsy or **core biopsy**

Define excisional biopsy.
Biopsy by removing the **entire** mass

Define incisional biopsy.
Biopsy by removing a **piece** of the mass

What is the orientation of incision for incisional biopsy of a suspected extremity sarcoma?
Longitudinal, not transverse, so that the incision can be incorporated in a future resection if biopsy for sarcoma is positive

Define core biopsy.
A large bore needle that takes a core of tissue (like an earth core sample)

What is a pseudocapsule and what is its importance?
It is the outer layer of a sarcoma that represents compressed malignant cells. Microscopic extensions of tumor cells invade through the pseudocapsule into adjacent structures. Thus, definitive therapy must include a wide margin of resection to account for this phenomenon and not just be "shelled-out" like a benign growth.

What is the most important factor in the prognosis?
Histologic grade of the primary lesion

What is the treatment?
Surgical resection and radiation (postoperative, ± preoperative)

What is the treatment of pulmonary metastasis?
Surgical resection for isolated lesions

What tests should be done in the follow up?
Physical exam, chest x-rays, repeat CT/MRI of the area of resection to look for recurrence

LYMPHOMA

How is the diagnosis made?
Cervical or axillary node excisional biopsy

What cell type is associated with the histology of Hodgkin's disease?
Sternberg-Reed cells

What are the four histopathologic types of Hodgkin's disease?
1. Nodular sclerosing (most common; about 50% of cases)
2. Mixed cellularity
3. Lymphocyte predominant (best prognosis)
4. Lymphocyte depleted

What are the indications for a "staging laparotomy" in Hodgkin's disease?
Controversial; usually performed for the low stages because they are treated differently than advanced stages
Some experts rely on CT scans and do not perform laparotomy

What is a staging laparotomy for Hodgkin's lymphoma?

A laparotomy to distinguish between advanced and low-stage disease to define proper therapy. It includes:

1. **Splenectomy**
2. Iliac crest bone aspiration
3. Biopsies of splenic hilar, celiac, mesenteric, porta hepatis, para-aortic, and iliac **lymph nodes**
4. **Liver biopsy**
5. **Oophoropexy**: if the patient is a woman of childbearing years, the ovaries are marked with metallic clips and then tacked behind the uterus for protection from the radiation field.

Define the stages (Ann Arbor) of Hodgkin's disease:

Stage I

Single lymph node region

Stage II

Two or more lymph node regions on **the same side of the diaphragm**

Stage III

Involvement on **both** sides of the diaphragm

Stage IV

Diffuse and/or disseminated involvement

What is stage A Hodgkin's?

Asymptomatic (think: **A**symptomatic = stage **A**)

What is stage B Hodgkin's?

Symptomatic; weight loss, fever, night sweats, etc.
Think, stage **B** = **B**ad

What treatments are used for low versus advanced stage Hodgkin's lymphoma?

Low stage: radiotherapy
Advanced stage: chemotherapy

What percentage of patients with Hodgkin's disease can be cured?

Approximately 80%

GI LYMPHOMA

What is it?	Non-Hodgkin's lymphoma arising in the GI tract
What are the signs/ symptoms?	Abdominal pain, obstruction, GI hemorrhage, GI tract perforation
What is the treatment of gastric lymphoma?	Resection and staging biopsies
What is the treatment of intestinal lymphoma?	Resection with removal of draining lymph nodes
What is the most common site of primary GI tract lymphoma?	The stomach

56 Skin Lesions

What are the most common skin cancers?
1. Basal cell carcinoma (75%)
2. Squamous cell carcinoma (20%)
3. Melanoma (4%)

What is the most common skin cancer that causes death?
Melanoma

What is malignant melanoma?
A redundancy! All melanomas are considered malignant

SQUAMOUS CELL CARCINOMA

What is it also known as?
Epidermoid carcinoma

What is it?
Carcinoma arising from epidermal cells

What are the most common sites?
Head, neck, and hands

What are the risk factors?
Sun exposure, pale skin, chronic inflammatory process, immunosuppression, xeroderma pigmentosum, arsenic

What are the signs/ symptoms?
Raised, slightly pigmented skin lesion; ulceration/exudate; chronic scab; itching

How is the diagnosis made?
Small lesion—excisional biopsy
Large lesions—needle or incisional biopsy

What is the treatment?
Small lesion < 1 cm: excise with 0.5 cm margin
Large lesion > 1 cm: resect with at least 1 cm margins of normal tissue (large lesions may require skin graft/flap)

What is the dreaded sign of metastasis?	Palpable lymph nodes (remove involved lymph nodes)
What is Marjolin's ulcer?	Squamous cell carcinoma that arises in an area of chronic inflammation (e.g., chronic fistula, burn wound, osteomyelitis)
What is the prognosis?	Excellent if totally excised (95% cure rate); most patients with positive lymph-node metastasis eventually die from metastatic squamous cell carcinoma

BASAL CELL CARCINOMA

What is it?	Carcinoma arising in the germinating basal cell layer of epithelial cells
What are the risk factors?	Sun exposure, fair skin, radiation, chronic dermatitis, xeroderma pigmentosum
What are the most common sites?	Head, neck, and hands
What are the signs/ symptoms?	Slow-growing skin mass, (chronic, scaly) scab, ulceration, with or without pigmentation
How is the diagnosis made?	Excisional or incisional biopsy
What is the treatment?	Resection with 1 cm margin (2 mm margin in cosmetically sensitive areas)
What is the risk of metastasis?	Very low (recur locally)

MISCELLANEOUS SKIN LESIONS

What is an epidermal inclusion cyst?	A benign subcutaneous cyst filled with epidermal cells (should be removed surgically)

What is a sebaceous cyst?

A benign subcutaneous cyst filled with sebum (waxy, paste-like substance) due to a blocked sweat gland (should be removed with a small area of skin that includes the blocked sweat gland); may become infected

What is actinic keratosis?

A premalignant skin lesion due to sun exposure; seen as a scaly skin lesion (surgical removal eliminates the 20% risk of cancer transformation)

What is Bowen's disease of the skin?

Squamous carcinoma in situ (should be removed surgically, thereby removing the problem)

What is seborrheic keratosis?

Benign pigmented lesion in the elderly; observe or treat by excision (especially if there is any question of melanoma), curettage, or topical agents

What is "MOHS" surgery?

MOHS technique or surgery: repeats thin excision until margins are clear by microscopic review

57 Melanoma

What is it?	Neoplastic disorder produced by malignant transformation of the melanocyte; melanocytes are derived from neural crest cells
Which patients are at greatest risk?	Occurs almost exclusively in the white population (classically: white patients with blonde/red hair, fair skin, and a history of easily sunburning)
What are the most common sites?	#1: Skin #2: Eyes #3: Anus Think: **SEA** = **S**kin, **E**yes, **A**nus
What is the most common site in African-Americans?	Palms of the hands, soles of the feet (acral lentiginous melanoma)
What characteristics are suggestive of melanoma?	Usually a pigmented lesion with an irregular border, irregular surface, and/or irregular coloration Other clues: darkening of a pigmented lesion, development of pigmented satellite lesions, irregular margins or surface elevations, notching, recent or rapid enlargement, erosion or ulceration of surface, pruritus
What are the "A,B,C,Ds" of melanoma?	**A: A**symmetry **B: B**order irregularity **C: C**olor variation **D: D**iameter greater than 6 mm and dark lesion
What are the associated risk factors?	Severe sunburn before age 18, giant congenital nevi, family history, race (white), ultraviolet radiation (sun), multiple dysplastic nevi

How does location differ in men and women?
Men get more lesions on the trunk; women get more on the extremities

Which locations are unusual?
Noncutaneous regions, such as mucous membranes of the vulva/vagina, anorectum, esophagus, and choroidal layer of the eye

What is the most common site of melanoma in men?
Back (one-third)

What is the most common site of melanoma in women?
Legs (one-third)

What are the four histologic types?
1. Superficial spreading
2. Lentigo maligna
3. Acral lentiginous
4. Nodular

Define the following terms:

Superficial spreading melanoma
Occurs in both sun-exposed and nonexposed areas
Superficial spread is the most common type (70% of melanomas)

Lentigo maligna melanoma
Malignant cells that are superficial, found usually in elderly patients on the head or neck
Called "Hutchinson's freckle," if noninvasive
Least aggressive type; very good prognosis
Accounts for less than 10% of melanomas

Acral lentiginous melanoma
Occurs on the palms, soles, subungual areas, and mucous membranes
Accounts for ≈ 5% of melanomas (most common melanoma in African-American patients ≈ 50%)

Nodular melanoma
Vertical growth predominates
Lesions are usually dark
Most aggressive type; worst prognosis
Accounts for ≈ 15% of melanomas

What is the most common type of melanoma?

Superficial spreading (> 70%)

What type of melanoma arises in Hutchinson's freckle?

Lentigo maligna melanoma

What is Hutchinson's freckle?

Lentigo melanoma in the radial growth phase without vertical extension (noninvasive); usually occurs on the faces of elderly women

STAGING

What is Clark's classification (microstaging of tumor) I?

Tumor confined to the epidermis; recurrence rate of 0% to 5%

II?

Tumor invading the papillary dermis; 5-year recurrence rate of < 5%

III?

Tumor cells up to the junction of the papillary and reticular dermis; 5-year recurrence rate of 33%

IV?

Invasion into the reticular dermis; 5-year recurrence rate of approximately 66%

V?

Invasion into subcutaneous fat; 5-year recurrence rate of approximately 75%

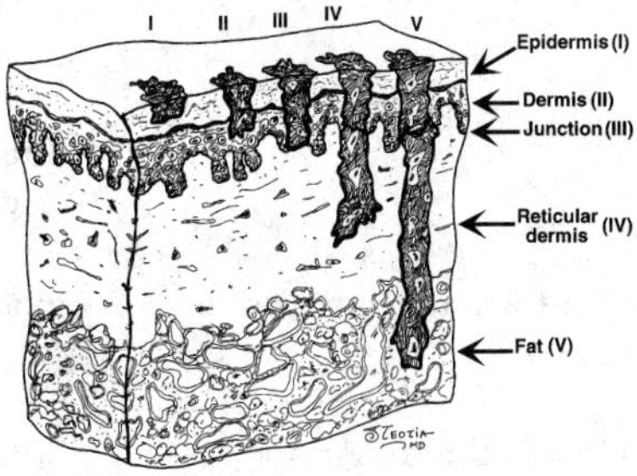

How can Clark's stages be remembered?

Think: **E**pidermis (I), **P**apillary dermis (II), **J**unction of papillary/reticular dermis (III), **R**eticular dermis (IV), and **F**at (V) = **E**very **P**igmented **J**unction **R**equires **F**ormalin

What is the Breslow classification (microstaging of tumor)?

Staging by actually measuring the depth of the lesion:
Less than 0.76 mm thickness has more than 90% cure with excision
More than 4.0 mm has at least an 80% risk of local recurrence or metastasis in 5 years

How can Breslow versus Clarke's classifications be remembered?

Think: Bres**low** = low = depth by measurement

Which tumor staging is more accurate in predicting survival?

The Breslow classification (a more consistent measure of tumor thickness)

What are the American Joint Committee on Cancer (AJCC) stages simplified:

I?

Less than 1.5 mm depth

II?

More than 1.5 mm depth

III?

Positive nodes (regional nodal basin)

IV?

Metastases (including NONregional nodal basin)

What are the common sites of metastasis?

Nodes local
Distant skin recurrence, lung, liver, bone, heart and brain
Melanoma has a specific attraction for small bowel mucosa and distant cutaneous sites
Brain metastases are a common cause of death

What are the metastatic routes?

Both lymphatic and hematogenous

How is the diagnosis made?

Excisional biopsy (complete removal leaving only normal tissue) or incisioned biopsy for very large lesions
(Early diagnosis is crucial)

What is the role of shave biopsy?

No role

When is elective lymph node dissection recommended?

Although further study is needed and underway, there is general agreement that tumors less than 0.76 mm thick have a low incidence of involved nodes and appear not to benefit from nodal dissection, and tumors more than 4.0 mm thick have little to gain from node dissection because most already have systemic disease. Remember, lymph node dissection is fraught with morbidity (e.g., lymphedema). Node dissection for intermediate-thickness melanoma is under debate and study.

How is the size of the surgical margin determined?

By depth of invasion:
0.5 cm margin if melanoma in situ
1 cm margin if less than 1 mm thick
2 cm margin if 1 to 4 mm thick
2 to 3 cm margin if more than 4 mm thick

What is the treatment of palpable lymph node metastasis?

Lymphadectomy

What factors determine the prognosis?

Depth of invasion and metastasis are the most important factors (Superficial spreading and lentigo maligna have a better prognosis because they have a longer horizontal phase of growth and are thus diagnosed at an earlier stage. Nodular has the worst prognosis because it grows predominantly vertically and metastasizes earlier.)

What is the workup to survey for metastasis in the patient with melanoma?

Physical exam, LFTs, CXR (bone scan/ CT/MRI reserved for symptoms)

What is the treatment of intestinal metastasis?

Surgical resection to prevent bleeding/ obstruction

What is the treatment of nodal metastasis?

Lymphadenectomy

What is the treatment of unresectable brain metastasis?	Radiation
What is the treatment of isolated adrenal metastasis?	Surgical resection
What is the treatment of isolated lung metastasis?	Surgical resection
What is the most common symptom of anal melanoma?	Bleeding
What is the treatment of anal melanoma?	APR or wide excision (no survival benefit from APR, but better local control)
What other therapy is available for metastatic disease?	1. IL-2 2. Interferon-α (15% response rate) 3. Monoclonal antibodies 4. Chemotherapy (e.g., dacarbazine)

58 Surgical Intensive Care

INTENSIVE CARE UNIT BASICS

How is an Intensive Care Unit note written?

The note is by **systems:**
- Neurologic (e.g., GCS, MAE, pain control)
- Pulmonary (e.g., vent settings)
- CVS (e.g., pressors, Swan numbers)
- Heme (CBC)
- FEN (e.g., Chem 10, nutrition)
- Renal (e.g., urine output, bun, cr)
- ID (e.g., T_{max}, WBC, antibiotics)
- Assessment
- Plan
- (FEN = fluids, electrolytes, nutrition); physical exam is included in each section

What are the possible causes of fever in the ICU?

Central line infection
UTI, urosepsis
Pneumonia
Intra-abdominal abscess
Sinusitis
DVT
Thrombophlebitis
Drug fever
Fungal infection, meningitis, wound infection

What is the most common bacteria in ICU pneumonia?

Gram-negative rods

INTENSIVE CARE UNIT FORMULAE/TERMS YOU SHOULD KNOW

What is CO?

Cardiac **O**utput: HR (heart rate) × SV (stroke volume)

What is the normal CO?

Between 4 and 8 L/min

What factors increase CO?	Increased contractility Increased heart rate Increased preload Decreased afterload
What is CI?	**C**ardiac **I**ndex: CO/BSA (body surface area)
What is the normal CI?	Between 2.5 and 3.5 $L/min/M_2$
What is SV?	**S**troke **V**olume: the amount of blood pumped out of the ventricle each beat; simply, end diastolic volume minus the end systolic volume **or** CO/HR
What is the normal SV?	Between 60 and 100 cc
What is CVP?	**C**entral **V**enous **P**ressure: indirect measurement of intravascular volume status
What is the normal CVP?	Between 4 and 11
What is PCWP?	**P**ulmonary **C**apillary **W**edge **P**ressure: indirectly measures left atrial pressure, which is an estimate of intravascular volume
What is the normal PCWP?	Between 5 and 15
What is anion gap?	$Na^{+} - (Cl^{-} + HCO^{-}_{3})$
What is the normal anion gap?	Between 10 and 14
What are the most common causes of high anion gap acidosis?	1. Lactic acidosis 2. Renal failure (failure to clear acids/uremia) (Also: DKA, ethanol, sepsis, methanol)
What is SVR?	**S**ystemic **V**ascular **R**esistance: MAP – CVP / CO × 80 (remember, P = FXR, **P**ower **F**o**R**ward; and calculating resistance: **R = P/F**)
What is SVRI?	**S**ystemic **V**ascular **R**esistance **I**ndex: SVR/BSA

What is the normal SVRI?	Between 1500 and 2400
What is MAP?	**M**ean **A**rterial **P**ressure: diastolic blood pressure + **1/3 (systolic – diastolic pressure)** Note: Not the mean between diastolic and systolic blood pressure because diastole lasts longer than systole
What is PVR?	**P**ulmonary **V**ascular **R**esistance: $PA_{(MEAN)}$ – PCWP / CO × 80 (PA is pulmonary artery pressure and LA is left atrial or PCWP pressure, again remember **P**ower **F**o**R**ward, **R = P/F**)
What is the normal PVR value?	100 ± 50
What is arterial oxygen content?	Hemaglobin × O_2 saturation (Sao_2)
What is Do_2?	Oxygen delivery: CO × (hemoglobin × Sao_2)
What factors can increase oxygen delivery?	Increased CO by increasing SV and/or HR, increased oxygen content by either increasing the hemoglobin and/or increasing Sao_2
What is mixed venous oxygen saturation?	SvO_2; simply, the O_2 saturation of the blood in the right ventricle; an indirect measure of peripheral oxygen supply and demand
Which lab values help assess adequate oxygen delivery?	SvO_2 (low with inadequate delivery), lactic acid (elevated with inadequate delivery), pH (acidosis with inadequate delivery)
What is FENa?	Fractional excretion of sodium: $U_{Na^+} \times P_{cr} / P_{Na^+} \times U_{cr} \times 100$ **Think: "You Need Pee" = You (Urine) Need (Na+) Pee (plasma);** therefore, $\mathbf{U_{Na^+}} \times \mathbf{P_{Cr}}$; and for the denominator switch everything, or $P_{Na^+} \times U_{Cr}$

What is the prerenal FENa value?	Less than 1.0; renal failure due to decreased renal blood flow (e.g., cardiogenic, hypovolemia, arterial obstruction, etc)
What is the formula for flow/pressure/resistance?	Remember **P**ower **F**o**R**ward: **P**ressure = **F**low × **R**esistance
What is the "10 for 0.08 rule" of acid-base?	For every increase of $Paco_2$ by 10 mm Hg, the pH falls by 0.08.
What is the "40, 50, 60 for 70, 80, 90 rule" for O_2 sats?	A PaO_2 of **40, 50, 60** corresponds roughly to an O_2 sat of **70, 80, 90,** respectively
One liter of O_2 via nasal cannula raises FiO_2 by how much?	Approximately 3% to 4%
What is pure respiratory acidosis?	**Low pH** (acidosis), **increased $Paco_2$**, nl bicarbonate (or high with compensation)
What is pure respiratory alkalosis?	**High pH** (alkalosis), **decreased $Paco_2$**, nl bicarbonate (or low with compensation)
What is pure metabolic acidosis?	**Low pH, low bicarbonate**, nl (or low with compensation) $Paco_2$
What is pure metabolic alkalosis?	**High pH, high bicarbonate**, nl (or high with compensation) $Paco_2$
What does MOF stand for?	**M**ultiple **O**rgan **F**ailure
What does SIRS stand for?	**S**ystemic **I**nflammatory **R**esponse **S**yndrome

SICU DRUGS

DOPAMINE

What is the site of action and effect at the following levels:

Low dose (1–3 μg/kg/min)?	++ Dopa agonist; **renal vasodilation** (A.K.A. "renal dose dopamine")

Intermediate dose (4–10 μg/kg/min)?	+ Alpha, ++ beta; positive inotropy and some vasoconstriction
High dose (> 10 μg/kg/min)?	+++ Alpha agonist; marked afterload increase due to arteriolar vasoconstriction

DOBUTAMINE

What is the site of action?	+++ $Beta_1$ agonist, ++ $beta_2$
What is the effect?	↑ inotropy; ↑ chronotropy, **decrease in systemic vascular resistance**

ISOPROTERENOL

What is the site of action?	+++ $Beta_1$ and $beta_2$ agonist
What is the effect?	↑ inotropy; ↑ chronotropy; (+ vasodilation of skeletal and mesenteric vascular beds)

EPINEPHRINE (EPI)

What is the site of action?	$Alpha_1$, $alpha_2$, $beta_1$, and $beta_2$ agonist
What is the effect?	↑ inotropy; ↑ chronotropy
What is the effect at high doses?	Vasoconstriction

NOREPINEPHRINE (NE)

What is the site of action?	$Alpha_1$, $alpha_2$, and $beta_1$ agonist
What is the effect?	↑ inotropy; ↑ chronotropy; ++ increase in blood pressure
What is the effect at high doses?	Severe vasoconstriction

NITROGLYCERINE (NTG)

What is the site of action?	+++ Venodilation; + arteriolar dilation

What is the effect? Increased venous capacitance, decreased preload, coronary arteriole vasodilation

SODIUM NITROPRUSSIDE (SNP)

What is the site of action? +++ Venodilation; +++ arteriolar dilation

What is the effect? Deceased preload; decreased afterload (allowing blood pressure titration)

What ICU IV medication bag must be covered with aluminum foil because it will be broken down by light? SNP

INTENSIVE CARE PHYSIOLOGY

Define the following terms:

Preload The load on the heart muscle that stretches it to end-diastolic volume (end-diastolic pressure) = **intravascular volume**

Afterload The load or resistance the heart must pump against = vascular tone = **SVR**

Contractility The force of heart muscle contraction

Compliance The distensibility of the heart by the preload

What is the Frank-Starling curve? Cardiac output increases with increasing preload up to a point

What is the clinical significance of the steep slope of the Starling curve relating end-diastolic volume to cardiac output? It demonstrates the importance of preload in determining cardiac output.

What factors influence the oxygen content of whole blood? Oxygen content is composed **largely** of that oxygen bound to hemoglobin, and is thus determined by the hemoglobin concentration and the arterial oxygen saturation; the partial pressure of oxygen dissolved in plasma plays a minor role.

What determines the oxygen delivery to the tissues?

The oxygen content of whole blood and the cardiac output

What factors influence mixed venous oxygen saturation?

Oxygen delivery (hemoglobin concentration, arterial oxygen saturation, cardiac output) and oxygen extraction

What lab test for tissue ischemia is based on the shift from aerobic to anaerobic metabolism?

Serum lactic acid levels

Define the following terms:

Dead space

That part of the inspired air that will not participate in gas exchange; it includes the anatomic dead space (the gas in the large airways/ET tube not in contact with capillaries) and the physiologic dead space (the alveolar gas that does not equilibrate with capillary blood)
Think: space = air

Shunt fraction

That fraction of pulmonary venous blood that did not participate in gas exchange
Think: shunt = blood

What causes increased dead space?

Overventilation (emphysema, excessive PEEP) or underperfusion (pulmonary embolus, low cardiac output)

What is the physiologic effect of increasing dead-space ventilation?

Progressive hypoxemia and hypercapnia

What causes increased shunt fraction?

Underventilation (pneumonia, pulmonary edema, respiratory distress syndrome, mucus plugging) or overperfusion (loss of pulmonary vascular autoregulation as in massive pulmonary embolus), SNP

What is the physiologic effect of increasing shunt fraction?

Initially, progressive hypoxemia, followed by late hypercapnia

At high shunt fractions, what is the effect of increasing FiO_2 on arterial PO_2?

At high shunt fractions (> 50%), changes in FiO_2 have almost **no effect** on arterial Po_2 because the blood that does "see" the O_2 is already at **maximal** O_2 absorption and, thus, increasing the FiO_2 has no effect (FiO_2 can be minimized to prevent oxygen toxicity).

At what concentration does O_2 toxicity occur?

FiO_2 of 60% × 48 hours; thus, try to keep FiO_2 below 50% at all times

What are the main causes of carbon dioxide retention?

Hypoventilation, increased dead space ventilation, and increased carbon dioxide production (as in hypermetabolic states)

Does hypoventilation affect oxygen saturation?

No; you can have an O_2 sat of 100% and a Pco_2 of 150!

Why are carbohydrates minimized in the diet/TPN of patients having difficulty with hypercapnia?

The respiratory quotient (RQ) is the ratio of carbon dioxide production to oxygen consumption, and is highest for carbohydrates (1.0) and lowest for fats (0.7); by minimizing carbohydrate consumption, the carbon dioxide production at any metabolic rate is minimized.

HEMODYNAMIC MONITORING

Why are indwelling arterial lines used for blood pressure monitoring in critically ill patients?

Because of the need for frequent measurements, the inaccuracy of frequently repeated cuff measurements, the inaccuracy of cuff measurements in hypotension, and the need for frequent arterial blood sampling/labs

Which pressures/values are obtained from a Swan-Ganz catheter?

CVP, PA pressures, PCWP, CO, PVR, SVR

Identify the Swan-Ganz waveforms.

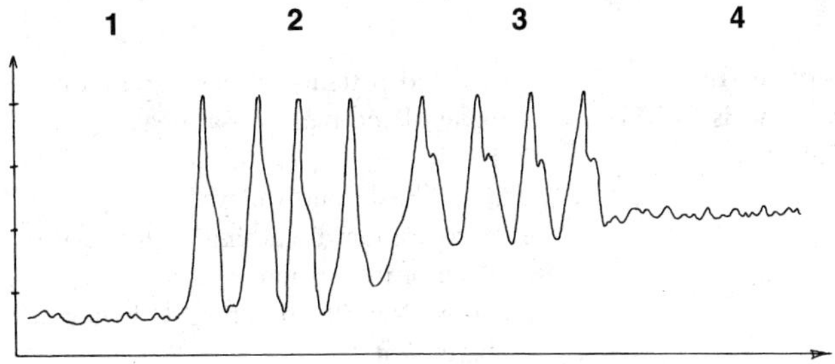

1. CVP/right atrium
2. Right ventricle
3. Pulmonary artery
4. Wedge

What is PCWP?

Pulmonary **C**apillary **W**edge **P**ressure: pulmonary capillary pressure after balloon occlusion of the pulmonary artery, which is equal to left atrial pressure because there are no valves in the pulmonary system. The left atrial pressure is essentially equivalent to left ventricular end diastolic pressure (LVEDP), left heart preload, and **intravascular volume status**

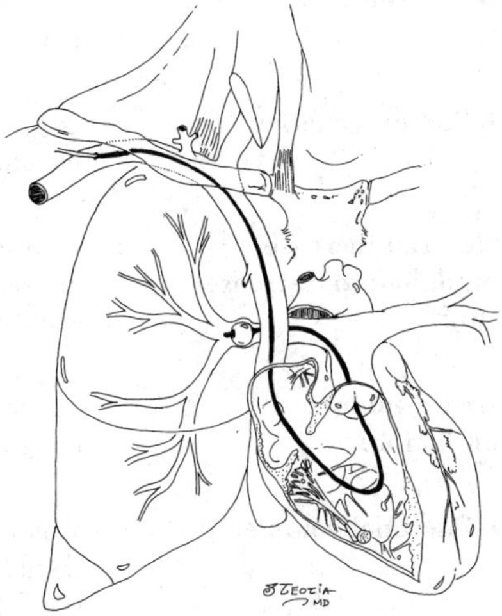

What is the primary use of the pulmonary capillary wedge pressure?

As an indirect measure of preload = intravascular volume

At what point in the respiratory cycle is PCWP most accurate?

Ventilated patient—at end expiration
Nonventilated patient—at peak inspiration
Think: "Peaks and valleys"
Peaks—**P**atient breathing on his own = **P**eak of inspiration
Valleys—**V**entilated patient = **V**alley of expiration

In which clinical situations is PCWP not an accurate estimate of preload?

Pulmonary disease, such as adult respiratory distress syndrome; pulmonary hypertension; valvular heart disease; ischemic heart disease with a noncompliant ventricle; high levels of PEEP; tamponade; PTX

How does thermodilution determine the cardiac output?

The temperature of a proximal saline injection is determined at a point distal (pulmonary artery) to its injection port. The temperature difference determines the amount of blood flow and, thus, cardiac output.

MECHANICAL VENTILATION

Define ventilation.

Air through the lungs; monitored by P_{CO_2}

Define oxygenation.

Oxygen delivery to the alveoli; monitored by O_2 sats and P_{O_2}

What can increase ventilation to decrease P_{CO_2}?

Increased respiratory rate (RR), increased tidal volume (minute ventilation)

What is minute ventilation?

Volume of gas ventilated through the lungs (RR × tidal volume)

Define tidal volume.

Volume delivered with each breath; should be 10 to 15 cc/kg on the ventilator

Are ventilation and oxygenation related?

No; you can have an O_2 sat of 100% and a P_{CO_2} of 150. O_2 sats do not tell you anything about the P_{CO_2}!(key point!)

What can increase P_{O_2} (oxygenation)in the ventilated patient?

Increased FiO_2
Increased PEEP

What can decrease P_{CO_2} in the ventilated patient?

Increased RR
Increased tidal volume
(i.e., increase minute ventilation)

Modes Defined

IMV?

Intermittent mandatory ventilation: mode with intermittent mandatory ventilations at a predetermined rate; patients can also breathe on their own above the mandatory rate **without** help from the ventilator

SIMV?

Synchronous IMV: mode of IMV that delivers the mandatory breath synchronously with patient's initiated effort; if no breath is initiated, the ventilator delivers the predetermined mandatory breath

A–C?

Assist–control ventilation: mode in which the ventilator delivers a breath when the patient initiates a breath, or the ventilator "assists" the patient to breathe; if the patient does not initiate a breath, the ventilator takes "control" and delivers a breath at a predetermined rate

In contrast to IMV, all breaths are by the ventilator.

CPAP?

Continuous **P**ositive **A**irway **P**ressure: positive pressure delivered **continuously** (during expiration and inspiration) by the ventilator, but no volume breaths (patient breathes on his own)

Pressure support?	Pressure is delivered **with an initiated breath** to assist breathing (pressure is NOT continuous—only with initiated breath)
What are the effects of positive pressure ventilation in a patient with hypovolemia or low lung compliance?	Venous return is decreased and cardiac output is decreased.
Define PEEP.	**P**ositive **E**nd **E**xpiration **P**ressure: positive pressure maintained at the end of a breath; keeps alveoli open
What is "physiologic PEEP"?	PEEP of 5 cm H_2O; thought to approximate normal pressure in normal nonintubated people caused by the closed glottis
What are the side effects of increasing levels of PEEP?	**Barotrauma** (injury to airway = pneumothorax), decreased CO due to decreased preload
What are the typical initial ventilator settings:	
Mode?	Intermittent mandatory ventilation
Tidal volume?	10 to 15 ml/kg
Ventilator rate?	10 breaths/min
FiO_2?	100% and wean down
PEEP?	5 cm H_2O From these parameters, change according to blood–gas analysis
What clinical situations cause an increase in airway resistance?	Airway or endotracheal tube obstruction, bronchospasm, ARDS, mucus plug, CHF (pulmonary edema)
What mechanical situations cause a decrease in respiratory compliance?	Pneumothorax, atelectasis, pneumonia, pulmonary edema, alveolar air trapping, ARDS

What are the presumed advantages of positive end expiratory pressure (PEEP)?

Prevention of alveolar collapse and atelectasis, improved gas exchange, increased pulmonary compliance, decreased shunt fraction

What are the possible disadvantages of PEEP?

Decreased cardiac output, especially in the setting of hypovolemia; decreased gas exchange; ↓compliance with high levels of PEEP, fluid retention, increased intracranial pressure, barotrauma

What parameters must be evaluated in deciding if a patient is ready to be extubated?

Gas exchange ($PaO_2 > 75$, $PaCO_2 < 45$), tidal volume (> 5 cc/kg), minute ventilation (< 10 L), negative inspiratory pressure (< –20 cm H_20 or more negative), $FiO_2 \leq 40\%$, PEEP 5

What is a possible source of fever in a patient with an NG tube or nasal endotracheal tube?

Sinusitis (diagnosed by sinus films/CT)

What is the 35–45 rule of blood gas values?

Normal vlaues:
pH = **7.35–7.45**
PCO = **35–45**

59

Vascular Surgery

What is atherosclerosis?

A diffuse disease process in arteries; atheromas containing cholesterol and lipid form within the intima and inner media, often accompanied by ulcerations and smooth muscle hyperplasia

What is the common theory of how atherosclerosis is initiated?

Endothelial injury→platelets adhere→growth factors released→ smooth muscle hyperplasia/plaque deposition

What are the risk factors for atherosclerosis?

Hypertension, **smoking,** diabetes mellitus, family history, hypercholesterolemia, obesity, and sedentary lifestyle

What are the common sites of plaque formation in arteries?

Branch points (carotid bifurcation), tethered sites (superficial femoral artery [SFA] in Hunter's canal in the leg)

What must be present for a successful arterial bypass operation?

1. Inflow (e.g., patent aorta)
2. Outflow (e.g., open distal popliteal artery)
3. Run off (e.g., patent trifurcation vessels down to the foot)

What is the major principle of safe vascular surgery?

Get **proximal and distal** control of the vessel to be worked on!

What does it mean to "POTTS" a vessel?

Place a vessel loop twice around a vessel so that if you put tension on the vessel loop, it will occlude the vessel

What is the suture needle orientation through graft versus diseased artery in a graft to artery anastomosis?

Needle "in to out" of the lumen in diseased artery to help **tack down the plaque** and the needle "out-to-in" on the graft

What are the layers of an artery?

1. Intima
2. Media
3. Adventia

Which arteries supply the blood vessel itself?

Vasovasorum

What is a true aneurysm?

Dilation (> 2x nl diameter) of all three layers of a vessel

What is a false (pseudo)aneurysm?

Dilation of artery not involving all three layers (e.g., hematoma with fibrous covering)

Often connects with vessel lumen and blood swirls inside the false aneurysm

PERIPHERAL VASCULAR DISEASE

Define the arterial anatomy.

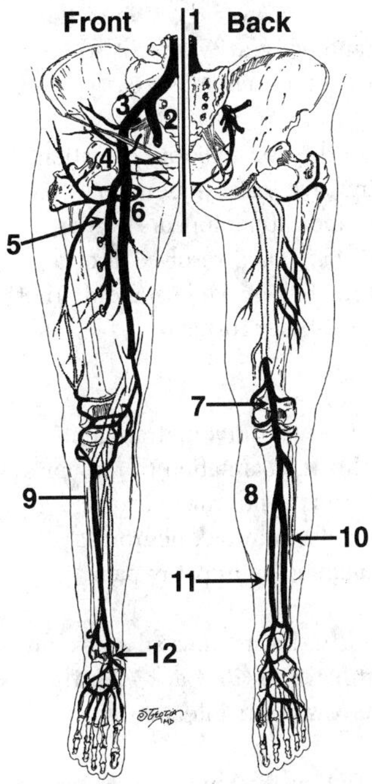

1. Aorta
2. Internal iliac (hypogastric)
3. External iliac
4. Common femoral artery
5. Profundi femoral artery
6. Superficial femoral artery (SFA)
7. Popliteal artery
8. Trifurcation
9. Anterior tibial
10. Peroneal artery
11. Posterior tibial artery
12. Dorsalis pedis artery

What is peripheral vascular disease (PVD)?

Occlusive atherosclerotic disease in the lower extremities

What is the most common site of arterial atherosclerotic occlusion in the lower extremities?	Occlusion of the SFA in Hunter's canal
What are the symptoms of PVD?	Intermittent claudication, rest pain, impotence, sensorimotor impairment, tissue loss
What is intermittent claudication?	Pain and/or cramping of the lower extremity, usually the calf muscle, after walking a specific distance; then the pain/cramping resolves after stopping for a specific amount of time while standing; this pattern is reproducible
What is rest pain?	Pain in the foot, usually over the distal metatarsals; this pain arises at rest (classically at night, awakening the patient)
What classically resolves rest pain?	Hanging the foot over the side of the bed or standing; gravity affords some extra flow to the ischemic areas
How can vascular causes of claudication be differentiated from nonvascular causes, such as neurogenic claudication or arthritis?	History (in the vast majority of patients) and noninvasive tests; remember, vascular claudication appears after a specific distance and resolves after a specific time of rest while standing (not so with most other forms of claudication)
What is the differential diagnosis of lower extremity claudication?	Neurogenic (e.g., nerve entrapment/discs), arthritis, coarctation of the aorta, popliteal artery syndrome, chronic compartment syndrome, neuromas, anemia, diabetic neuropathy pain
What are the signs of PVD?	Absent pulses, bruits, muscular atrophy, decreased hair growth, thick toenails, tissue necrosis/ulcers/infection
What is the site of a PVD ulcer versus venous stasis ulcer?	PVD arterial insufficiency ulcer—usually on the toes/foot Venous stasis ulcer—medial malleolus (ankle)

What is the ABI?	The **A**nkle to **B**rachial **I**ndex (ABI); simply, the ratio of the systolic blood pressure at the ankle to the systolic blood pressure at the arm (brachial artery) A:B; ankle pressure taken with Doppler; the ABI is noninvasive
What ABIs are associated with normals, claudicators, and rest pain?	Normal ABI—$\geq$ 1.0 Claudicator ABI—< 0.7 Rest pain ABI—< 0.4
Who gets false ABI readings?	Patients with calcified arteries, especially those with diabetes
What are PVRs?	**P**ulse **V**olume **R**ecordings; pulse wave forms are recorded from lower extremities representing volume of blood per heart beat at sequential sites down leg A large wave form means good collateral blood flow. (Noninvasive using pressure cuffs)
Prior to surgery for chronic PVD, what diagnostic test will every patient receive?	**A-gram** (arteriogram: dye in vessel and x-rays) maps disease and allows for best treatment option (i.e., angioplasty vs. surgical bypass vs. endarterectomy) Gold standard for diagnosing PVD
What is the bedside management of a patient with PVD?	1. Sheep skin (easy on the heels) 2. Foot cradle (keeps sheets/blankets off the feet) 3. Skin lotion to avoid further cracks in the skin that can go on to form a fissure and then an ulcer
What are the indications for surgical treatment in PVD?	1. Rest pain 2. Tissue necrosis 3. Infection 4. Severe claudication refractory to conservative treatment that affects quality of life/livelihood (e.g., can't work due to the claudication)
What is the treatment of claudication?	For the vast majority, conservative treatment, including exercise, smoking cessation, treatment of HTN, diet, aspirin, with or without Trental (pentoxifylline)

How does aspirin work?

Inhibits platelets (inhibits cyclo-oxygenase)

How does Trental (pentoxifylline) work?

Results in increased RBC deformity and flexibility (think: pento**X**ifylline = RBC fle**X**ibility)

What is the risk of limb loss with claudication?

Five percent limb loss at 5 years (think: 5 in 5)

What is the risk of limb loss with rest pain?

More than 50% of patients will have amputation of the limb at some point

In the patient with PVD, what is the main postoperative concern?

Cardiac status, because most patients with PVD have coronary artery disease and about 20% have an AAA

MI is the most common cause of postoperative death after a PVD operation

What is Leriche's syndrome?

Impotence, buttock claudication, and gluteus muscle atrophy due to occlusive disease of the iliacs/distal aorta

Think **C.I.A.:**

C: Claudication

I: Impotence

A: Atrophy

What are the treatment options for severe PVD?

1. Surgical graft bypass
2. Angioplasty—balloon dilation
3. Endarterectomy—remove diseased intima and media
4. Surgical patch angioplasty (place patch over stenosis)

What is a FEM POP bypass?

Bypass SFA occlusion with a graft from the femoral artery to the popliteal artery

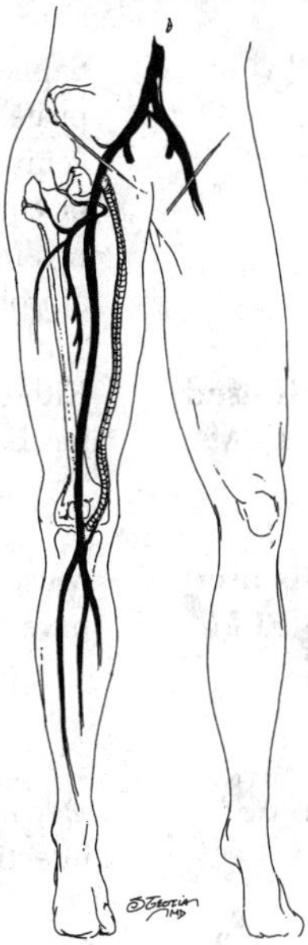

What is a FEM DISTAL bypass?

Bypass from the femoral artery to a distal artery (peroneal artery, anterior tibial artery, or posterior tibial artery)

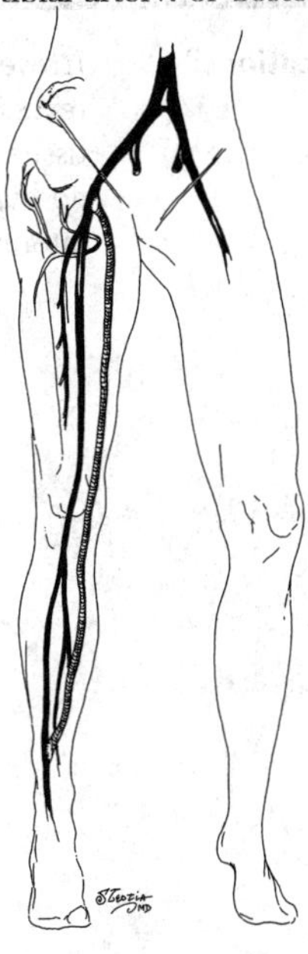

What graft material has the longest patency rate?

Autologous vein graft

What is an "in situ" vein graft?

Saphenous vein is more or less left in place, all branches are ligated, and the vein valves are broken with a small hook or cut out. A vein can also be used if reversed so that the valves do not cause a problem.

What type of graft is used for above-the-knee FEM POP bypass?

Either vein or Gortex® graft; vein still has better patency

What type of graft is used for below the knee FEM POP or FEM distal bypass?

Must use vein graft; prosthetic grafts have a prohibitive thrombosis rate

What is DRY gangrene?

Dry necrosis of tissue without signs of infection ("mummified tissue")

What is WET gangrene?

Moist necrotic tissue with signs of infection

LOWER EXTREMITY AMPUTATIONS

What are the indications?

Irreversible tissue ischemia (no hope for revascularization bypass) and necrotic tissue, severe infection, severe pain with no bypassable vessels, or if patient is not interested in a bypass procedure

Identify the level of the following amputations:

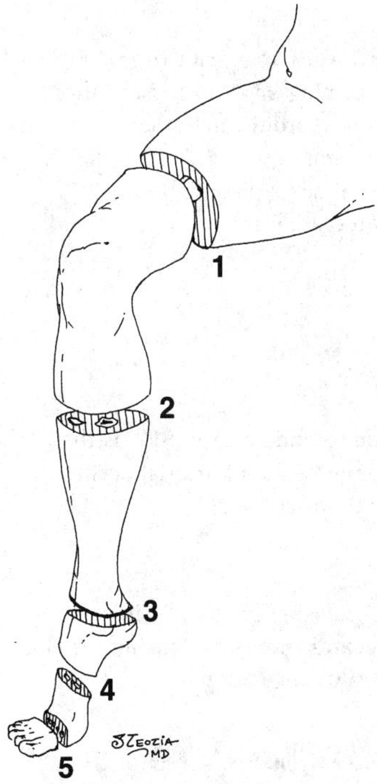

1. Above-the-knee amputation (AKA)
2. Below-the-knee amputation (BKA)
3. Symes amputation
4. Transmetatarsal amputation
5. Toe amputation

What is a Ray amputation? Removal of toe and head of metatarsal

ACUTE ARTERIAL OCCLUSION

What is it? Acute occlusion of an artery, usually by embolization; other causes include acute thrombosis of an atheromatous lesion, vascular trauma

What are the classic signs/symptoms of acute arterial occlusion? The "six P's": pain, paralysis, pallor, paresthesia, polar (some say poikilothermia—you pick), pulselessness (you **must** know these!)

What is the classic timing of pain with acute arterial occlusion due to an embolus? Acute onset; the patient can classically tell you exactly when and where it happened

What is the immediate preoperative management?

1. Anticoagulate with IV heparin (bolus followed by constant infusion)
2. A-gram

What are the sources of emboli?

1. Heart—85% (e.g., clot from AFib, clot forming on dead muscle after MI, endocarditis, myxoma)
2. Aneurysms
3. Atheromatous plaque (atheroembolism)

What is the most common cause of embolus from the heart?

AFib

What is the most common site of arterial occlusion by an embolus?

Common femoral artery (SFA is the most common site of arterial occlusion due to atherosclerosis)

Diagnostic studies?

1. A-gram
2. EKG (looking for MI, AFib)
3. Echocardiogram (±) looking for clot, MI, valve vegetation

What is the treatment?

Surgical embolectomy via cutdown and Fogarty balloon (bypass is reserved for embolectomy failure)

What is a Fogarty?

Fogarty balloon catheter—catheter with a balloon tip that can be inflated with saline; used for embolectomy/thrombectomy by insinuating the catheter with the balloon deflated past the embolus and then inflating the balloon and pulling the catheter out; the balloon brings the embolus with it

How many mm in diameter is a 12 French Fogarty catheter?

Simple; to get mm from French measurements, divide the French number by pi or 3.14; thus, a 12 French catheter is 12/3 = 4 mm in diameter

What must you look for postoperatively after reperfusion of a limb?

Compartment syndrome, hyperkalemia, renal failure due to myoglobinuria, MI

What is compartment syndrome?

The leg (calf) is separated into compartments by very unyielding fascia; **tissue swelling** due to reperfusion can cause an increase in the intracompartmental pressure, resulting in decreased capillary flow, ischemia, and myonecrosis; myonecrosis may occur after the intracompartment pressure reaches only 30 mm Hg

What are the signs/ symptoms of compartment syndrome?

Classic signs include pain, especially after passive flexing/extension of the foot, paralysis, paresthesias, and pallor; **pulses are present** in most cases because systolic pressure is much higher than the minimal 30 mm Hg needed for the syndrome!

Can a patient have a pulse and compartment syndrome?

YES!

How is the diagnosis made?

History/suspicion, compartment pressure measurement

What is the treatment of compartment syndrome?

Treatment includes opening compartments via bilateral calf- incision fasciotomies of all 4 compartments in the calf.

ABDOMINAL AORTIC ANEURYSMS

What is it also known as?

AAA, or "triple A"

What is it?

An abnormal dilation of the abdominal aorta (> 1.5–2x normal), forming a true aneurysm

What is the common etiology?

CONTROVERSIAL; believed to be **atherosclerotic** in 95% of cases, although the cause is thought to be multifactorial

Common underlying defect is a vessel-wall weakness secondary to loss of elastin/collagen.

What is the most common site?	Infrarenal (95%)
What is the incidence?	Five percent of all adults over 60 years of age; approximately 4% of white men (highest risk group) About 1 in 5 patients with PVD will have an AAA; thus, rule out AAA in all your patients with PVD!
What are the risk factors?	**Atherosclerosis,** hypertension, smoking, male gender, advanced age
What are the symptoms?	Most AAAs are **asymptomatic** and are discovered during routine abdominal exam by primary care physicians; in the remainder, symptoms range from vague epigastric discomfort to back/abdominal pain
What are the signs of rupture?	Classic triad of ruptured AAA: 1. **Abdominal pain** 2. **Pulsatile abdominal mass** 3. **Hypotension** Pulsatile mass is usually left of the midline and above the umbilicus. Severe back or flank pain and signs of blood loss suggests ruptured/leaking AAA; if a patient has the classic triad, take him straight to the OR.
What are the risk factors for rupture?	Recent rapid expansion, large diameter, hypertension, COPD, symptomatic
By how much each year do AAAs grow?	Approximately 2 to 4 mm/year on average (larger AAAs grow faster than smaller AAAs)
Why do larger AAAs rupture more often and grow faster than smaller AAAs?	Probably because of Laplace's law (wall tension = pressure x diameter)
What is the risk of rupture per year based on AAA diameter size:	
Less than 5 cm?	4%

Between 5 and 7 cm? 7%

More than 7 cm? 20%

What is the risk of rupture within 5 years based on AAA diameter:

Less than 5 cm? 20% rupture

Between 5 and 7 cm? 33%

More than 7 cm? More than 90%

Where does the aorta bifurcate? At the level of the **umbilicus;** therefore, when palpating for an AAA, palpate above the umbilicus and below the xiphoid process

What is the differential diagnosis? Acute pancreatitis, aortic dissection, mesenteric ischemia, MI, perforated ulcer, diverticulosis, renal colic, etc.

What are the diagnostic tests? Use U/S to follow AAA clinically; other tests involve contrast CT and A-gram; A-gram will assess lumen patency and iliac/renal involvement.

What is the limitation of A-gram? AAAs often have large mural thrombi, which result in a falsely reduced diameter because only the patent lumen is visualized.

What are the signs of AAA on AXR? Calcification in the aneurysm wall, best seen on lateral projection (A.K.A. egg-shell calcifications)

What are the indications for surgical repair of AAA? **AAA more than 5 cm** in diameter, if the patient does not have any overwhelming contraindications to surgery; also, rupture of the AAA, rapid growth, symptoms

What is the treatment? Prosthetic graft placement, with rewrapping of the native aneurysm adventitia around the prosthetic graft after the thrombus is removed; when rupture is strongly suspected, start IV fluids, cross match blood, and **proceed to immediate laparotomy; there is no time for diagnostic tests!**

Why wrap the graft in the native aorta?
To reduce the incidence of enterograft fistula formation

What type of repair should be performed with AAA and iliacs severely occluded or iliac aneurysm(s)?
Aortobi-iliac or aortobifemoral graft replacement (bifurcated graft)

What is the treatment if the patient has abdominal pain, pulsatile abdominal mass, and hypotension?
OR, for emergent AAA repair

What is the treatment if the patient has known AAA and new onset of abdominal pain or back pain?
Straight to the OR for surgical repair

What is the mortality rate associated with the following types of AAA treatment:

Elective?
Good; less than 4% operative mortality

Ruptured?
Poor; more than 50% operative mortality (including those who die prior to reaching the hospital, the mortality of a ruptured AAA is about **90%**)

What is the leading cause of postoperative death in a patient undergoing elective AAA treatment?
Myocardial infarction

What are the other etiologies of AAA?
Inflammatory (connective tissue diseases), mycotic (a misnomer because most are due to bacteria, **not** fungi)

What is the mean normal abdominal aortic diameter?
2 cm

What are the possible operative complications?
Atheroembolism, declamping hypotension, acute renal failure (especially if aneurysm involves the renal arteries), ureteral injury, hemorrhage

Why is colonic ischemia a concern in the repair of AAAs?

Often the IMA is sacrificed during surgery, which relies on collateral circulation to perfuse the left colon; if the collaterals are not adequate, the patient will have colonic ischemia

What are the signs of colonic ischemia?

Heme-positive stool, or bright red blood per rectum (BRBPR)

What is the study of choice to diagnose colonic ischemia?

Colonoscopy

When is colonic ischemia seen postoperatively?

Usually in the first week

What is the treatment of necrotic sigmoid colon due to colonic ischemia?

1. Resection of necrotic colon
2. Hartmann's pouch or mucus fistula
3. End colostomy

What is the possible long-term complication that often presents with both upper/lower GI bleeding?

Aortoenteric fistula (fistula between aorta and duodenum)

What are the other possible postoperative complications?

Impotence (sympathetic plexus injury), retrograde ejaculation, aortovenous fistula (to IVC), graft infection, **anterior spinal syndrome**

What is the anterior spinal syndrome?

Classically:

1. Paraplegia
2. Loss of bladder/bowel control
3. Loss of pain/temperature sensation below level of involvement
4. **Sparing of proprioception**

Anterior spinal syndrome is due to spinal cord ischemia from cross clamping of the aorta (higher incidence with ruptured AAA)

Which artery is involved in anterior spinal cord syndrome?

Artery of **Adamkiewicz**—supplies the anterior spinal cord

What are the most common bacteria involved in aortic graft infections?

1. *Staphylococcus aureus*
2. *Staphylococcus epidermidis* (usually late)

How is a graft infection and an aortoenteric fistula treated?

Perform an **extraanatomic bypass** with resection of the graft

What is an extraanatomic bypass graft?

Axillofemoral bypass graft—**graft not in a normal vascular path;** usually, the graft goes from the axillary artery to the femoral artery and then from one femoral artery to the other (fem-fem bypass)

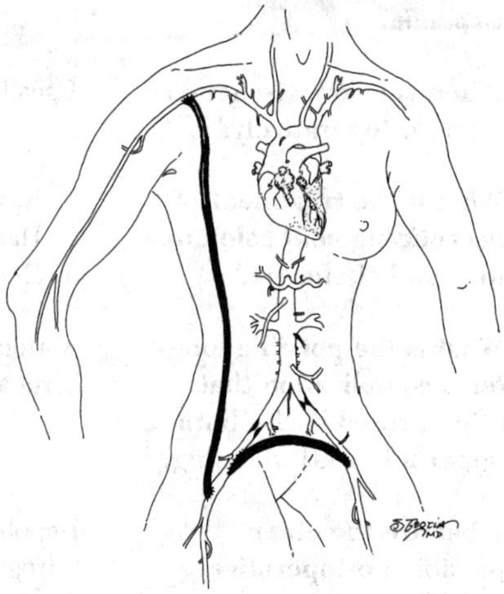

CLASSIC INTROP QUESTIONS DURING AAA REPAIR

Which vein crosses the neck of the AAA proximally?

The renal vein

What part of the small bowel crosses in front of the AAA?

The duodenum

Which large vein runs to the left of the AAA?

IMV

Which artery comes off the middle of the AAA and runs to the left?

IMA

Which vein runs behind the RIGHT common iliac artery?

The **LEFT** common iliac vein

MESENTERIC ISCHEMIA

CHRONIC MESENTERIC ISCHEMIA

What is it?

Chronic intestinal ischemia due to long-term occlusion of the intestinal arteries; most commonly due to atherosclerosis; usually in two or more arteries because of the extensive collaterals

What are the symptoms?

Weight loss, postprandial abdominal pain, anxiety/fear of food because of postprandial pain, ± heme occult, ± diarrhea/vomiting

What is "intestinal angina"?

Postprandial pain due to gut ischemia

What are the signs?

Abdominal bruit is commonly heard

How is the diagnosis made?

A-gram

What supplies blood to the gut?

1. SMA
2. IMA
3. Celiac axis vessels

What is the classic finding on A-gram?

Two of the three mesenteric arteries are occluded and there is atherosclerotic narrowing of the third patent artery

What are the treatment options?

Bypass, endarterectomy

ACUTE MESENTERIC ISCHEMIA

What is it?

Acute onset of intestinal ischemia

What are the causes?

1. **Emboli** to a mesenteric vessel from the heart
2. **Acute thrombosis** of long-standing atherosclerosis of mesenteric artery

What are the causes of emboli from the heart?

AFib, MI, cardiomyopathy, valve disease/endocarditis, mechanical heart valve

What drug has been associated with acute intestinal ischemia?	Digitalis
To which intestinal artery do emboli preferentially go?	Superior mesenteric artery (SMA)
What are the signs/symptoms of acute mesenteric ischemia?	Severe pain—classically "**pain out of proportion to physical exam,**" no peritoneal signs until necrosis, vomiting/diarrhea/hyperdefecation, ± heme stools
What is the classic triad of acute mesenteric ischemia?	1. Acute onset of pain 2. Vomiting and/or diarrhea 3. History of AFib or heart disease
How is the diagnosis made?	History/physical exam → A-gram (waste no time!)
What is the treatment of a mesenteric embolus?	Perform Fogarty catheter embolectomy, resect obviously necrotic intestine, and leave marginal-looking bowel until a second-look laparotomy is performed 24–72 hours postop
What is the treatment of acute thrombosis?	**Papaverine** vasodilator via A-gram catheter until **patient is in the OR;** then, most surgeons would perform a supraceliac aorta graft to the involved intestinal artery or endarterectomy; intestinal resection/second-look as needed

MEDIAN ARCUATE LIGAMENT SYNDROME

What is it?	Mesenteric ischemia due to narrowing of the celiac axis vessels by extrinsic compression by the median arcuate ligament
What are the symptoms?	Postprandial pain, weight loss
What are the signs?	Abdominal bruit in almost all patients
How is the diagnosis made?	A-gram
What is the treatment?	Release arcuate ligament surgically

CAROTID VASCULAR DISEASE

ANATOMY

Identify the following structures:

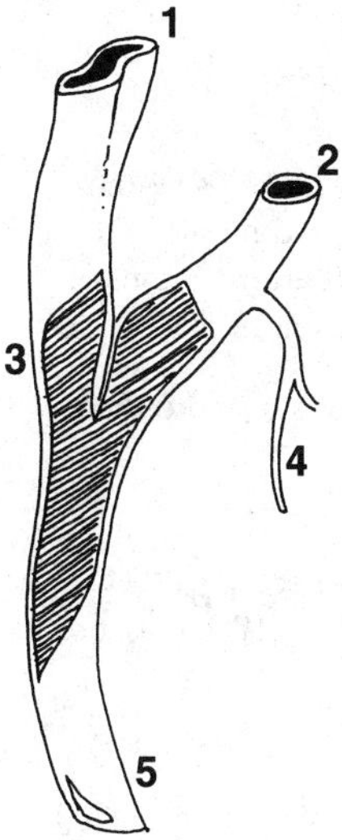

1. Internal carotid artery
2. External carotid artery
3. Carotid "bulb"
4. Superior thyroid artery
5. Common carotid artery

Shaded area: common site of plaque formation

What are the signs/ symptoms?

Amaurosis fugax, TIA, RIND, CVA

Define the following terms:

Amaurosis fugax

Temporary monocular blindness ("curtain coming down"): seen with microemboli to the retina; an example of a TIA

TIA

Transient **I**schemic **A**ttack: focal neurologic deficit with resolution of all symptoms within 24 hours

RIND

Reversible **I**schemic **N**eurologic **D**eficit: transient neurologic impairment (without any lasting sequelae) lasting 24 to 72 hours

CVA

Cerebro**V**ascular **A**ccident (stroke): neurologic deficit with permanent brain damage

What is the risk of a CVA in patients with TIA?
About 10% a year

What is the noninvasive method of evaluating carotid disease?
Carotid ultrasound/Doppler: gives general location and degree of stenosis

What is the gold standard invasive method of evaluating carotid disease?
A-gram

What is the surgical treatment of carotid stenosis?
Carotid endarterectomy (CEA): the removal of the diseased intima and media of the carotid artery, often performed with a shunt in place

What are the indications for CEA in the ASYMPTOMATIC patient?
Carotid artery stenosis of more than 60%

What are the indications for CEA in the SYMPTOMATIC (CVA, TIA, RIND) patient?
Carotid stenosis greater than 70%
> 50% stenosis and multiple episodes of TIAs
"Ulcerative" plaque
Multiple TIAs
(this list is controversial and evolving)

Before performing a CEA in the symptomatic patient, what study other than the A-gram should be performed?
Head CT

In bilateral high-grade carotid stenosis, on which side should the CEA be performed in the asymptomatic, right-handed patient?
Left CEA first, to protect the dominant hemisphere and speech center

What is the dreaded complication after a CEA?
Stroke

What are the possible postoperative complications after a CEA?
Stroke (CVA), MI, hematoma, wound infection, hemorrhage, hypo/hypertension, thrombosis, vagus nerve injury (change in voice), hypoglossal nerve injury (tongue deviation toward side of injury—"wheelbarrow" effect), intracranial hemorrhage

What is the mortality rate after CEA?	About 1%
What is the stroke rate after CEA?	Between 1% and 5% (higher in the symptomatic patient)
What is the risk of ipsilateral stroke after a CEA in the asymptomatic patient?	0.5%/year (1/200)
What is the risk of ipsilateral stroke after a CEA in the symptomatic patient?	About 2%
What is the postoperative medication?	Aspirin (inhibits platelets by inhibiting cyclo-oxygenase)

CLASSIC CEA INTRAOP QUESTIONS

What thin muscle is cut right under the skin in the neck?	Platysma muscle
What are the extracranial branches of the internal carotid artery?	None
Which vein crosses the carotid bifurcation?	The facial vein
What is the first branch of the external carotid?	The superior thyroidal artery
Which muscle crosses the common carotid proximally?	Omohyoid muscle
Which muscle crosses the carotid artery distally?	Digastric muscle
Which nerve crosses approximately 1 cm distal to the carotid bifurcation?	**Hypoglossal** nerve; cut it and you get a tongue deviating toward the side of the injury (the "wheelbarrow effect")

Which nerve crosses the internal carotid near the ear?

Facial nerve (marginal branch)

What is in the carotid sheath?

1. Carotid
2. Internal jugular vein
3. **Vagus** nerve lies posteriorly in 98% of patients and anterior in 2%)

SUBCLAVIAN STEAL SYNDROME

What is it?

Arm fatigue and vertebrobasilar insufficiency due to obstruction of the left subclavian artery or innominate proximal to the vertebral artery branch point; ipsilateral arm movement causes increased blood flow demand, which is met by retrograde flow from the vertebral artery, thereby "stealing" from the vertebrobasilar arteries

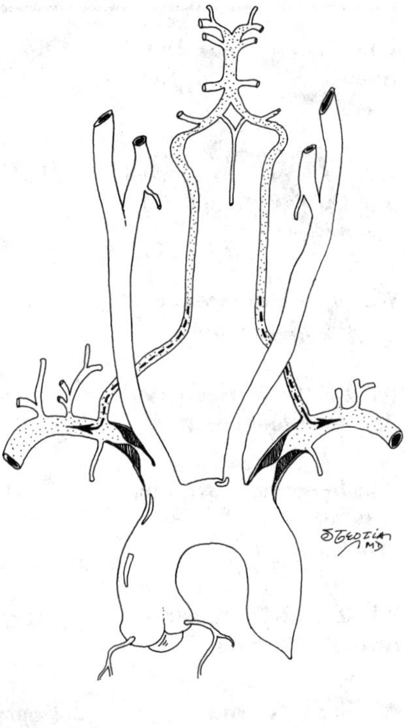

Which artery is most commonly occluded?

Left subclavian

What are the signs/ symptoms?

Upper extremity claudication and signs of vertebrobasilar insufficiency: syncopal attacks, vertigo, confusion, dysarthria, blindness, or ataxia

What are the signs?

Upper extremity blood pressure discrepancy, bruit (above the clavicle)

What is the treatment?

Surgical bypass

RENAL ARTERY STENOSIS

What is it?

Stenosis of the renal artery, resulting in decreased perfusion of the juxtaglomerular apparatus and subsequent activation of the aldosterone–renin–angiotensin system (i.e., hypertension due to renal artery stenosis)

What is the incidence?

~ 10% to 15% of the US population has HTN; of these, approximately 4% have potentially correctable renovascular HTN

Also note that 30% of malignant HTN has a renovascular etiology

What is the etiology of the stenosis?

~ two-thirds are due to atherosclerosis (men > women), ~ one-third are due to fibromuscular dysplasia (women > men, average age 40 years, and 50% with bilateral disease)

Note: another rare cause is hypoplasia of the renal artery

What is the classic profile of a patient with renal artery stenosis due to fibromuscular dysplasia?

A young woman with hypertension

What are the associated risks/clues?

Family history, early onset of HTN, HTN that is refractory to medical treatment

What are the signs/ symptoms?

Most patients are asymptomatic, but may have headache, **diastolic** HTN, flank bruits (present in 50%), and decreased renal function

What are the diagnostic tests?

A-gram: maps artery and extent of stenosis; gold standard
IVP: 80% of patients have delayed nephrogram phase (i.e., delayed filling of contrast)
Renal vein renin ratio (RVRR): if sampling of renal vein renin levels shows ratio between the two kidneys $\geq$ 1.5, then diagnostic for a unilateral stenosis
Captopril provocation test: Will show a drop in BP

Are renin levels in serum ALWAYS elevated?

No; systemic renin levels may also be measured but are only increased in malignant HTN, as the increased intravascular volume dilutes the elevated renin level in most patients

What is the invasive nonsurgical treatment?

Percutaneous renal transluminal angioplasty (PRTA)
- Much better results with fibromuscular dysplasia, but also good for isolated short-segment atherosclerotic lesions away from the ostium of the renal artery
- With FM dysplasia: 85% to 100% success rate using PRTA and 5% restenosis rate
- With atherosclerosis: 40% to 90% success using PRTA and about one-fourth restenosis

What is the surgical treatment?

Resection, bypass, vein/graft interposition, or endarterectomy

What antihypertensive medication is CONTRAINDICATED in patients with hypertension due to renovascular stenosis?

ACE inhibitors (result in renal insufficiency)

SPLENIC ARTERY ANEURYSM

What is it? Aneurysm of the splenic artery

What are the causes? Women—medial dysplasia
Men—atherosclerosis

How is the diagnosis made? Usually by abdominal pain → U/S, in the OR after rupture, or incidentally by **egg-shell calcifications seen on AXR**

What is the risk factor for rupture? Pregnancy

POPLITEAL ARTERY ANEURYSM

What is it? Aneurysm of the popliteal artery caused by atherosclerosis and, rarely, bacterial infection

How is the diagnosis made? Usually by physical exam → A-gram, U/S

Why examine the contralateral popliteal artery? Half of all patients with a popliteal artery aneurysm have a popliteal artery aneurysm in the contralateral popliteal artery

Why examine the rest of the arterial tree (especially the abdominal aorta)? **Three-fourths of all patients with popliteal aneurysms have additional aneurysms elsewhere;** over half of these are located in the abdominal aorta/iliacs.

MISCELLANEOUS

Define the following terms:

"Milk leg" A.K.A. phlegmasia alba dolens (alba = white): often seen in pregnant women with occlusion of iliac vein due to extrinsic compression by the uterus (thus, the leg is "white" because of subcutaneous edema)
In comparison, phlegmasia cerulea dolens is secondary to severe venous outflow obstruction and results in a cyanotic leg. The extensive venous thrombosis results in arterial inflow impairment.

Raynaud's phenomenon

Vasospasm of digital arteries with color changes of the digits; usually initiated by cold/emotion

White (spasm), then blue (cyanosis), then red (hyperemia)

Takayasu's arteritis

Arteritis of the aorta and aortic branches, resulting in stenosis/ occlusion/aneurysms

Seen mostly in women

Buerger's disease

A.K.A. thromboangiitis obliterans: occlusion of the small vessels of the hands and feet

Seen in **young men who smoke**

Often results in digital gangrene→amputations

Section III

Subspecialty Surgery

60

Pediatric Surgery

What is the motto of pediatric surgery?
"Children are NOT little adults!"

PEDIATRIC IV FLUIDS AND NUTRITION

What is the estimated blood volume of infants and children?
About 8% of body weight (more than adults), or approximately 80 cc/kg

What is the maintenance IV fluid for children?
D5 1/4 NS + 20 mEq KCl

Why 1/4 NS?
Children (especially < 4) cannot concentrate their urine—clear the sodium)

How are maintenance fluid rates calculated in children?
4, 2, 1 per hour:
- **4 cc/kg for the first 10 kg of body weight**
- **2 cc/kg for the second 10 kg of body weight**
- **1 cc/kg for every kilogram over the first 20** (e.g., the rate for a 25 kg child is 4 × 10 = 40 plus 2 × 10 = 20 plus 1 × 5 = 5, for an IVF rate of 65 cc/hr)

What is the minimal urine output for children?
From 1 to 2 ml/kg/hr

What is the best way to present urine output measurements on rounds?
Urine Output/kg/hr

What is the major difference between adult and pediatric nutritional needs?
Premature infants/infants/children need more calories and protein/kg/day

What are the caloric requirements by age for the following patients:

Premature infants?	80 Kcal/kg/day and then go up
Children less than 1 year old?	Approximately 100 Kcal/kg/day (90–120)
Children aged 1 to 7?	Approximately 85 Kcal/kg/day (75–90)
Children aged 7 to 12?	Approximately 70 Kcal/kg/day (60–75)
Youths aged 12 to 18	Approximately 40 Kcal/kg/day (30–60)

What are the protein requirements by age for the following patients:

Children less than 1 year?	3 g/kg/day (2–3.5)
Children aged 1 to 7?	2 g/kg/day (2–2.5)
Children aged 7 to 12?	2 g/kg/day
Youths aged 12 to 18?	1.5 grams/kg/day

FETAL CIRCULATION

What is the number of umbilical veins?	1 (usually)
What is the number of umbilical arteries?	2
Which umbilical vessel carries oxygenated blood?	Umbilical vein
The oxygenated blood travels through the liver to the IVC through which structure?	Ductus venosus
Oxygenated blood passes from the right atrium to the left atrium through which structure?	Foreman ovale

Unsaturated blood goes from the right ventricle to the descending aorta through which structure?	Ductus arteriosus
What are the ADULT structures of the following fetal structures:	
Ductus venosus?	Ligamentum venosus
Umbilical vein?	Ligamentum teres
Umbilical artery?	Medial umbilical ligament
Ductus arteriosus	Ligamentum arteriosis
Urachus?	Median umbilical ligament
Tongue remnant of thyroid's descent?	Foramen cecum
Persistent remnant of vitelline duct?	Meckel's diverticulum

ECMO

What is ECMO?	**E**xtra**C**orporeal **M**embrane **O**xygenation chronic cardiopulmonary bypass—for complete respiratory support
What are the types of ECMO?	Venovenous: Blood from vein→oxygenated→back to vein Venoarterial: Blood from vein (IJ)→oxygenated→back to artery (carotid)
What are the indications?	Severe hypoxia, usually due to: congenital diaphragmatic hernia, meconium aspiration, persistent pulmonary hypertension, sepsis
What are the contraindications?	Weight less than 2 kg, IVH (intraventricular hemorrhage in brain contraindicated due to heparin in line)

NECK

What is the major differential diagnosis of a pediatric neck mass?

Thyroglossal duct cyst (midline), branchial cleft cyst (lateral), lymphadenopathy, abscess, cystic hygroma, hemangioma, teratoma/dermoid cyst, thyroid nodule, lymphoma/leukemia, (also, parathyroid tumors, neuroblastoma, histiocytosis X, rhabdomyosarcoma, salivary gland tumors, neurofibroma)

THYROGLOSSAL DUCT CYST

What is it?

Remnant of the diverticulum formed by the migration of thyroid tissue; normal development involves migration of thyroid tissue from the foramen cecum at the base of the tongue through the hyoid bone to its final position around the tracheal cartilage

What is the average age at diagnosis?

Usually presents around 5 years of age

How is the diagnosis made?

Ultrasound

What are the complications?

Enlargement, infection, and fistula formation between oropharynx or salivary gland; aberrant thyroid tissue may masquerade as a thyroglossal duct cyst, and if it is not cystic, deserves a thyroid scan

What is the anatomic location?

Almost always in the **midline**

What is the treatment?

Antibiotics if infection is present, then excision, which must include the midportion of the hyoid bone and the entire tract to foramen cecum (Sistrunk procedure)

BRANCHIAL CLEFT ANOMALIES

What is it?

Remnant of the primitive branchial clefts in which epithelium forms a sinus tract between the pharynx (second cleft),

	or the external auditory canal (first cleft), and the skin of the anterior neck; if the sinus ends blindly, a cyst may form
What is the common presentation?	Infection because of communication between the pharynx and external ear canal
What is the anatomic position?	Second cleft anomaly—**lateral to the midline** along the anterior border of the sternocleidomastoid, anywhere from the angle of the jaw to the clavicle First cleft anomaly—not as common as second cleft anomalies; tend to be located higher under the mandible
What is the most common cleft remnant?	Second; thus, these are found most often laterally versus thyroglossal cysts, which are found centrally (key point)
What is the treatment?	Antibiotics if infection is present, then surgical excision of cyst and tract once inflammation is resolved
What is the major anatomic difference between thyroglossal cyst and branchial cleft cyst?	Thyroglossal cyst = **midline** Branchial cleft cyst = **lateral**

STRIDOR

What is it?	Harsh noise heard on breathing caused by obstruction of the trachea or the larynx; often accounted for in the newborn by congenital malformations causing airway obstruction
What are the signs/ symptoms?	Dyspnea, cyanosis, difficulty with feedings
What is the differential diagnosis?	Laryngomalacia—Leading cause of stridor in infants; results from inadequate development of supporting structures of the larynx; usually self-limited and treatment is expectant unless respiratory compromise is present

Tracheobronchomalacia—similar to laryngomalacia, but involves the entire trachea
Vascular rings and slings—abnormal development or placement of thoracic large vessels resulting in obstruction of trachea/bronchus

What are the symptoms of vascular rings?
Stridor, dyspnea on exertion, or dysphagia

How is the diagnosis of vascular rings made?
Barium swallow revealing typical configuration of esophageal compression
Echo/arteriogram

What is the treatment of vascular rings?
Surgical division of the ring, if the patient is symptomatic

CYSTIC HYGROMA

What is it?
Congenital abnormality of lymph sac resulting in lymphangioma

What is the anatomic location?
Occurs in sites of primitive lymphatic lakes and can occur virtually anywhere in the body, most commonly in the floor of mouth, under the jaw, in the neck, in the axilla, or in the thorax

What is the treatment?
Early total surgical removal because they tend to enlarge; sclerosis may be needed if the lesion is unresectable

What are the possible complications?
Enlargement in critical regions, such as the floor of the mouth or paratracheal region, may cause obstruction of the airway; also, they tend to insinuate onto major structures (although not malignant), making them difficult and hazardous to excise

ASPIRATED FOREIGN BODY (FB)

Which bronchus do FBs go into more commonly (left or right)?
Less than age 4—50–50
Age 4 and up—most go into the right bronchus because it develops into a straight shot (less of an angle)

What is the most commonly aspirated object?

Peanut

What is the associated risk with peanut aspiration?

Lipoid pneumonia

How can an FB result in "air trapping and hyperinflation"?

By forming a "ball valve" (i.e., air in, no air out) as seen on CXR as a hyperinflated lung on expiratory film

How can you tell on A-P CXR if a coin is in the esophagus or the trachea?

Coin in **esophagus** results in the coin lying "en face" with the face of the coin viewed as a **round object** due to compression by the anterior and posterior structures

If the coin is in the **trachea,** it is viewed as **a side projection** due to the U-shaped cartilage with membrane posteriorly

What is the treatment of tracheal or esophageal FB?

Remove FB with **rigid** bronchoscope or **rigid** esophagoscope

CHEST

What is the differential diagnosis of a lung mass?

Bronchial adenoma (carcinoid is most common), pulmonary sequestration, pulmonary blastoma, rhabdomyosarcoma, chondroma, hamartoma, leiomyoma, mucus gland adenoma, metastasis

What is the differential diagnosis of mediastinal tumor/mass?

1. Neurogenic tumor (ganglioneuromas, neurofibromas)
2. Teratoma
3. Lymphoma
4. Thymoma

(T's: teratoma, terrible lymphoma, thymoma, thyroid tumor)

Rare: pheochromocytoma, hemangioma, rhabdomyosarcoma, osteochondroma

PECTUS DEFORMITY

What heart abnormality is associated with pectus abnormality?

Mitral valve prolapse (many patients receive preoperative echocardiogram)

PECTUS EXCAVATUM

What is it?	Chest wall deformity with sternum caving inward (think: ex**CAV**atum = **CAVE**)
What is the cause?	Abnormal, unequal overgrowth of rib cartilage
What are the signs/ symptoms?	Many patients are asymptomatic; mental distress, dyspnea on exertion, chest pain
What is the treatment?	Open perichondrium, remove abnormal cartilage, place substernal strut; new cartilage grows back in the perichondrium in normal position; remove strut 6 months later

PECTUS CARINATUM

What is it?	Chest wall deformity with sternum outward (pectus = chest, carinatum = pigeon); much less common than pectus excavatum
What is the cause?	Abnormal, unequal overgrowth of rib cartilage
What is the treatment?	Open perichondrium and remove abnormal cartilage. Place substernal strut. New cartilage grows into normal position. Remove strut 6 months later.

ESOPHAGEAL ATRESIA WITHOUT TRACHEOESOPHAGEAL (TE) FISTULA

What is it?	Blind-ending esophagus due to atresia
What are the signs?	Excessive oral secretions and inability to keep food down
How is the diagnosis made?	Inability to pass NG tube; plain x-ray shows tube coiled in the upper esophagus and absence of gas in the abdomen

What is the primary treatment?

Suction blind pouch, IVFs, (gastrostomy to drain stomach if prolonged preoperative esophageal stretching is planned)

What is the definitive treatment?

Surgical with 1° anastomosis, often with preoperative stretching of blind pouch (other options include colonic or jejunal interposition graft or gastric tube formation if esophageal gap is long)

ESOPHAGEAL ATRESIA WITH TRACHEOESOPHAGEAL FISTULA

What is it?

Esophageal atresia occurring with a fistula to the trachea; occurs in more than 90% of esophageal atresia

What is the incidence?

One in 1500 to 3000 births

Define the following types of fistulas/atresias:

Type A?

Esophageal atresia without TE fistula (8%)

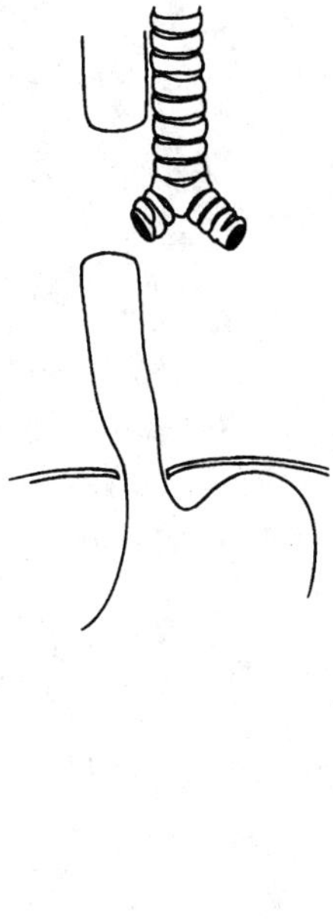

Type B?

Proximal esophageal atresia with proximal TE fistula (1%)

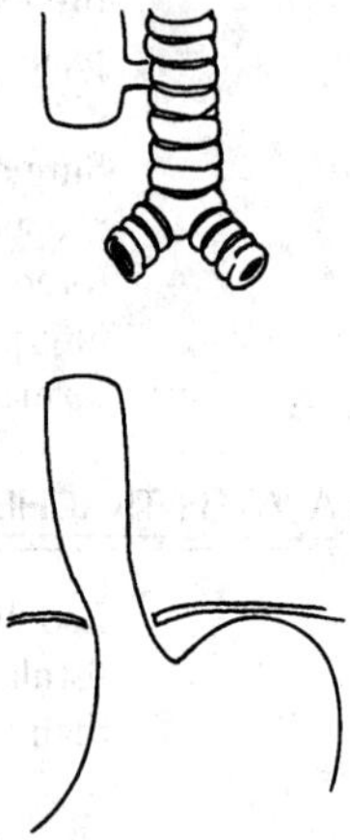

Type C?

Proximal esophageal atresia with distal TE fistula (85%); **most common type**

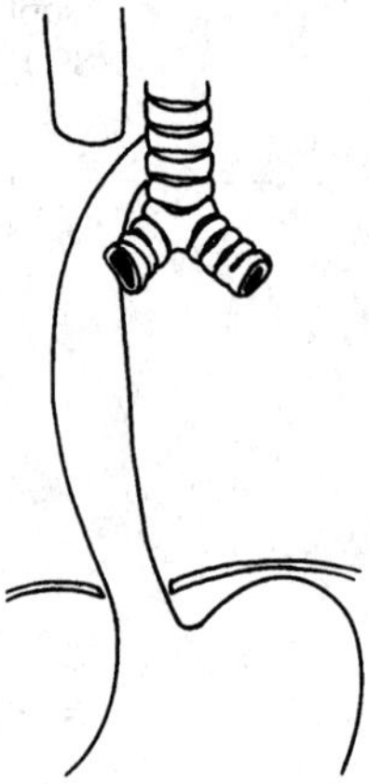

Type D?

Proximal esophageal atresia with both proximal and distal TE fistulas (2%)

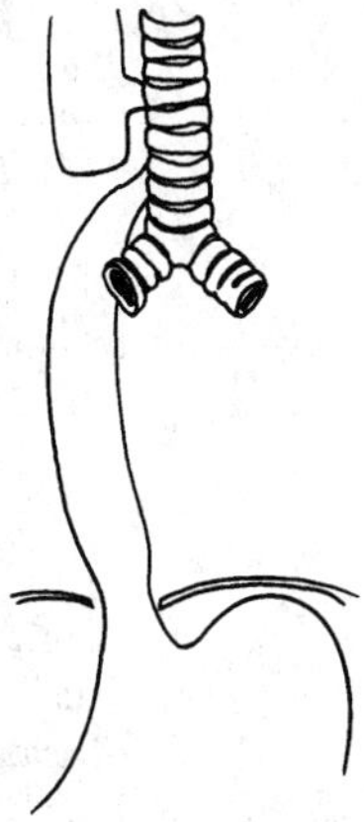

Type E?

"H-type" TE fistula without esophageal atresia (4%)

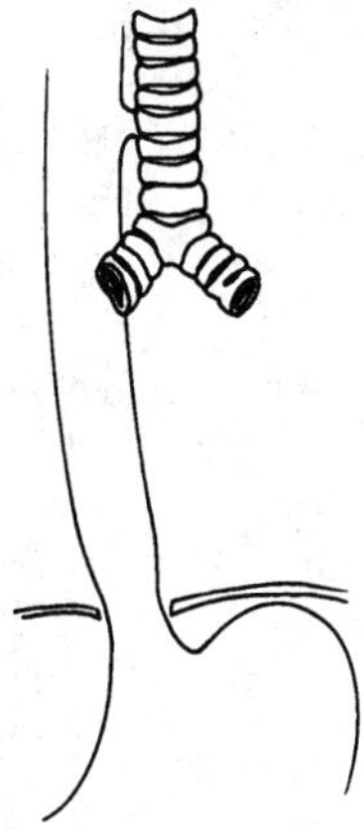

How do you remember which one is the most common type?

Simple: the most **C**ommon type = type **C**

What are the symptoms?

Excessive secretions caused by an accumulation of saliva (may not occur with type E)

What are the signs?

Obvious respiratory compromise, aspiration pneumonia, postprandial regurgitation, gastric distention as air enters the stomach directly from the trachea

How is the diagnosis made?

Failure to pass an NG tube (although this will not be seen with type E); plain film demonstrates tube coiled in the upper esophagus; "pouchogram" (contrast in esophageal pouch); gas on AXR (tracheoesophageal fistula)

What is the initial treatment?

Directed toward minimizing complications from aspiration:
1. Suction blind pouch (NPO/TPN)
2. Upright position of child
3. Prophylactic antibiotics

What is the definitive treatment?

Surgical correction via a thoracotomy, usually through the right chest with division of fistula and end-to-end esophageal anastomosis, if possible

What can be done to lengthen the proximal esophageal pouch?

Delayed repair: with or without G-tube and daily **stretching** of the proximal pouch

Which type should be fixed via a right neck incision?

"H-Type" (type E) is high in the thorax and can most often be approached via a right neck incision.

What are the associated anomalies?

Vacterl cluster (present in about 10% of cases):

Vertebral or vascular, **A**norectal, **C**ardiac, **TE** fistula, **E**sophageal atresia, **R**adial limb and renal abnormalities, **L**umbar and limb

Previously known as **VATER:** **V**ertebral, **A**nus, **TE** fistula, **R**adial

What is the significance of a "gasless" abdomen on AXR?

No air to the stomach and, thus, no tracheoesophageal fistula

CONGENITAL DIAPHRAGMATIC HERNIA

What is it?

Failure of complete formation of the diaphragm, leading to a defect through which abdominal organs herniate

What is the incidence?

One in 2100 live births; males are more commonly affected

What are the types of hernias?

Bochdalek and Morgagni

What are the associated positions?

Bochdalek—posterolateral with L > R (think: "Bochdalek = back to the left")
Morgagni—anterior parasternal hernia, relatively uncommon

What are the signs?

Respiratory distress as the presence of bowel in the thorax impedes lung development with lung hypoplasia in both lungs and pulmonary hypertension; dyspnea, tachypnea, retractions and cyanosis; at birth, swallowed air further distends the intestine, compressing the lung and causing a mediastinal shift, impeding venous return to the thorax and ventilation of the contralateral lung; may also auscultate bowel sounds in the chest

What is the treatment?

NG tube, ET tube, stabilization, and if the patient is stable, surgical repair; if the patient is unstable, to the ECMO then to the OR, when deemed feasible

PULMONARY SEQUESTRATION

What is it?

Abnormal benign lung tissue with separate blood supply that **DOES NOT** communicate with the normal tracheobronchial airway

Define the following terms:

Interlobar

Sequestration in the normal lung tissue covered by normal visceral pleura

Extralobar

Sequestration not in the normal lung covered by its own pleura

What are the signs/ symptoms?

Asymptomatic, recurrent pneumonia

How is the diagnosis made?

CXR, chest CT, A-gram, U/S with Doppler flow to ascertain blood supply

What is the treatment of each type:

Extralobar — Surgical resection

Intralobar — Lobectomy

What is the major risk during operation for sequestration? — Anomalous blood supply from below the diaphragm (can be cut and retract into the abdomen and result in exsanguination!); always document blood supply by A-gram or U/S with Doppler flow

ABDOMEN

What is the differential diagnosis of pediatric upper GI bleeding? — Gastritis, esophagitis, gastric ulcer, duodenal ulcer, esophageal varices, foreign body, epistaxis, coagulopathy, vascular malformation, duplication cyst

What is the differential diagnosis of pediatric lower GI bleeding? — Upper GI bleeding, anal fissures, NEC (premature infants), midgut volvulus (usually children < 1 yr old), strangulated hernia, intussusception, Meckel's diverticulum, infectious diarrhea, polyps, IBD, hemolytic uremic syndrome, Henoch-Schonlein purpura, vascular malformation, coagulopathy

What is the differential diagnosis of neonatal bowel obstruction? — Malrotation with volvulus, intestinal atresia, duodenal web, annular pancreas, imperforate anus, Hirschsprung's disease, NEC, intussusception (rare), Meckel's diverticulum, incarcerated hernia, meconium ileus, meconium plug, maternal narcotic abuse (ileus), maternal hypermagnesemia (ileus), sepsis (ileus)

What is the differential diagnosis of infant constipation? — Hirschsprung's disease, cystic fibrosis, anteriorly displaced anus, polyps

INGUINAL HERNIA

What is the most commonly performed procedure by pediatric surgeons in the United States? — Indirect inguinal hernia repair

What is the most common inguinal hernia in children?

Indirect

What is an indirect inguinal hernia?

Hernia lateral to Hesselbach's triangle into the internal inguinal ring and down the inguinal canal (think: through the abdominal wall indirectly into the internal ring and out through the external inguinal ring)

What is Hesselbach's triangle?

1. Epigastric vessels
2. Inguinal ligament
3. Lateral border of the rectus sheath

What type of hernia goes through Hesselbach's triangle?

A direct hernia due to a weak abdominal floor; rare in children (0.5% of all inguinal hernias)

What is the incidence of indirect inguinal hernia in all children?

Approximately 3%

What is the incidence in premature infants?

Up to 25%

What is the male:female ratio?

6:1

What are the risk factors for an indirect inguinal hernia?

Male gender, ascites, V-P shunt, prematurity, family history, meconium ileus, abdominal wall defect elsewhere, hypo/epispadias, connective tissue disease, bladder exstrophy, undescended testicle, cystic fibrosis

Which side is affected more commonly?

Right (about 60%:40%)

What percentage are bilateral?

Approximately 15%

What percentage have a family history of indirect hernias?

Approximately 10%

What are the signs/ symptoms?	Groin bulge, scrotal mass, thickened cord, silk glove sign
What is the silk glove sign?	The hernia sac rolls under the finger like the finger of a silk glove
Why should it be repaired?	Risk of incarcerated/strangulated bowel or ovary; will not go away on its own in the vast majority of cases
How is a pediatric inguinal hernia repaired?	High ligation of the hernia sac (no repair of the abdominal wall floor, which is a big difference between the procedure in children and adults; high refers to high position on the sac neck next to the peritoneal cavity)
Which infants need overnight apnea monitoring/observation?	Premature infants; infants less than 3 months of age
What is the risk of wound infection after an indirect hernia repair?	Approximately 1%
What is the risk of recurrence after high ligation of an indirect pediatric hernia?	Approximately 1%
Describe the steps in the repair of an indirect inguinal hernia from skin to skin.	Cut skin, then fat, then Scarpa's fascia, then external oblique fascia through the external inguinal ring, find hernia sac anteriomedially and bluntly separate from the other cord structures, ligate sac high at the neck at the internal inguinal ring, resect sac and allow sac stump to retract into the peritoneal cavity, close external oblique, close Scarpa's fascia, close skin
Define the following terms:	
Cryptorchidism	Failure of the testicle to descend into the scrotum

Hydrocele — Fluid-filled sac (i.e., fluid in a patent processus vaginalis or in the tunica vaginalis around the testicle)

Communicating hydrocele — Hydrocele that communicates with the peritoneal cavity and thus fills and drains peritoneal fluid or gets bigger, then smaller

Noncommunicating hydrocele — Hydrocele that does not communicate with the peritoneal cavity; stays about the same size

Can a hernia be ruled out if a inguinal mass transilluminates? — NO; baby bowel is very thin and will often transilluminate

CLASSIC INTRAOPERATIVE QUESTIONS DURING REPAIR OF AN INDIRECT INGUINAL HERNIA

From what abdominal muscle layer is the cremaster muscle derived? — Internal oblique muscle

From what abdominal muscle layer is the inguinal ligament (A.K.A. Poupart's ligament) derived? — External oblique muscle

What nerve travels with the spermatic cord? — Ilioinguinal nerve

What is in the spermatic cord (5 structures)?

1. Cremasteric muscle fibers
2. Vas deferens
3. Testicular artery
4. Testicular pampiniform venous plexus
5. With or without hernia sac

What is the hernia sac made of? — Basically peritoneum or a patent processus vaginalis

What is the name of the fossa between the testicle and epididymis? — Fossa of Geraldi

What attaches the testicle to the scrotum?
The gubernaculum

How can the opposite side be assessed for a hernia intraoperatively?
Many surgeons operatively explore the opposite side when they repair the affected side.
A laparoscope is placed into the abdomen via the hernia sac and the opposite side internal inguinal ring is examined.

Name the remnant of the processus vaginalis around the testicle?
Tunica vaginalis

What is an inguinal Richter's hernia?
Hernia with only a bowel side wall incarcerated

What is a Littre's inguinal hernia?
Hernia with a Meckel's diverticulum in the hernia sac

What may a yellow/orange tissue that is not fat be on the spermatic cord/ testicle?
Adrenal rest

What is the most common organ in an inguinal hernia sac in boys?
Small intestine

What is the most common organ in an inguinal hernia sac in girls?
Ovary/fallopian tube

What lies in the inguinal canal in girls instead of the vas?
Round ligament

Where in the inguinal canal does the hernia sac lie in relation to the other structures?
Anteriomedially

What is a "cord lipoma"?
Preperitoneal fat on the cord structures (pushed in by the hernia sac); not a real lipoma
Should be removed surgically, if feasible

Within the spermatic cord, do the vessels or the vas lie medially?	The vas is medial to the testicular vessels.
What is a small outpouching of testicular tissue off of the testicle?	Testicular appendage (A.K.A. the appendix testes); should be removed with electrocautery
What is a "blue dot sign"?	A blue dot on the scrotal skin due to a twisted testicular appendage
How is a transected vas treated?	Repair with primary anastomosis
How do you treat a transected ilioinguinal nerve?	Should not be repaired; many surgeons place a metallic clip on it to inhibit neuroma formation
What happens if you cut the ilioinguinal nerve?	Loss of sensation to the medial aspect of the inner thigh and scrotum/labia; loss of cremasteric reflex

MISCELLANEOUS

Define the following terms:	
Phimosis	Fibrous attachment of the foreskin to the underlying penile glans; the foreskin will not retract
Paraphimosis	Inability to place the foreskin over the glans of the penis (foreskin stays retracted) (Think: Para = around)
Posthitis	Foreskin infection
What is the disadvantage of a foreskin?	Associated with: phimosis, paraphimosis, posthitis, hygiene, UTIs, penile cancer (very small, but real, risk)

TESTICULAR TORSION

What is it?	Torsion (twist) of the spermatic cord resulting in venous outflow obstruction and subsequent arterial occlusion→infarction of the testicle

What is the classic history?
Acute onset of scrotal pain after vigorous activity or minor trauma

What is a "Bell clapper" deformity?
Bilateral nonattachment of the testicles by the gubernaculum to the scrotum (like the clappers of a bell)

What are the symptoms?
Pain in the scrotum, suprapubic pain

What are the signs?
Very tender, swollen, elevated testicle; nonillumination

What is the differential diagnosis?
Testicular trauma, inguinal hernia, epididymitis, appendage torsion

How is the diagnosis made?
Surgical exploration, U/S (solid mass) and Doppler flow study, cold Tc-99m scan

What is the treatment?
Surgical detorsion and bilateral orchiopexy to scrotum

Within how much time from the onset of symptoms must the testicle be detorsed?
Less than 6 hours will yield the best results

GERD

What is it?
Gastro **E**sophageal **R**eflux **D**isease

What are the causes?
LES malfunction/malposition, hiatal hernia, gastric outlet obstruction, partial bowel obstruction, common in cerebral palsy

What are the signs/symptoms?
Spitting up, emesis, bronchitis, pneumonia, laryngospasm due to aspiration of gastric contents into the tracheobronchial tree

How is the diagnosis made?
UGI, bronchoscopy

What cytologic aspirate finding on bronchoscopy can diagnose aspiration of gastric contents?
Lipid-laden macrophages (from phagocytosis of fat)

What is the medical/ conservative treatment?

H_2 blockers
Cisapride
Small meals
Elevation of head

What is the surgical treatment?

Nissen 360° fundoplication, with or without G tube

CONGENITAL PYLORIC STENOSIS

What is it?

Hypertrophy of the smooth muscle of the pylorus, resulting in obstruction of outflow

What are the associated risks?

Family history, **firstborn** males are affected most commonly, decreased incidence in African-American population

What is the incidence?

One in 500 to 750 births, male:female ratio = 4:1

What is the average age at onset?

Usually from 2 weeks after birth to about 2 months (2 to 2)

What are the symptoms?

Increasing frequency of regurgitation, leading to eventual nonbilious projectile vomiting, weight loss or lack of gain, decreasing frequency of stools

What are the signs?

Abdominal mass or "olive" in the epigastric region (85%), hypokalemic hypochloremic metabolic alkalosis, icterus (10%), visible gastric peristalsis, paradoxic aciduria, hematemesis (< 10%)

What is the differential diagnosis?

Pylorospasm, milk allergy, increased ICP, hiatal hernia, GE reflux, adrenal insufficiency, uremia, malrotation, duodenal atresia, annular pancreas, duodenal web

How is the diagnosis made?

Usually by history and physical exam alone
U/S—demonstrates elongated (> 15 mm) pyloric channel and thickened muscle wall (> 3.5 mm)
If U/S is nondiagnostic, then barium swallow—shows "string sign" or "double railroad track sign"

What is the initial treatment?
Hydration and correction of alkalosis with D10 NS plus 20 to 40 meq of KCl; *Note:* the infant's liver glycogen stores are very small, therefore use D10; Cl^- and hydration will correct the alkalosis

What is the definitive treatment?
Surgical, via Fredet-Ramstedt pyloromyotomy (division of circular muscle fibers without entering the lumen/mucosa)

What are the postoperative complications?
Unrecognized incision through the duodenal mucosa, bleeding, wound infection, aspiration pneumonia

What is the appropriate postoperative feeding?
Between 6 and 12 hours postoperative feeding with sugar water, advanced to full-strength formula over 24 hours

Which vein crosses the pylorus?
Vein of Mayo

DUODENAL ATRESIA

What is it?
Complete obstruction or stenosis of duodenum caused by an ischemic insult during development, or failure of recanalization

What is the anatomic location?
Eighty-five percent are distal to the ampulla of Vater, 15% are proximal to the ampulla of Vater (these present with nonbilious vomiting)

What are the signs?
Bilious vomiting (if distal to the ampulla), epigastric distention

What is the differential diagnosis?
Malrotation with Ladd's bands, annular pancreas

How is the diagnosis made?
Plain abdominal film revealing "double bubble," with one air bubble in the stomach and the other in the duodenum

What is the treatment?
Duodenoduodenostomy or duodenojejunostomy

What are the associated abnormalities?	Between 50% and 70% have cardiac, renal, or other gastrointestinal defects; 30% have trisomy 21

JEJUNAL ATRESIA

What is it?	Obstruction due to atresia or stenosis resulting from a late mesenteric vascular accident caused by intrauterine volvulus, malrotation, internal hernia, intussusception, or strangulation in an abdominal wall defect
What are the classifications:	
Type I?	Mucosal web or diaphragm
Type II?	Atretic cord between two blind ends with intact mesentery
Type IIIa?	Complete separation with "V-shaped" mesentery defect (**most common type**)
Type IIIb?	"Apple peel" or "Christmas tree" deformity
Type IV?	Instances of multiple atresia characterized by "string of sausage" appearance
What are the signs?	Bilious vomiting, abdominal distention, failure to pass meconium (possibly), 3 to 4 air-fluid bubbles on plain films, jaundice (40%), microcolon due to disuse, history of polyhydramnios (35%)
What is the primary treatment?	NG tube, fluid resuscitation
What is the definitive treatment?	Surgical resection of atretic loop with reanastomosis, with possible tapering of dilated proximal loop

ILEAL ATRESIA

What is it?	Similar process to jejunal atresia, but involving the ileum

What are the classifications?

Same as jejunal atresia; type IIIa is the most common variant

What are the signs/ symptoms?

Same as jejunal atresia

What is the definitive treatment?

Same as jejunal atresia

What are the possible complications?

Meconium peritonitis secondary to perforation in about 10% of cases

MECONIUM ILEUS

What is it?

Intestinal obstruction due to solid meconium concretions

What is the incidence?

Occurs in about 15% of infants with cystic fibrosis, although almost all patients with meconium ileus have cystic fibrosis (CF)

What percentage of patients with meconium ileus have CF?

More than 95%

What are the signs/ symptoms?

Bilious vomiting, abdominal distention, failure to pass meconium, Neuhauser's sign (i.e., ground-glass appearance in the right lower quadrant representing viscid meconium mixed with air), peritoneal calcifications

What is Neuhauser's sign?

A.K.A. "soap bubble" sign: on AXR, the meconium mixes with air and appears like ground glass

How is the diagnosis made?

Family history of CF, plain abdominal films showing significant dilation of similar-sized bowel loops, but few if any air-fluid levels, BE may demonstrate "microcolon" and inspissated meconium pellets in the terminal ileum

What is the treatment?	Nonoperative clearance of meconium using Gastrografin enema, which is hypertonic and therefore draws fluid into the lumen, separating meconium pellets from the bowel wall (60% success rate)
What is the surgical treatment?	If enema is unsuccessful, then enterotomy with intraoperative catheter irrigation using acetylcysteine (Mucomyst)
What is the long-term medical treatment?	Pancreatic enzyme replacement
What is cystic fibrosis (CF)?	Inherited disorder of epithelial Cl^- transport defect affecting sweat glands, airways, and GI tract (pancreas, intestine); diagnosed by sweat test (elevated levels of NaCl > 60 mEq/liter), and genetic testing

MECONIUM PERITONITIS

What is it?	A sign of **intrauterine** bowel perforation; sterile meconium leads to an intense local inflammatory reaction with eventual formation of calcifications
What are the signs?	Calcifications on plain films

MECONIUM PLUG SYNDROME

What is it?	Colonic obstruction due to unknown factors that dehydrate meconium, forming a "plug"
What are the signs/ symptoms?	Abdominal distention and **failure to pass meconium within first 24 hours of life;** plain films demonstrate many loops of distended bowel and air-fluid levels
What is the treatment?	Contrast enema is both diagnostic and therapeutic; demonstrates "microcolon" to the point of dilated colon (usually in transverse colon) and reveals copious intraluminal material.

What is the major differential diagnosis?	Hirschsprung's disease
Is meconium plug highly associated with cystic fibrosis?	No; less than 5% of patients have CF, in contrast to meconium ileus, in which nearly all have CF (95%)

ANORECTAL MALFORMATIONS

What are they?	Malformations of the distal GI tract in the general categories of anal atresia, imperforate anus, and rectal atresia

IMPERFORATE ANUS

What is it?	Congenital absence of normal anus (complete absence or fistula)
Define a "high" imperforate anus?	Rectum patent to level above puborectalis sling
Define "low" imperforate anus?	Rectum patent to below puborectalis sling
Which type is much more common in women?	Low
What are the associated anomalies?	**V**ertebral abnormalities, **A**nal abnormalities, **TE** fistulas, **R**adial/**R**enal abnormalities, **L**umbar abnormalities (**VACTERL;** most commonly TE fistula)
What are the signs/symptoms?	No anus, fistula to anal skin, fistula to bladder, UTI, fistula to vagina, fistula to urethra, bowel obstruction, distended abdomen, hyperchloremic acidosis
Why is hyperchloremic acidosis associated with imperforate anus?	Colon absorbs Cl^- from urine from a bladder/urethra fistula
How is the diagnosis made?	Physical exam, the classic Cross table "invertogram" plain x-ray to see level of rectal gas (not very accurate), perineal ultrasound

What is the treatment of the following conditions:

Low imperforate anus with anal fistula? Dilatation of anal fistula and subsequent anoplasty

High imperforate anus? Diverting colostomy and mucus fistula; neoanus is usually made at 1 year of age

HIRSCHSPRUNG'S DISEASE

What is it also known as? Aganglionic megacolon

What is it? Neurogenic form of intestinal obstruction in which obstruction is due to inadequate relaxation and peristalsis; **absence of normal ganglion cells** of the rectum and colon

What are the associated risks? Family history; 5% chance of having a second child with the affliction

What is the male:female ratio? 4:1

What is the anatomic location? Aganglionosis begins at the anorectal line and involves rectosigmoid in 80% of cases (10% have involvement to splenic flexure and 10% have involvement of entire colon).

What are the signs/symptoms? Abdominal distention and bilious vomiting; more than 95% present with failure to pass meconium in the first 24 hours; can also present later with constipation, diarrhea, and decreased growth

What is the classic history? Failure to pass meconium in the first 24 hours of life

What is the differential diagnosis? Meconium plug syndrome, meconium ileus, sepsis with adynamic ileus, colonic neuronal dysplasia, hypothyroidism, maternal narcotic abuse, maternal hypermagnesemia (tocolysis)

How is the diagnosis made?	**AXR:** reveals dilated colon **Unprepared barium enema:** reveals constricted aganglionic segment with dilated proximal segment, but this picture may not develop for 3 to 6 weeks; BE will also demonstrate retention of barium for 24 to 48 hours (normal evacuation = 10 to 18 hours) **Rectal biopsy:** for definitive diagnosis, submucosal suction biopsy is adequate in 90% of cases; otherwise, full-thickness biopsy should be performed to evaluate Auerbach's plexus
What is the "colonic transition zone"?	The transition (taper) from aganglionic small colon into the large dilated normal colon seen on BE
What is the initial treatment?	In neonates, a colostomy proximal to the transition zone prior to correction, to allow for pelvic growth and dilated bowel to return to normal size
What is a "leveling" colostomy?	The colostomy performed for Hirschsprung's disease at the **level** of normally innervated ganglion cells as ascertained on frozen section intraoperatively

Describe the following procedures:

Swenson

Primary anastomosis between the anal canal and healthy bowel (rectum removed)

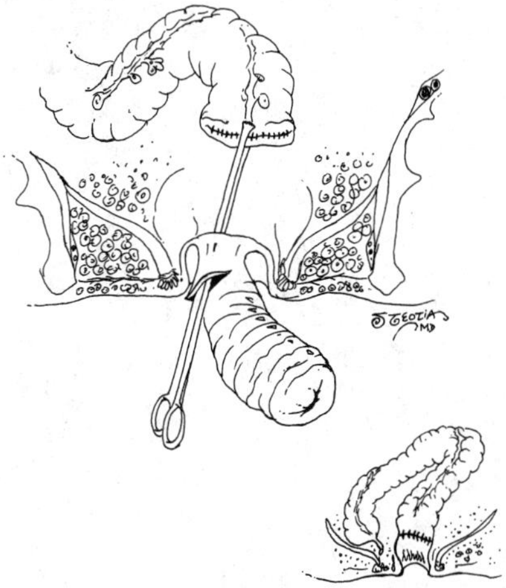

Duhamel

The anterior, aganglionic region of the rectum is preserved and anastomosed to a posterior portion of healthy bowel; a functional rectal pouch is thereby created (**think:** duha = dual barrels side by side)

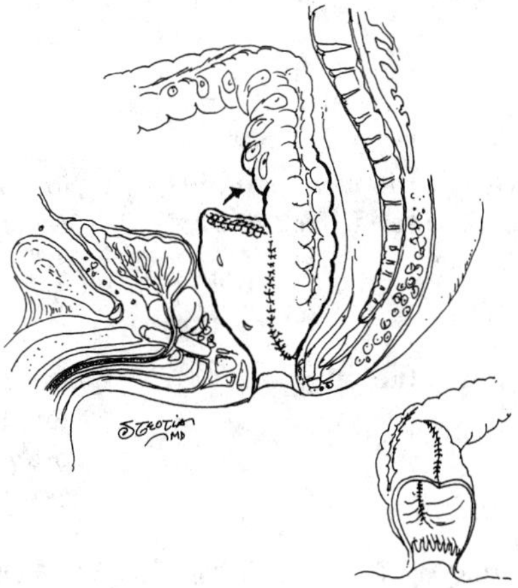

Soave

(A.K.A. endorectal pull-through); this procedure involves bringing proximal normal colon through the aganglionic rectum, which has been stripped of its mucosa but otherwise present (think: **soave** = **save** the rectum, lose the mucosa)

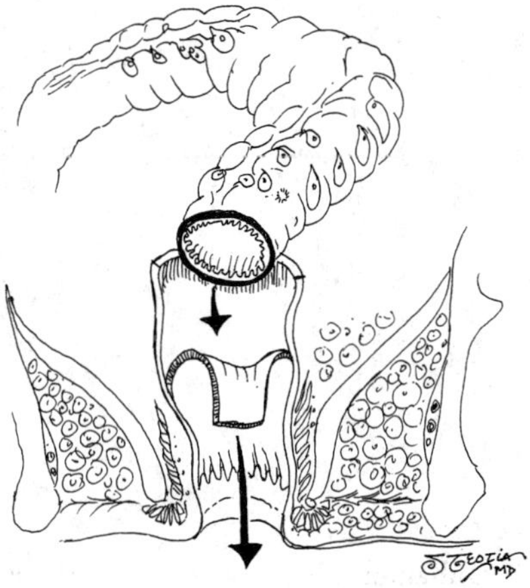

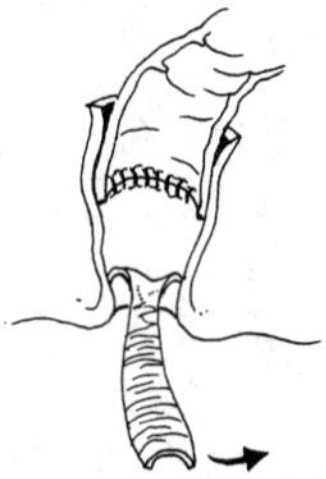

What is the new trend in surgery for Hirschsprung's disease?

No colostomy; remove aganglionic colon (as confirmed on frozen section) and perform pull-through anastomosis at the same time (Boley modification)

What is the prognosis?

Overall survival rate is greater than 90%; more than 96% are continent and postoperative symptoms improve with age

MALROTATION AND MIDGUT VOLVULUS

What is it?

Failure of the normal bowel rotation, with resultant abnormal intestinal attachments and anatomic positions

Where is the cecum?	With malrotation, the cecum usually ends up in the left upper quadrant
What are Ladd's bands?	Fibrous bands that extend from the abnormally placed cecum in the right upper quadrant, often crossing over the duodenum and causing obstruction
What is the usual age at onset?	One-third present in the first week of life, three-fourths by one month of life, and 90% are diagnosed by 1 year of age.
What is the usual presentation?	Sudden onset of bilious vomiting **(bilious vomiting in an infant is malrotation until proven otherwise!)**
How is the diagnosis made?	Upper GI series with follow-through; BE showing abnormal position of the cecum in the upper abdomen
What are the possible complications?	Volvulus with midgut infarction, leading to death or necessitating massive enterectomy **(rapid diagnosis is essential!)**
What is the treatment?	IV antibiotics and fluid resuscitation with LR, followed by emergent laparotomy with LADD's procedure; second-look laparotomy if the bowel is severely ischemic in 24 hours to determine if the remaining bowel is viable
What is the Ladd's procedure?	1. Counterclockwise reduction of midgut volvulus 2. Splitting of Ladd's bands 3. Division of peritoneal attachments to the cecum, ascending colon 4. Appendectomy
How is the volvulus reduced?	Rotation of the bowel in a **counterclockwise** direction
Where is the cecum after reduction?	In the left lower quadrant

What is the cause of bilious vomiting in an infant until proven otherwise?	Malrotation with midgut volvulus

OMPHALOCELE

What is it?	Defect of the abdominal wall at the umbilical ring; extruded viscera are **covered** by sac
What comprises the "sac"?	Peritoneum and amnion
What organ is often found protruding from an omphalocele, but is almost never found with a gastroschisis?	The liver
What is the incidence?	Approximately 1 in 5000 births
How is the diagnosis made?	Prenatal U/S
What are the possible complications?	Malrotation of the gut, anomalies
What is the treatment?	1. NG tube for decompression 2. IV fluids 3. Prophylactic antibiotics 4. Surgical repair of the defect
What is the treatment of a small defect (< 2 cm)?	Closure of abdominal wall
What is the treatment of a medium defect (2–10 cm)?	Removal of outer membrane and placement of a silicone patch to form a "silo," temporarily housing abdominal contents; the silo is then slowly decreased in size over 4 to 7 days, as the abdomen accommodates the viscera; then the defect is closed

What is the treatment of large defects (> 10 cm)?

Skin flaps or treatment with Betadine spray, mercurochrome, or silver sulfadiazine (Silvadene) over the defect, allowing an eschar to form, which epithelializes over time, allowing opportunity for future repair months to years later

What are the associated abnormalities?

Fifty percent of cases occur with often severe abnormalities of the GI tract, cardiovascular system, GU tract, musculoskeletal system, CNS, and chromosomes.

Of what "pentalogy" is omphalocele a part?

Pentalogy of Cantrell

What is the pentalogy of Cantrell?

"D COPS":
Diaphragmatic defect (hernia)

Cardiac abnormality
Omphalocele
Pericardium malformation/absence
Sternal cleft

GASTROSCHISIS

What is it?

Defect of the abdominal wall; extruded viscera is not covered by the sac

Where is the defect?

Lateral to the umbilicus (right > left)

On what side of the umbilicus is the defect found?

The right (think: right = gastroschisis)

What is the usual size of the defect?

Between 2 and 4 cm

What are the possible complications?

Thick edematous peritoneum due to exposure to amnionic fluid; malrotation of the gut
Other complications include: hypothermia; hypovolemia due to third-spacing; sepsis; and metabolic acidosis due to hypovolemia and poor perfusion, NEC, prolonged ileus

How is the diagnosis made? Prenatal U/S

What is the treatment? Primary—NG tube decompression, IV fluids (D10 LR), and IV antibiotics
Definitive—surgical reduction of viscera and abdominal closure; may require staged closure with silo

What is a "silo"? Silastic silo is a temporary housing for external abdominal contents; silo is slowly tightened over time; *Note:* a prolonged postoperative adynamic ileus requiring TPN for adequate caloric support may be present

What is the prognosis? More than 90% survival rate

What are the associated anomalies? Unlike omphalocele, relatively uncommon except for intestinal atresia, which occurs in 10%–15% of cases

What are the major differences compared with omphalocele? No membrane coverings
Uncommon associated abnormalities

POWER REVIEW

What are the differences between omphalocele and gastroschisis in terms of the following characteristics:

Anomalies? Common in omphalocele (50%), uncommon in gastroschisis

Peritoneal/amnion covering (sac)? Always with omphalocele, never with gastroschisis

Position of umbilical cord? On the sac with omphalocele, from skin to the left of the gastroschisis defect

Thick bowel? Common with gastroschisis, rare with omphalocele (unless sac ruptures)

Protrusion of liver? Common with omphalocele, almost never with gastroschisis

Large defect? Omphalocele

APPENDICITIS

What is it?	Obstruction of the appendiceal lumen (fecalith, lymphoid hyperplasia), producing a closed loop with resultant inflammation that can lead to necrosis and perforation
What is its claim to fame?	Most common surgical disease requiring emergency surgery in children
What is the affected age?	Very rare before age 3
What is the usual presentation?	Onset of referred or **periumbilical pain** followed by **anorexia,** nausea, and vomiting; Note: unlike gastroenteritis, **pain precedes vomiting;** pain then migrates to the **right lower quadrant,** where it becomes more intense and localized due to local peritoneal irritation If the patient is hungry and can eat, seriously question the diagnosis of appendicitis.
How is the diagnosis made?	History and physical exam
What are the signs/symptoms?	Signs of peritoneal irritation may be present—guarding, muscle spasm, rebound tenderness, obturator and Psoas signs, low-grade fever rising to high grade if perforation occurs
What is the differential diagnosis?	Intussusception, volvulus, Meckel's diverticulum, Crohn's disease, ovarian torsion, cyst, tumor, perforated ulcer, pancreatitis, PID, ruptured ectopic pregnancy, mesenteric lymphadenitis
What is the common bacterial cause of mesenteric lymphadenitis?	*Yersinia enterocolitica*
What are the associated lab findings?	Increased WBC (> 10,000 per mm^3 in > 90% of cases, with a left shift in most)

What is the role of urinalysis?

To evaluate for possible pyelonephritis or renal calculus, but mild hematuria and pyuria are common in appendicitis due to ureteral inflammation

What is the "hamburger" sign?

Ask patients with suspected appendicitis if they would like a hamburger or their favorite food; if they can eat, seriously question the diagnosis.

What radiographic studies may be performed?

Often none; CXR to rule out RML or RLL pneumonia; abdominal films are usually nonspecific, but calcified fecalith is present in 5% of cases; ultrasound to evaluate for ovarian/gynecologic pathology

What is the treatment?

Nonperforated—prompt appendectomy and cefoxitin to avoid perforation
Perforated—triple antibiotics, fluid resuscitation, and prompt appendectomy; all pus is drained and cultures obtained, with postoperative antibiotics continued for 5 to 7 days, +/− drain

How long should antibiotics be administered if nonperforated?

24 hours

How long if perforated?

Usually 5 to 7 days, or until WBCs are normal and patient is afebrile

If a normal appendix is found upon exploration, what must be examined/ruled out?

Meckel's diverticulum, Crohn's disease, intussusception, gynecologic disease

What is the approximate risk of perforation?

~ 25% after 24 hours from onset of symptoms
~ 50% by 36 hours
~ 75% by 48 hours

INTUSSUSCEPTION

What is it?

Obstruction caused by bowel telescoping into the lumen of adjacent distal bowel; may result when a "leadpoint" is carried downstream by peristalsis

What is the usual age at presentation?

Disease of infancy; 60% present from 4 to 12 months, 80% by age 2 years

What is the most common site?

Terminal ileum involving ileocecal valve and extending into the ascending colon

What is the most common cause?

Hypertrophic Peyer's patches, which act as a lead point; many patients have prior viral illness

What are the signs/ symptoms?

Alternating lethargy and irritability (colic), bilious vomiting, "currant jelly" stools, right lower quadrant mass on plain abdominal film, empty right lower quadrant on palpation (Dance's sign)

What is the intussuscipiens?

The recipient segment of bowel (think: "recipiens" = intussus "cipiens")

What is the intussusceptum?

The leading point or bowel that enters the intussuscipiens

Identify locations 1 and 2 on the following illustration:

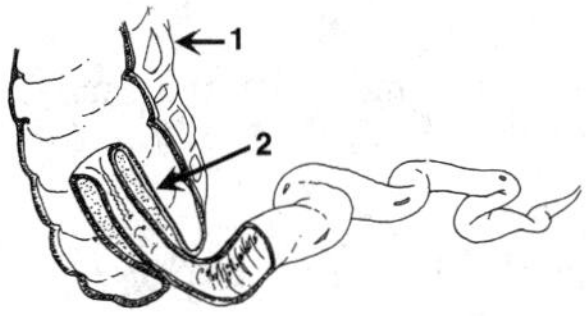

1. Intussuscipiens
2. Intussusceptum

How can the spelling of intussusception be remembered?

Intussusception—two "s's," followed by one "s." Think: the United States ship the U.S. = U.S.S. U.S. (analogous to the ship the U.S.S. Constitution)

What is the treatment?

Air or barium enema; 85% reduce with hydrostatic pressure (i.e., meter elevation); if unsuccessful, then laparotomy and reduction by "milking" the ileum from the colon should be performed

Note: most surgeons also perform appendectomy at that time; if these measures fail, then resection with end-to-end anastomosis should be performed

What are the causes of intussusception in older patients?	Meckel's diverticulum, polyps, and tumors, all of which act as a lead point

MECKEL'S DIVERTICULUM

What is it?	Remnant of the omphalomesenteric duct/vitelline duct, which connects the yolk sac with the primitive midgut in the embryo
What is the usual location?	Between 45 and 90 cm proximal to the ileocecal valve on the antimesenteric border of the bowel
What is the major differential diagnosis?	Appendicitis
Is it a true diverticulum?	Yes; all layers of the intestine are found in the wall
What is the incidence?	2% of the population at autopsy, but more than 90% of these are asymptomatic
What is the gender ratio?	Two to three times more common in males
What is the usual age at onset of symptoms?	Most frequently in the first 2 years of life, but can occur at any age
What are the possible complications?	**Intestinal hemorrhage** (painless)—50% Accounts for half of all lower GI bleeding in patients younger than 2 years; bleeding is due to ectopic gastric mucosa secreting acid → ulcer → bleeding **Intestinal obstruction**—25% Most common complication in adults; includes volvulus and intussusception **Inflammation** (+/- perforation)—20%
What percentage of cases have heterotopic tissue?	More than 50%; usually gastric mucosa (85%), but duodenal, pancreatic, and colonic mucosa have been described

What is the most common ectopic tissue in a Meckel's diverticulum?

Gastric mucosa

What other pediatric disease entity can also present with GI bleeding secondary to ectopic gastric mucosa?

Enteric duplications

What is the most common cause of lower GI bleeding in children?

Meckel's diverticulum with ectopic gastric mucosa

What is the "rule of 2s"?

2% are symptomatic
Found about **2 feet** from the ileocecal valve
Found in **2%** of the population
Majority of symptoms occur before age **2**
One of **2** will have ectopic tissue
Most diverticula are about **2** inches long
Male:female ratio = 2:1

What is a Meckel's scan?

Scan for ectopic gastric mucosa in Meckel's diverticulum; uses technetium **pertechnetate** IV, which is preferentially taken up by gastric mucosa

NECROTIZING ENTEROCOLITIS

What is it also known as?

NEC

What is it?

Necrosis of intestinal mucosa often with bleeding; may progress to transmural intestinal necrosis, shock/sepsis, and death

What are the predisposing conditions?

PREMATURITY
Stress: shock, hypoxia, RDS, apneic episodes, sepsis, exchange transfusions, PDA and cyanotic heart disease, hyperosmolar feedings, polycythemia, indomethacin

What is the pathophysiologic mechanism?

Probable splanchnic vasoconstriction with decreased perfusion, mucosal injury, and probable bacterial invasion

What is its claim to fame?
Most common cause of emergent laparotomy in the neonate

What are the signs/ symptoms?
Abdominal distention, vomiting, heme positive or gross rectal bleeding, fever or hypothermia, jaundice, abdominal wall erythema (consistent with perforation and abscess formation)

What are the radiographic findings?
Fixed, dilated intestinal loops; pneumatosis intestinalis (air in the bowel wall); free air; and portal vein air (sign of advanced disease)

What are the lab findings?
Low Hct, low glucose, low platelets

What is the treatment?
Seventy-five percent are managed medically:
1. Cessation of feedings
2. OG tube
3. IV fluids
4. IV antibiotics
5. Ventilator support, as needed

What are the surgical indications?
Free air in the abdomen revealing perforation and positive peritoneal tap revealing transmural bowel necrosis

Is portal vein gas or pneumatosis intestinalis by themselves an indication for an operation with NEC?
No

What are the indications for peritoneal tap?
Severe thrombocytopenia, distended abdomen, abdominal wall erythema, unexplained clinical downturn

What are the possible complications?
Occur commonly and include further bowel necrosis, gram-negative sepsis, DIC, wound infection, cholestasis, short bowel syndrome, and strictures
Long term complications: small bowel obstruction

What is the prognosis?
Greater than 80% overall survival rate

BILIARY TRACT

What is "physiologic jaundice"?
Hyperbilirubinemia in the first 2 weeks of life due to inadequate conjugation of bilirubin

What enzyme is responsible for the conjugation of bilirubin?
Glucouronyl transferase

How is hyperbilirubinemia due to "physiologic jaundice" treated?
UV light

BILIARY ATRESIA

What is it?
Obliteration of the extrahepatic biliary tree

What is the incidence?
One in 16,000 births

What are the signs/ symptoms?
Persistent jaundice (nl physiologic jaundice resolves in < 2 weeks), hepatomegaly, splenomegaly, ascites and other signs of portal hypertension, acholic stools, biliuria

What are the lab findings?
Mixed jaundice is always present (i.e., both direct and indirect bilirubin increased), elevated serum alkaline phosphatase

What is the "rule of 5s" of indirect bilirubinemia?
Bizarre but true: with progressive hyperbilirubinemia, jaundice progresses by levels of 5 from the head to toes: 5 mg/dl= jaundice of head, 10 mg/dl = jaundice of trunk, 15 mg/dl = jaundice of leg/feet

What is the differential diagnosis?
Neonatal hepatitis (TORCH); biliary hypoplasia

How is the diagnosis made?
1. U/S to rule out choledochal cyst and to examine extrahepatic bile ducts and gallbladder
2. HIDA scan—shows no excretion into the GI tract (with phenobarbitol preparation)
3. Operative cholangiogram and liver biopsy

What is the treatment?
Early laparotomy by 2 months of age with a modified form of the Kasai hepatoportoenterostomy

How does a Kasai work?
The anastomosis of the porta hepatis and the small bowel allows drainage of bile via many microscopic bile ducts in the fibrous structure of the porta hepatis.

What if the Kasai fails?
Revise or liver transplantation

What are the possible postoperative complications?
Cholangitis (manifested as decreased bile secretion, fever, leukocytosis, and recurrence of jaundice), progressive cirrhosis (manifested as portal hypertension with bleeding varices, ascites, hypoalbuminemia, hypothrombinemia, and fat-soluble vitamin K, A, D, E deficiencies)

What are the associated abnormalities?
Between 25% and 30% have other anomalies including annular pancreas, duodenal atresia, malrotation, polysplenic syndrome, situs inversus, and preduodenal portal vein; 15% have congenital heart defects

CHOLEDOCHAL CYST

What is it?
Cystic enlargement of the bile ducts; most commonly arises in the extrahepatic ducts, but can also arise in intrahepatic ducts

What is the usual presentation?
Fifty percent present with intermittent jaundice, right upper quadrant mass, and abdominal pain; may also present with pancreatitis

What are the possible complications?
Cholelithiasis, cirrhosis, carcinoma, and portal HTN

What are the anatomic variants:

I?

Dilation of common hepatic and common bile duct, with cystic duct entering the cyst; most common type (90%)

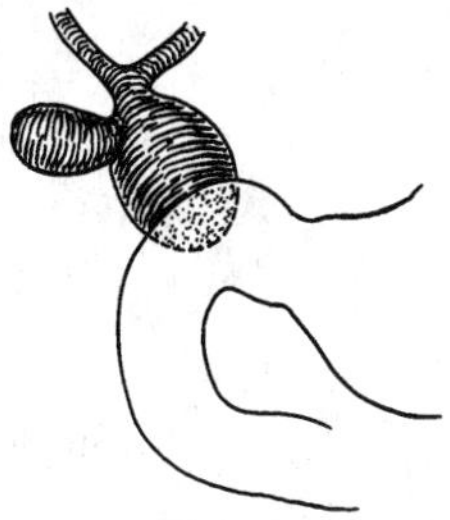

Type I

II?

Lateral saccular cystic dilation

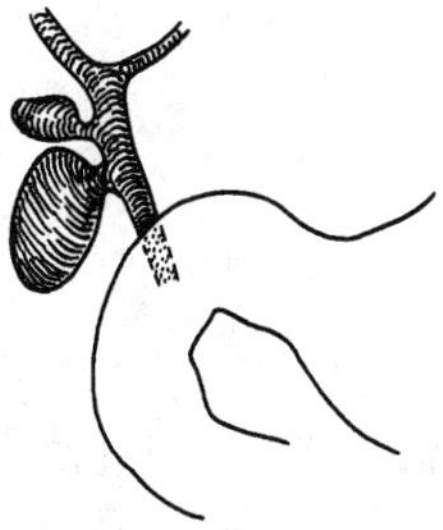

Type II

III?

Choledochocele represented by an intraduodenal cyst

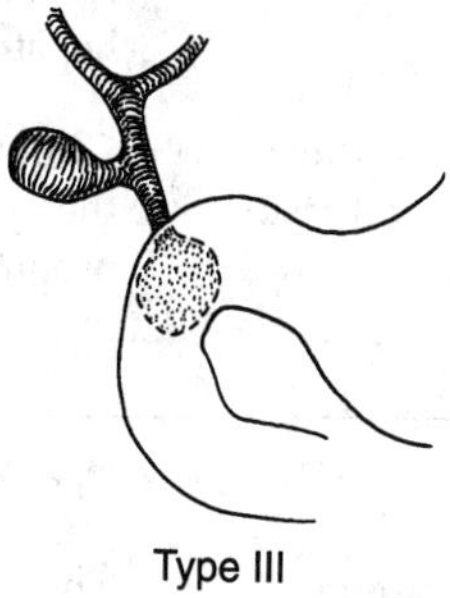

Type III

IV?

Multiple extrahepatic cysts, intrahepatic cysts, or both

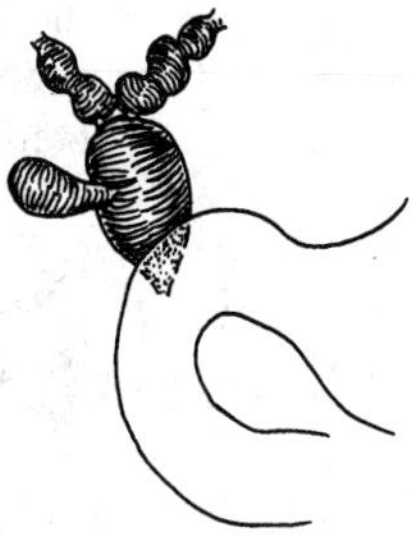

Type IV

V?

Single or multiple intrahepatic cysts

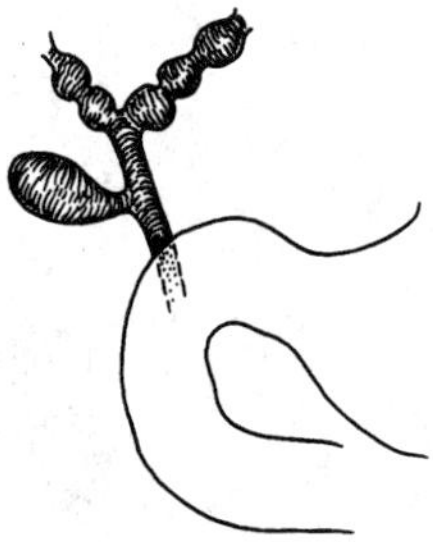

Type V

How is the diagnosis made?

U/S

What is the treatment?

Operative cholangiogram to clarify pathologic process and delineate the pancreatic duct, followed by complete resection of the cyst and a Roux-en-Y hepatojejunostomy

What condition are these patients at increased risk of developing?

Cholangiocarcinoma often arises in the cyst; therefore, treat by the complete prophylactic resection of the cyst.

CHOLELITHIASIS

What is it?

The formation of gallstones

What are the common causes in children?

The etiology differs somewhat from that of adults; the most common cause is cholesterol stones, but there is an increased percentage of pigmented stones due to hemolytic disorders.

What is the differential diagnosis?
Hereditary spherocytosis, thalassemia, pyruvate kinase deficiency, Sickle cell disease, cystic fibrosis, long-term parenteral nutrition, idiopathic

What are the associated risks?
Use of oral contraceptives, teenage pregnancy, positive family history

How is the diagnosis made?
U/S and ERCP when indicated

What is the treatment?
Cholecystectomy is recommended for **all** children with gallstones

ANNULAR PANCREAS

What is an annular pancreas?
Congenital pancreatic abnormality with complete encirclement of the duodenum by the pancreas

What are the symptoms of annular pancreas?
Duodenal obstruction

What is the treatment of annular pancreas?
Duoduodenostomy bypass of obstruction (do not resect the pancreas!)

TUMORS

What is the differential diagnosis of pediatric abdominal mass?
Wilms' tumor, neuroblastoma, hernia, intussusception, malrotation with volvulus, mesenteric cyst, duplication cyst, liver tumor (hepatoblastoma/hemangioma), rhabdomyosarcoma, teratoma

WILMS' TUMOR

What is it?
Embryonal tumor of **renal** origin

What is the incidence?
Very rare: 500 new cases in the United States per year

What is the average age at diagnosis?
Usually between 2 and 4 years of age

What are the symptoms?
Usually asymptomatic except for abdominal mass; 20% of patients present with minimal blunt trauma to mass

What are the signs?

Abdominal mass (most do not cross the midline); hematuria (10%–15%); hypertension in 20% of cases, related to compression of juxtaglomerular apparatus; signs of Beckwith-Wiedemann syndrome

How is the diagnosis made?

Physical exam, abdominal CT with IV contrast to evaluate collecting system, CXR to rule out lung metastases, U/S

Define the stages:

Stage I

Limited to the kidney and completely resected

Stage II

Extends beyond the kidney, but completely resected; capsule invasion and perirenal tissues may be involved

Stage III

Residual tumor confined to **the abdomen**

Stage IV

Hematogenous metastases (lung, distal lymph nodes, and brain)

Stage V

Bilateral renal involvement

What are the best indicators of survival?

Stage and histologic subtype of tumor; 85% of patients have favorable histology (FH); 15% have unfavorable histology (UH); overall survival for FH is 90% for all stages

What is the treatment?

Radical resection of affected kidney with evaluation for staging, followed by chemotherapy (low stages), and radiation (higher stages)

What are the associated abnormalities?

Aniridia, hemihypertrophy, Beckwith-Wiedemann syndrome, neurofibromatosis, and horseshoe kidney

What is the Beckwith-Wiedemann syndrome?

Syndrome of:

1. Umbilical defect
2. Macroglossia (big tongue)
3. Gigantism
4. Visceromegaly (big organs)

(think **W**ilms' = Beckwith-**W**iedemann)

NEUROBLASTOMA

What is it?	Embryonal tumor of neural crest origin
What are the anatomic locations?	**Adrenal medulla—50%** Paraaortic abdominal paraspinal ganglia—25% Posterior mediastinum—20% Neck—3% Pelvis—3%
With which type of tumor does a patient with Horner's syndrome present ?	Neck, superior mediastinal tumors
What is the incidence?	One in 7000 to 10,000 live births; most common solid malignant tumor of infancy; most common solid tumor in children outside the CNS
What is the average age at diagnosis?	Approximately 50% are diagnosed by 2 years of age Approximately 90% are diagnosed by 8 years of age
What are the symptoms?	Vary by tumor location—anemia, failure to thrive, weight loss, and poor nutritional status with advanced disease
What are the signs?	Asymptomatic abdominal mass (palpable in 50% of cases), respiratory distress (mediastinal tumors), Horner's syndrome (upper chest or neck tumors), proptosis (with orbital metastases), subcutaneous tumor nodules, HTN (20%–35%)
How is the diagnosis made?	Physical exam; 24-hour urine to measure VMA, HVA, and metanephines (elevated in > 85%); plain x-rays (may show calcifications); CXR; CT; Mibg scan (I-Metaiodobenzylguanide as used in pheochromocytoma); and bone marrow biopsy to rule out metastases, ferritin, neuron-specific enolase, N-*myc* oncogene, DNA ploidy

What is the difference in position of tumors in neuroblastoma versus Wilms' tumors?	Neuroblastoma may cross the midline, but Wilms' tumors do so only rarely
What is the treatment?	Depends on staging
Define the stages:	
Stage I	Tumor confined to the organ of origin
Stage II	Tumor that extends beyond the organ of origin, **but not** across the midline
Stage III	Tumor that extends **across the midline**
Stage IV	Metastatic disease
Stage IVS	Localized primary tumor not crossing the midline, but with **remote disease** confined to the liver, subcutaneous tissues, and bone marrow
What is the treatment of each stage:	
Stage I?	Surgical resection
Stage II?	Resection and chemotherapy
Stage III?	Resection and chemotherapy
Stage IV?	Resection and chemotherapy, with or without radiation therapy
What is the survival rate of each stage:	
Stage I?	Approximately 90%
Stage II?	Approximately 80%
Stage III?	Approximately 40%
Stage IV?	Approximately 15%

Stage IV S?	**Survival rate is more than 80%!** *Note:* these tumors are basically stage I or II with metastasis to the liver, subcutaneous tissue, or bone marrow; most of these patients, if under 1 year of age, have a spontaneous cure. (think: stage IV **S** = **S**pecial condition)
What are the laboratory prognosticators?	Aneuploidy is favorable! The lower the number of N-*myc* oncogene copies, the better the prognosis.
Which oncogene is associated with neuroblastoma?	N-*myc* oncogene Think: **N**-myc = **N**euroblastoma

RHABDOMYOSARCOMA

What is it?	Highly malignant **striated muscle** sarcoma
What is its claim to fame?	Most common sarcoma in children
What are the most common sites?	1. Head and neck (40%) 2. GU tract (20%) 3. Extremities (20%) Other sites: abdomen, anus, retroperitoneum, pelvis, thorax
What are the signs/ symptoms?	Mass
How is the diagnosis made?	Tissue biopsy, CT, MRI, bone marrow, plain x-rays
Define the stages:	
Stage I	Localized, completely excised tumor
Stage II	Microscopic residual disease
Stage III	Gross residual disease
Stage IV	Distant metastases
What is the treatment?	Surgical excision, chemotherapy, and radiation therapy

What is the 3-year survival rate at each stage:	
Stage I?	Approximately 80%
Stage II?	Approximately 70%
Stage III?	Approximately 50%
Stage IV?	Approximately 25% 55% at 5 years

HEPATOBLASTOMA

What is it?	Malignant tumor of the liver (derived from embryonic liver cells)
What is the average age at diagnosis?	Presents in the first 3 years of life
What is the male:female ratio?	2:1
How is the diagnosis made?	Physical exam—abdominal distention; right upper quadrant mass that moves with respiration Elevated serum α-fetoprotein and ferritin (can be used as tumor markers) CT scan of the abdomen, which often predicts resectability
What percentage will have an elevated α-fetoprotein level?	Approximately 90%
What is the treatment?	Resection by lobectomy or trisegmentectomy is the treatment of choice; large tumors may require preoperative chemotherapy and **subsequent** hepatic resection
What is the overall survival rate?	Approximately 50%
What is the major difference in age presentation between hepatoma and hepatoblastoma?	Hepatoblastoma presents at less than 3 years of age; hepatoma presents at more than 3 years of age and in adolescents.

OTHER PEDIATRIC SURGERY QUESTIONS

What is bilious vomiting in an infant?
Malrotation, until proven otherwise! (about 90% of patients with malrotation present before the first year of life)

What does TORCHES stand for?
Nonbacterial fetal and neonatal infections: **T**oxoplasmosis, **R**ubella, **C**ytomegalovirus (CMV), **He**rpes, **S**yphilis

What is the common pediatric sedative?
Chloral hydrate

What are the contraindications to circumcision?
Hypospadias, etc., because the foreskin might be needed for future repair of the abnormality

When should an umbilical hernia be repaired?
If the patient is older than 2 years of age and the hernia defect is more than 1.5 cm in diameter; otherwise observe, because most close spontaneously; repair before school age if it persists

What is the cancer risk in the cryptorchid testicle?
More than ten times the normal testicular cancer rate

When should orchidopexy be performed?
All patients with undescended testicle undergo orchidopexy after 1 year of life.

What are the signs of child abuse?
Cigarette burns, rope burns, scald to posterior thighs and buttocks, multiple fractures/old fractures, genital trauma, delay in accessing health care system

What is the treatment of child abuse?
Admit the patient to the hospital

How are the vast majority of splenic injuries treated in children?
Bedrest (i.e., nonoperatively)

What is the role of DPL in children?
Much less than with adults, because most centers go to the CT scanner to evaluate the abdomen

What is a common simulator of peritoneal signs in the blunt pediatric trauma victim?

Gastric distention (place an NG tube)

What is Dance's sign?

Empty right lower quadrant in patients with ileocecal intussusception

What is the treatment of hemangioma?

Observation, because most regress spontaneously

What are the indications for operation in hemangiomas?

Severe thrombocytopenia, congestive heart failure, functional impairment (vision, breathing)

What are the treatment options for hemangiomas?

Steroids, radiation, surgical resection, angiographic embolization

What is the most common benign liver tumor in children?

Hemangioma

What is Eagle-Barret's syndrome?

A.K.A. prune belly; congenital inadequate abdominal musculature (very lax and thin)

What are the most common cancers in children?

1. Leukemia
2. CNS tumors
3. Lymphomas

What is the most common solid neoplasm in infants?

Neuroblastoma

What is the most common solid tumor in children?

CNS tumors

What syndrome must you consider in the patient with abdominal pain, hematuria, history of joint pain and a purpuric rash?

Henoch-Schonlein syndrome; patient may also have melena (50%), or at least guaiac-positive stools (75%)

What is Apley's law?

The farther a chronically recurrent abdominal pain is from the umbilicus, the greater the likelihood of an organic cause for the pain.

What is the most common cause of SBO in children?

Hernias

What is a patent urachus?

Persistence of the urachus, a communication between the bladder and the umbilicus; presents with urine out of the umbilicus and recurrent UTIs

What is a "Replogle tube"?

10 French sump pump NG tube for babies (originally designed by Dr. Replogle for suction of the esophageal blind pouch of esophageal atresia)

What are "A's and B's"?

Apnea and **B**radycardia episodes in babies

What is the "Double Bubble" sign on AXR?

Gastric bubble and DUODENAL BUBBLE on AXR; seen with duodenal obstruction (web, annular pancreas, malrotation with volvulus, duodenal atresia, etc.)

What is Poland's syndrome?

Absence of pectoralis muscle
Absence of pectoralis minor muscle
Often associated with ipsilateral hand malformation
Nipple/breast/right-breast hypoplasia

What is the treatment of ATYPICAL mycobacterial lymph node infection?

Surgical removal of the node

What is the Pentology of Cantrell?

"D COPS":
Diaphragmatic defect (hernia)

Cardiac abnormality
Omphalocele
Pericardium malformation/absence
Sternal cleft

What chromosomal abnormality is associated with duodenal web/atresia/stenosis?

Trisomy 21

How many calories in breast milk?

20 kcal/30 cc (same as most formulas)

POWER REVIEW

What is the age at presentation of the following conditions:	
Pyloric stenosis?	From 2 weeks to 2 months
Intussusception?	From 4 months to 2 years (> 80%)
Wilms' tumor?	Between 1 and 4 years
Malrotation?	Birth to 1 year (> 85%)
Neuroblastoma?	Approximately 50% present by age 2 and more than 80% present by age 8 years
Hepatoblastoma?	Less than 3 years of age
Appendicitis?	More than 3 years of age

61

Plastic Surgery

Define the following terms:

Syndactyly	Webbed fingers
Polydactyly	Extra fingers
Mammoplasty	Breast surgery (reduction/augmentation)
Facelift	Removal of excess facial skin via hairline/chin/ear incisions
Blepharoplasty	Eyelid surgery—removing excess skin/fat
Rhinoplasty	Nose surgery, after trauma or cosmetic
STSG	**S**plit **T**hickness **S**kin **G**raft
Langer's lines	The natural direction/alignment of connective tissue in the dermis (e.g., transverse lines across the abdomen); incisions perpendicular to Langer's lines result in larger scars than incision parallel to the lines

WOUND HEALING

What are the phases of wound healing?

1. Inflammation
2. Epithelialization
3. Fibroplasia
4. Contraction

What are the actions of the following phases:

Inflammation?	Vasoconstriction followed by vasodilation, capillary leak
Epithelialization?	Epithelial coverage of wound

Fibroplasia?	Fibroblasts and accumulation of collagen, elastin, and reticulin
Wound contraction?	Myofibroblasts contract wound
What is the maximal contraction of wound in mm/day?	Less than 0.75 mm/day

EPITHELIALIZATION

What degree of bacterial contamination prevents epithelialization?	More than 100,000 organisms/gm tissue (10^5)
What structures does the epithelium grow in from superficial burns/wounds?	Sweat glands and hair follicles
In full-thickness burns?	From wound margins, grows in less than 1 cm from wound edge because no sweat glands or hair remains; this epithelium has no underlying dermis
What malignant ulcer is associated with a long-standing scar/burn?	Marjolin's ulcer (A.K.A. burn scar carcinoma)

WOUND CONTRACTION

What are myofibroblasts?	Specialized fibroblasts that behave like smooth muscle cells to pull the wound edges together following granulation
How can this contraction be slowed?	Split-thickness skin grafts (STSG)
How can it be stopped?	Full-thickness skin grafts (FTSG)
Which contracts more: an STSG or an FTSG?	An STSG contracts up to 41% in surface area, whereas an FTSG contracts little, if at all.
What is granulation tissue?	Within 4 to 6 days after an open wound, development of capillary beds and fibroblasts provides a healthy base for epithelial growth from wound edges; this tissue also resists bacterial infection.

Name the local factors that impair wound healing.	Hematoma, seroma, infection, tight sutures, tight wrap
What generalized conditions inhibit wound healing?	Anemia Malnutrition Steroids Cancer Radiation Hypoxia Sepsis
What helps wound healing in patients on steroids?	Vitamin A is thought to counteract the deleterious effect of steroids on wound healing.
When does a wound gain more than 80% of its maximal tensile strength?	After approximately 6 weeks
Define the following terms:	
Laceration	Torn/mangled/cut wound
Abrasion	Superficial skin removal
Contusion	Bruise without a break in the skin
Keloid	Hypertrophic scar
Why not clean lacerations with Betadine?	Betadine is harmful to and inhibits normal healthy tissue
What is the best way to clean out a laceration?	H_2O irrigation

SKIN GRAFTS

What is an STSG?	Includes the epidermis and a variable amount of the dermis
How thick is it?	Between 12/1000 and 18/1000 of an inch
What is an FTSG?	Involves the entire epidermis and dermis

What are the prerequisites for a skin graft to take?

The bed must be vascularized; a graft to a bone or tendon will not take.
Bacteria must be less than 100,000.
Shearing motion and fluid beneath the graft must be minimized.

What is a better bed for a skin graft: fascia or fat?

Fascia (much better blood supply)

What is "tie-over bolus dressing"?

In an area that does not lend itself to circumferential wrapping, a tie-over dressing provides continuous compression to skin grafts in concave wounds.
The skin graft is fixed to the recipient site with long sutures and then is covered with xeroform.
A bolus of cotton is then applied and the sutures on the opposite side are pulled together to hold the packing in place.

FLAPS

Where does a random skin flap get its blood supply?

From the dermal–subdermal plexus

Where does an axial skin flap get its blood supply?

It is vascularized by direct cutaneous arteries

Name some axial flaps and their arterial supply.

Forehead flap—superficial temporal artery; often used for intraoral lesions
Deltopectoral flap—second, third, and fourth anterior perforators of the internal mammary artery; often used for head and neck wounds
Groin flap—superficial circumflex iliac artery; allows coverage of hand and forearm wounds

What is a "free flap"?

A flap separated from all vascular supply that requires microvascular anastomosis (microscope)

What is a TRAM flap?

Transverse **R**ectus **A**bdominis **M**yocutaneous flap

What is a "Z-plasty"?

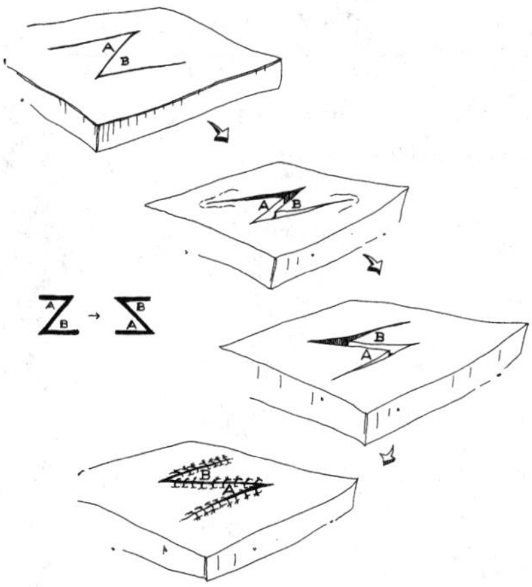

HANDS

What are the bones of the hand?	Phalanges (fingers) Metacarpal bones Carpal bones
What is the distal finger joint?	Distal interphalangeal (DIP) joint
What is the middle finger joint?	Proximal interphalangeal (PIP) joint
What is the proximal finger joint?	Metacarpal phalangeal (MP) joint
What is the name of the "intrinsic" hand muscles?	Lumbricales
Where is "no man's land"?	Flexor hand lacerations anywhere from the middle of the middle phalanx to the distal palmer crease; must be repaired by a hand expert

SENSORY SUPPLY TO THE HAND

What is the ulnar nerve distribution?

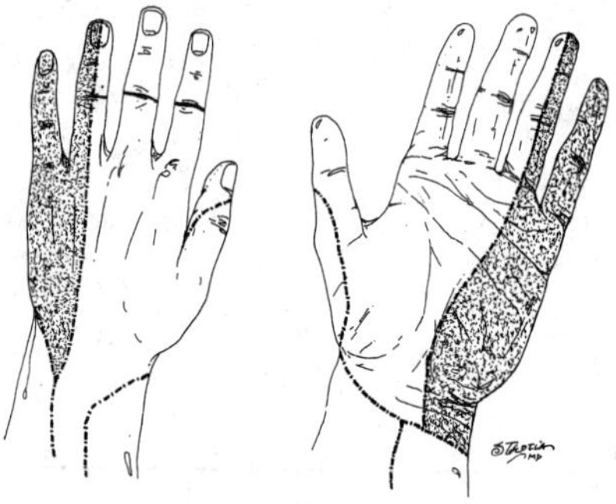

What is the radial nerve distribution?

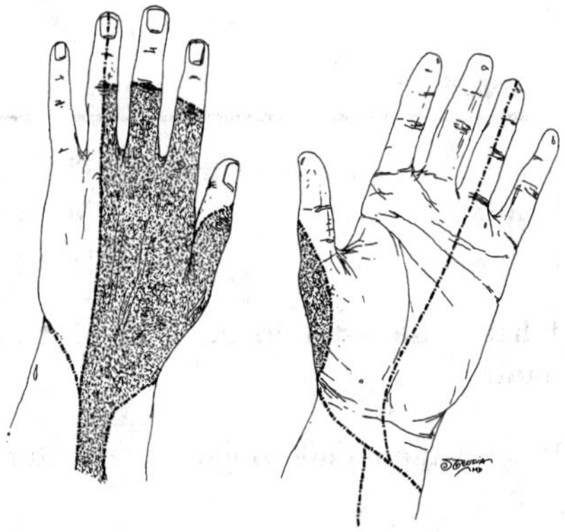

What is the median nerve distribution?

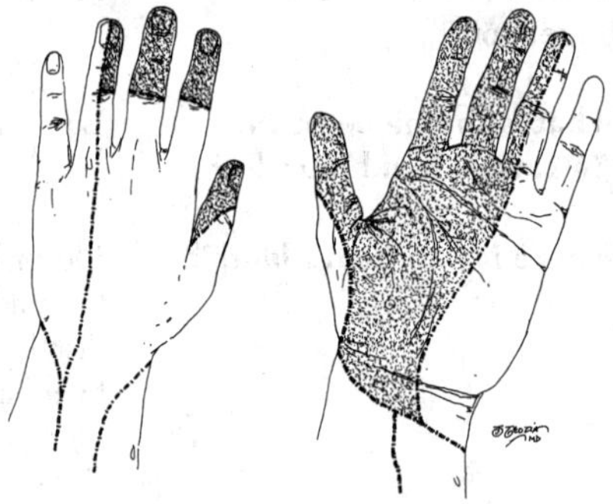

How can the radial nerve motor function be tested? Extend the wrist against resistance

How can the ulnar nerve motor function be tested? Spread fingers apart against resistance

How can the median nerve function be tested?

1. Touch the thumb to the pinky (distal median nerve)
2. Squeeze examiner's finger (proximal median nerve)

How can the flexor digitorum profundus apparatus be tested?

Isolated flexion of the finger DIP joint

How can the flexor digitorum superficialis apparatus be tested?

Isloated flexion of the finger at the MP joint

Where do the digital arteries run?

On both sides of the digit

What hand laceration should be left unsutured?

Lacerations due to human bites

Should a clamp ever be used to stop a laceration bleeder?

No; use pressure and then tourniquet for definitive repair if bleeding does not cease, because **nerves run with blood vessels!**

What is a felon?

Infection in **the tip** of the finger pad (think: felon = fingerprints = infection in pad); treat by drainage

What is a paronychia?

Infection on the **side** of the finger nail; treat by drainage

What is tenosynovitis?

Tendon sheath infection

What are Kanavel's signs?

Four signs of tenosynovitis:

1. Affected finger held in slight **flexion**
2. **Pain** over volar aspect of affected finger tendon upon **palpation**
3. **Swelling** of affected finger
4. **Pain on passive extension** of affected finger

How is a human hand bite treated?

Debridement/irrigation/administration of antibiotics

What is the most common hand/wrist tumor?

Ganglion cyst

What is an extremely painful type of subungual tumor?

Glomus tumor

What is a "boxer's fracture"?

Fracture of the fourth or fifth metacarpal

What is the classic deformity resulting from laceration of the extensor tendon over the DIP joint?

Mallet finger

What is the classic deformity resulting from laceration of the extensor tendon over the PIP joint?

Boutonniere deformity

Which fracture causes pain in the "anatomic snuffbox"?

Scaphoid fracture; often not seen on x-ray at presentation, usually seen at a later date (2 weeks) on x-ray

Can result in avascular necrosis.

Place in a cast if clinically suspected, regardless of x-ray findings.

What is the "safe position" of hand splinting?

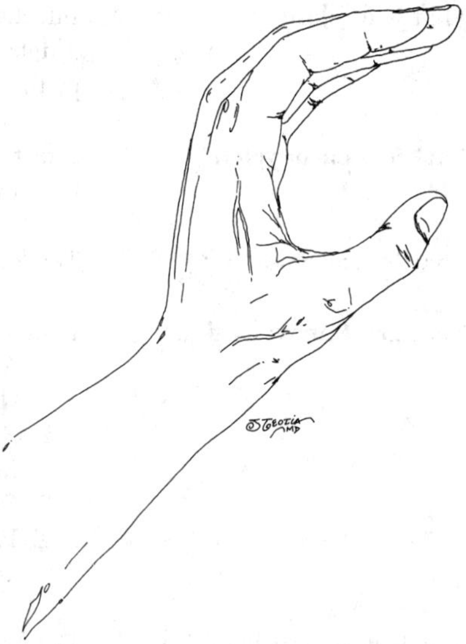

What is Dupuytren's contracture?

Fibrosis of the palmar fascia, resulting in contracture of the digits and inability to extend digits

What is Gamekeeper's thumb?

Injury to the ulnar collateral ligament of the thumb

How should a subungual (i.e., under the nail) hematoma be treated?

Release pressure by burning a hole in the nail (use hand-held disposable battery-operated coagulation probe)

62

Otolaryngology: Head and Neck Surgery

ANATOMY

Define the cranial nerves:	
I	Olfactory nerve
II	Optic nerve
III	Oculomotor nerve
IV	Trochlear nerve
V	Trigeminal nerve
VI	Abducens nerve
VII	Facial nerve
VIII	Vestibulocochlear nerve
IX	Glossopharyngeal nerve
X	Vagus nerve
XI	Accessory nerve
XII	Hypoglossal nerve
Define motor/sensory actions of the following cranial nerves:	
I	Smell
II	Sight
III	Eyeball movement, pupil sphincter, ciliary muscle
IV	Superior oblique muscle movement

V	Sensory to teeth, sinuses, face muscles of chewing (mastication)
VI	Lateral rectus muscle (lateral gaze)
VII	Motor: facial muscles, lacrimal/sublingual/submandibular glands Sensory: anterior tongue/soft palate
VIII	Hearing, positioning
IX	Motor: stylopharyngeus, parotid, pharynx Sensory: posterior tongue, pharynx, middle ear
X	Motor: vocal cords, heart, bronchus, GI tract Sensory: bronchus, heart, GI tract, larynx, ear
XI	Motor: trapezius muscle, sternocleidomastoid muscle
XII	Motor: tongue, strap muscles (ansa cervicalis branch)

What are the three divisions of the trigeminal nerve (cranial nerve V)?

1. Ophthalmic
2. Maxillary
3. Mandibular

What happens when the hypoglossal nerve (cranial nerve XII) is cut?

When the patient sticks out the tongue, it deviates to the same side as the injury (wheelbarrow effect)

Name the duct of the submandibular gland.

Wharton's duct

Name the duct of the parotid gland.

Stenson's duct

What is the source of blood supply to the nose?

1. Internal carotid artery: anterior and posterior ethmoidal arteries via ophthalmic artery
2. External carotid artery: superior labial artery (via facial artery) and **sphenopalatine artery** (via internal maxillary artery)

Name the three bones that make up the posterior nasal septum.

1. Ethmoid (perpendicular plate)
2. Vomer (latin for plow)
3. Palatine

(Some also include maxillary crest.)

Name the seven bones of the bony eyeball orbit.

1. Frontal
2. Zygoma
3. Maxillary
4. Lacrimal
5. Ethmoid
6. Palatine
7. Sphenoid

Which sinus is fully formed at birth?

Ethmoid sinus

Name the four strap muscles.

1. Sternothyroid
2. Omohyoid
3. Thyrohyoid
4. Sternohyoid

Which muscle crosses the external and internal carotid arteries?

Digastric muscle

In a neck incision, what is the first muscle incised?

Platysma

Which nerve supplies the strap muscles?

Ansa cervicalis (XII)

Which nerve runs with the carotid in the carotid sheath?

Vagus

Which nerve crosses the internal carotid artery at approximately 1 to 2 cm above the bifurcation?

Hypoglossal nerve

Name the three auditory ossicle bones.

1. Malleus
2. Incus
3. Stapes

What comprises the middle ear?

Eustachian tube, ossicle bones, tympanic membrane ("ear drum"), mastoid air cell

What comprises the inner ear?	Cochlea, semicircular canals, internal auditory canal

EAR

OTITIS EXTERNA (SWIMMER'S EAR)

What is it?	Generalized infection involving the external ear canal and often the tympanic membrane
What is the usual cause?	Prolonged water exposure and damaged squamous epithelium of the ear canal (i.e., swimming, hearing aid use)
What are the typical pathogens?	Most frequently *Pseudomonas;* may be *Proteus, Staphylococcus,* occasionally fungi (*Aspergillus, Candida*), or virus (herpes zoster or herpes simplex)
What are the signs/ symptoms?	Ear pain (otalgia), external ear and/or ear canal swelling, erythema, pain on manipulation of the auricle, debris in canal
What is the treatment?	Most importantly, keep the ear dry; mild infections respond to cleaning and dilute acetic acid drops. Most infections require complete removal of all debris and topical antibiotics with or without hydrocortisone (antiinflammatory); consider antifungal drops for otomycosis.

MALIGNANT OTITIS EXTERNA (MOE)

What is it?	Fulminant **bacterial** otitis externa
Who is affected?	Most common scenario: an elderly, poorly controlled diabetic (other forms of immunosuppression do not appear to predispose patients to MOE)
What are the causative organisms?	Usually *Pseudomonas aeruginosa*
What is the classic feature?	A nub of granulation tissue on the floor of the external ear canal at the bony-cartilaginous junction

What are the other signs/ symptoms?

Severe ear pain, excessive purulent discharge, and usually **exposed bone**

What are the diagnostic tests?

1. CT scan: shows erosion of bone, inflammation
2. Technetium-99 scan: temporal bone inflammatory process
3. Gallium tagged white blood cell scan: to follow and document resolution

What are the complications?

Invasion of surrounding structures to produce a cellulitis, osteomyelitis of temporal bone, mastoiditis; later, a facial nerve palsy, meningitis, or brain abscess

What is the treatment?

Control of diabetes, meticulous local care with extensive debridement, hospitalization and IV antibiotics (anti-*Pseudomonas:* usually an aminoglycoside plus a penicillin)

TUMORS OF THE EXTERNAL EAR

What are the most common types?

Squamous cell is most common; occasionally, basal cell carcinoma or melanoma

From what location do they usually arise?

The auricle, but occasionally from the external canal

What is the associated risk factor?

Excessive sun exposure

What is the treatment of the following conditions:

Cancers of the auricle?

Usually treated by wedge excision

Extension to the canal?

May require excision of the external ear canal, or partial temporal bone excision

Middle ear involvement?

Best treated by en bloc temporal bone resection

TYMPANIC MEMBRANE (TM) PERFORATION

What is the etiology?
Usually the result of trauma (direct or indirect) or secondary to middle ear infection; often occurs secondary to slap to the side of the head (compression injury)

What are the symptoms?
Pain, conductive hearing loss, tinnitus

What are the signs?
Bleeding from the ear, clot in the meatus, visible tear in the TM

What is the treatment?
Keep dry; use systemic antibiotics if there is evidence of infection or contamination

What is the prognosis?
Most (90%) heal spontaneously, though larger perforations may require surgery (e.g., fat plug, temporalis fascia tympanoplasty)

CHOLESTEATOMA

What is it?
An epidermal inclusion cyst of the middle ear or mastoid, containing desquamated keratin debris; may be acquired or congenital

What are the causes?
Negative middle ear pressure due to eustachian tube dysfunction (primary acquired; typically in attic) or direct growth of epithelium through a TM perforation (secondary acquired)

What other condition is it often associated with?
Chronic middle ear infection

What is the usual history?
Chronic ear infection with chronic, malodorous drainage

What is the appearance?
Grayish-white, shiny keratinous mass behind or involving the TM; often described as a "pearly" lesion

What are the associated problems?

Ossicular erosion, producing conductive hearing loss; also, local invasion resulting in:
- Vertigo/sensorineural hearing loss
- Facial paresis/paralysis
- CNS dysfunction/infection

What is the treatment?

Surgery (tympanoplasty/mastoidectomy) aimed at eradication of disease and reconstruction of the ossicular chain

BULLOUS MYRINGITIS

What is it?

A vesicular infection of the TM and adjacent deep canal

What are the causative agents?

Unknown; viral should be suspected because of frequent association with viral URI (in some instances, *Mycoplasma pneumoniae* has been cultured)

What are the symptoms?

Acute, severe ear pain; low-grade fever; and bloody drainage

What are the findings on otoscopic examination?

Shows large, reddish blebs on the TM and/or the wall of the meatus

Is hearing affected?

Not usually; occasional reversible sensorineural loss

What is the treatment?

Oral antibiotics (erythromycin if *Mycoplasma* is suspected), topical analgesics may be used, with resolution of symptoms usually occurring in 36 hours

ACUTE SUPPURATIVE OTITIS MEDIA (OM)

What is it?

A bacterial infection of the middle ear, often following a viral upper respiratory infection; may be associated with a middle ear effusion

What is the cause?

Dysfunction of the eustachian tube that allows bacterial entry from nasopharynx; often associated with an occluded eustachian tube, although it is uncertain whether this is a cause or a result of the infection

What are the predisposing factors?

Young age, male gender, bottle feeding, crowded living conditions (i.e., daycare), cleft palate, Down's syndrome, cystic fibrosis

What is the etiology?

1. *Streptococcus pneumoniae* (one-third of cases)
2. *Haemophilus influenzae*
3. *Moraxella catarrhalis*
4. *Staphylococcus*
5. β-hemolytic strep
6. Viral/no culture

What is the etiology in infants less than 6 months old?

1. *Staphylococcus aureus*
2. *E. coli*
3. *Klebsiella*

What are the symptoms?

Otalgia, fever, decreased hearing, infant pulls on ear, increased irritability; as many as 25% of patients are asymptomatic

What are the signs?

Early, redness of the TM; later, TM bulging with loss of the normal landmarks and finally impaired TM mobility on pneumatic otoscopy

What are the complications?

TM perforation, acute mastoiditis, meningitis, brain abscess, extradural abscess, labyrinthitis; if recurrent or chronic, OM may have adverse effects on **speech** and cognitive development due to decreased hearing

What is the treatment?

Ten-day course of antibiotics; amoxicillin is the first-line agent; if the patient is PCN allergic, trimethoprim-sulfamethoxazole or erythromycin should be administered

What is the usual course?

Symptoms usually resolve in 24 to 36 hours

What are the indications for myringotomy and PE tube placement?

1. Persistent middle ear effusion over 3 months
2. Debilitated or immunocompromised patient
3. More than three episodes over 6 months (especially if bilateral)

What is a PE tube?	**P**neumatic **E**qualization tube (tube placed across tympanic membrane)
What is a Bezold's abscess?	Abscess behind the superior attachment of the sternocleidomastoid muscle resulting from extension of a mastoiditis infection

SEROUS OTITIS MEDIA

What is it?	Usually an acute response to temporary ventilatory dysfunction of the eustachian tube
What are the precipitating factors?	Nasopharyngeal inflammation; often allergic rhinitis or the common cold
What more serious lesion may have similar presentation?	Nasopharyngeal carcinoma; be especially suspicious in the adult with prolonged unilateral serous otitis
What are the symptoms?	Sensation of otic fullness, tinnitus, hearing loss
What are the findings on exam?	Amber-colored TM and often a visible fluid line or air bubbles behind the TM, which may be retracted with decreased mobility
What is the treatment?	Most cases resolve without treatment; antihistamines may help; myringotomy with aspiration of fluid has a high certainty of cure but is rarely necessary

MUCOID OTITIS MEDIA

What age group is most often affected?	Usually seen in children
What other condition is it associated with?	Chronic dysfunction of the eustachian tube, a common sequela of acute OM
What is the most common sequela?	Acquired **hearing loss** in children

What are the symptoms?
Often asymptomatic, though impaired hearing is common

What are the findings on exam?
Otoscopy may reveal a dull, retracted, immobile TM

What is the treatment?
Search for underlying etiology; antihistamine-decongestant combinations are not efficacious; watch for 2 to 3 months for spontaneous resolution; myringotomy with tube insertion is necessary if there is no resolution; audiogram is indicated to document hearing loss

OTOSCLEROSIS

What is it?
A genetic disease characterized by abnormal spongy and sclerotic bone formation in the temporal bone around the footplate of the stapes, thus preventing its normal movement

What is the inheritance pattern?
Autosomal dominant with incomplete one-third penetrance

What are the symptoms?
Painless, progressive hearing loss (may be unilateral or bilateral), tinnitus

What is the usual age of onset?
Second through fourth decade

How is the diagnosis made?
Normal TM with conductive hearing loss and no middle-ear effusion (though may be mixed or even sensorineural if bone of cochlea is affected)

What is Schwartze's sign?
Erythema around the stapes due to hypervascularity of new bone formation

What is the treatment?
Frequently surgical (stapedectomy with placement of prosthesis), hearing aids, or observation; sodium fluoride may be used if a sensorineural component is present or for preoperative stabilization

FACIAL NERVE PARALYSIS

How is the defect localized?

Supranuclear—paralysis of lower face only, forehead muscles are spared because of bilateral corticobulbar supply
Intratemporal bone—paralysis of upper and lower face, decreased tearing, altered taste, absent stapedius reflex
Distal to stylomastoid foramen—paralysis of facial muscles only

What are the causes?

Usually from lesions of the nerve within its course through the temporal bone:
- Bell's palsy
- Trauma
- Cholesteatoma with erosion of facial canal
- Tumor (carcinoma, glomus jugulare)
- Herpes zoster inflammation of geniculate ganglion (Ramsey-Hunt syndrome)
- Peripheral lesions are usually parotid gland tumors or facial laceration

What is the most common cause of bilateral facial nerve palsy?

Lyme disease (Borrelia burgdorferi)

BELL'S PALSY

What is it?

Sudden onset, unilateral facial weakness, or paralysis in absence of CNS, ear, or cerebellopontine angle disease (i.e., no identifiable cause)

What is the clinical course?

Acute onset, with greatest muscle weakness reached within 3 weeks

What is the incidence?

Most common cause of **unilateral** facial weakness/paralysis

What is the pathogenesis?

Unknown; most widely accepted hypothesis is viral etiology (Herpes virus); ischemic and immunologic factors are also implicated

What is the common preceding event?

Upper respiratory tract infection

What are the signs/ symptoms?	Pathology is related to swelling of the facial nerve; may present with total facial paralysis, altered lacrimation, increased tearing on affected side, change in taste if region above chorda tympani is affected, dry mouth, and hyperacusis
What is the treatment?	Usually none is required, as most resolve spontaneously in 1 month; protect eye with drops if it cannot be closed; most otolaryngologists advocate steroids and acyclovir. Surgical decompression of CN VII is indicated if paralysis progresses or tests indicate deterioration
What is the prognosis?	Overall, 90% of patients recover completely; if paralysis is incomplete, 95% to 100% will recover without sequelae

SENSORINEURAL HEARING LOSS

What is it?	Hearing loss caused by a lesion occurring in the cochlea or acoustic nerve rather than the external or middle ear
What are the symptoms?	Distortion of hearing, impaired speech discrimination, tinnitus
What are the signs?	Air conduction is better than bone conduction (positive Rinne test), Weber lateralizes to the side without the defect; audiogram varies, but most commonly shows greatest loss in high-frequency tones
What are the causes?	Aging (presbycusis)—leading cause Acoustic injury from sudden or prolonged exposure to loud noises Perilymph fistula Congenital (TORCH: maternal toxoplasmosis, rubella, CMV, Herpes, and syphilis) Meniere's disease Drug/toxin-induced (antibiotics, especially aminoglycosides; aspirin; quinine; anticancer medications such as cisplatin; loop diuretics)

Acoustic neuroma
Pseudotumor cerebri
CNS disease (e.g., meningitis, multiple sclerosis)
Endocrine disorders (e.g., diabetes, hypothyroid)
Sarcoidosis
Metabolic disorders (e.g., hyperlipoproteinemia, chronic renal failure)
Chronic otitis media

What is the most common cause in children?
Meningitis (bacterial)

What is the treatment?
Treatment of underlying cause, hearing aids, lip reading, cochlear implant

VERTIGO

What is it?
The sensation of head movement, usually rotational

What is the cause?
Asymmetric neuronal activity between right and left vestibular systems

What is the history?
Must attempt to differentiate between central and peripheral disease

- Peripheral: severe vertigo, nausea, vomiting, always accompanied by horizontal or rotatory nystagmus (fast component almost always to side opposite disease), other evidence of inner ear disease (tinnitus, hearing loss); frequently associated with a previously operated ear, a chronic draining ear, barotrauma, or abdominal or head trauma
- Central (brainstem or cerebellum): insidious onset, less intense and more subtle sensation of vertigo; difficulty describing the symptoms; occasionally, vertical nystagmus

What are the steps in diagnostic evaluation?
Depends on probability of central versus peripheral; careful neurologic and otologic examinations are required

May need FTA/VDRL (syphilis), temporal bone scans/CT/MRI, ENG, position testing, audiometric testing

What is the most common etiology?

Benign paroxysmal positional vertigo (BPPV); history of brief spells of severe vertigo with specific head positions

What is the differential diagnosis?

Central: vertebral basilar insufficiency (often in older patients with DJD of spine), Wallenberg syndrome, MS, epilepsy, migraine
Peripheral: Benign paroxysmal positional vertigo, motion sickness, syphilis, Meniere's disease, vestibular neuronitis, labyrinthitis, acoustic neuroma, syphilis, perilymph fistula

What is Tullio's phenomenon?

Induction of vertigo by loud noises. Classically due to otosyphilis

MENIERE'S DISEASE

What is it?

Disorder of the membranous labyrinth causing fluctuating sensorineural hearing loss, episodic vertigo, nystagmus, tinnitus, and aural fullness

What is the classic triad?

Hearing loss, tinnitus, vertigo (H, T, V)

What is the pathophysiology?

Obscure, but most experts believe excessive production/defective resorption of endolymph

What is the treatment?

Primarily medical: salt restriction, diuretics (thiazides), antinausea agents; occasionally diazepam is added; 80% of patients respond to medical management
Surgery is offered to those who fail medical treatment or who have incapacitating vertigo (60%–80% effective)

VESTIBULAR NEURITIS

What is it?

Severe attack(s) of prolonged vertigo; thought to have a viral origin

What is the typical history?

Healthy adult (age 30–60 years) who has had a URI or sinusitis prior to an acute vestibular crisis characterized by severe vertigo, nausea, vomiting, and nystagmus

What is the course?

Symptoms usually last 3 to 7 days, with progressive improvement noted following a single episode; recurrences (usually less severe) may occur in the ensuing weeks

What is the treatment?

IV phenothiazine given slowly will usually stop severe vertigo, nausea, and vomiting; diazepam or meclizine (vestibulosuppressives) may be helpful; mainstay of treatment is early, aggressive vestibular rehabilitation exercises once symptoms have been controlled

GLOMUS TUMORS

What are they?

Benign, slow-growing tumors arising in glomus bodies found in the adventitial layer of blood vessels; often associated with cranial nerves IX and X in the middle ear

What is the usual location?

Middle ear, jugular bulb, course of CN X

What percentage are bilateral?

Ten percent

How common are they?

Most common benign tumor of the temporal bone

What are the symptoms?

By location: pulsatile tinnitus, hearing loss, vertigo, cranial nerve palsy

What are the signs?

Conductive hearing loss, mass behind the ear drum, CN deficit

What are the steps in evaluation?

Exam, audiogram, CT, MRI, A-gram

What is the treatment?

Surgical resection, radiation therapy for poor operative candidates or for recurrences

POSTERIOR FOSSA TUMORS

What are they?
Most commonly (90%) acoustic neuromas, which are benign schwannomas of CN VIII; less common primary tumors are meningioma, cholesteatoma, arachnoid cyst, cholesterol granuloma

Which site is most commonly affected?
Cerebellopontine angle

What are the early symptoms?
Tinnitus, hearing loss, vertigo

What symptoms occur later?
May involve CN IX, X, XI (caudal tumor growth), cerebellum by compression

How is the diagnosis made?
Audiometry, brainstem-evoked potentials, radiology (CT and MRI). T1 MRI with contrast (gadolinium) is the gold standard

What is the treatment?
Surgical resection
Gamma knife for poor operative candidates

NOSE AND PARANASAL SINUSES

EPISTAXIS

What is it?
Bleeding from the nose

What are the predisposing factors?
Trauma, "nose picking," sinus infection, allergic or atrophic rhinitis, blood dyscrasias, tumor, environmental extremes (hot, dry climates, winters)

What is the usual cause?
Rupture of superficial mucosal blood vessels (Kiesselbach's plexus if anterior, sphenopalatine artery if posterior)

What is the most common type?
Anterior (90% of all epistaxis); usually due to trauma

Which type is more serious?	Posterior; usually occurs in the elderly or is associated with a systemic disorder (hypertension, arteriosclerosis)
What is the treatment?	Direct pressure; if this fails, proceed to anterior nasal packing with gauze strips, followed if necessary by posterior packing with Foley catheter or lamb's wool; packs must be removed in less than 5 days to prevent infectious complications
What infectious disease syndrome is seen with nasal packing?	Toxic shock syndrome: fever, shock, **rash** due to exotoxin from *Staphylococcus aureus*
Treatment?	Supportive with removal of nasal packing, IV hydration, oxygen, and anti-staphylococcal antibiotics

ACUTE RHINITIS

What is it?	Inflammation of nasal mucous membrane
What is the most common cause?	Upper respiratory tract infection; rhinovirus is the most common agent in adults (other nonallergic causes: nasal deformities and tumors, polyps, atrophy, immune diseases, vasomotor problems)
What are the symptoms?	Nasal stuffiness, rhinorrhea, sneezing, mild fever, headache, and general malaise; obstruction and thickened/purulent nasal discharge may follow
What are the findings on physical exam?	Swollen, erythematous nasal mucosa with a watery mucous discharge
What is the course/treatment?	Usually lasts 5 to 7 days; antihistamines and decongestants may help symptoms

ALLERGIC RHINITIS

What are the symptoms?	Nasal stuffiness; watery rhinorrhea; paroxysms of morning sneezing; and itching of nose, conjunctiva, or palate

How is the condition characterized?

Early onset (before age 20), familial tendency, presence of other allergic disorders (eczema, asthma), elevated serum IgE, eosinophilia on nasal smear

What are the findings on physical exam?

Pale, boggy, bluish nasal turbinates coated with thin, clear secretions; in children, a transverse nasal crease is sometimes caused by repeated "allergic salute"

What is the treatment?

Allergen avoidance, antihistamines, decongestants; steroids or sodium cromylate in severe cases; desensitization via allergen immunotherapy is the only "cure"

ACUTE SINUSITIS

What is the typical history?

Previously healthy patient with unrelenting progression of a viral URI or allergic rhinitis beyond the normal 5- to 7-day course

What are the symptoms?

Periorbital pressure/pain, nasal obstruction, nasal/postnasal mucopurulent discharge, fatigue, fever, headache

What are the signs?

Tenderness over affected sinuses, pus in the nasal cavity; may also see reason for obstruction (septal deviation, spur, tight osteomeatal complex); transillumination is unreliable

What is the pathophysiology?

Thought to be secondary to decreased ciliary action of the sinus mucosa and edema causing obstruction of the sinus ostia, lowering intrasinus oxygen tension and predisposing patients to bacterial infection

What are the causative organisms?

Up to 50% of patients have negative cultures and are presumably (initially) viral; pneumococcus, *S. aureus*, group A streptococci, and *H. influenzae* are the most common bacteria cultured

What is the treatment?

Fourteen-day course of antibiotics (penicillin G, amoxicillin, Ceclor, and Augmentin are commonly used), topical and systemic decongestants, and saline nasal irrigation

CHRONIC SINUSITIS

What is it?

Infection of nasal sinuses lasting longer than 4 weeks, or pattern of recurrent acute sinusitis punctuated by brief asymptomatic periods

What is the pathology?

Permanent mucosal changes secondary to inadequately treated acute sinusitis, consisting of mucosal fibrosis, polypoid growth, and inadequate ciliary action, hyperostosis (increased bone density on CT scan)

What are the symptoms?

Chronic nasal obstruction, postnasal drip, mucopurulent rhinorrhea, low-grade facial and periorbital pressure/pain

What are the causative organisms?

Usually anaerobes (such as *Bacteroides, Veillonella, Rhinobacterium*); also *H. influenzae, Streptococcus viridans, Staphylococcus aureus, Staphylococcus epidermidis*

What is the treatment?

Medical management with decongestants, mucolytics, topical steroids, and antibiotics; if this approach fails, proceed to endoscopic or external surgical intervention

What is FESS?

Functional **E**ndoscopic **S**inus **S**urgery

What are the complications of sinusitis?

Orbital cellulitis (if ethmoid sinusitis), meningitis, epidural or brain abscess (frontal sinus), cavernous sinus thrombosis (ethmoid or sphenoid), osteomyelitis (A.K.A. Pott's puffy tumor if frontal)

CANCER OF THE NASAL CAVITY AND PARANASAL SINUSES

What are the usual locations?
Maxillary sinus (two-thirds)
Nasal cavity
Ethmoid sinus
Rarely in frontal or sphenoid sinuses

What are the associated cell types?
Squamous cell (80%)
Adenocellular (15%)
Uncommon: sarcoma, melanoma

What rare tumor arises from olfactory epithelium?
Esthesioneuroblastoma; usually arises high in the nose (cribriform plate) and is locally invasive

What are the signs/ symptoms?
Early—nasal obstruction, blood-tinged mucus, epistaxis
Late—localized pain, cranial nerve deficits, facial/palate asymmetry, loose teeth

How is the diagnosis made?
CT can adequately identify extent of the disease and local invasion. MRI is often also used to evaluate soft-tissue disease.

What is the treatment?
Surgery, with or without x-ray therapy

What is the prognosis?
Five-year survival for T1 or T2 lesions approaches 70%

JUVENILE NASOPHARYNGEAL ANGIOFIBROMA

What is it?
The most commonly encountered vascular mass found in the nasal cavity; locally aggressive but nonmetastasizing

What is the usual history?
Adolescent males who present with nasal obstruction, recurrent severe epistaxis, possibly anosmia

What is the usual location?
Site of origin is the roof of the nasal cavity at the superior margin of sphenopalatine foramen

What can the mass transform into?
Fibrosarcoma (rare cases reported)

How is the diagnosis made?
Carotid arteriography, CT; biopsy is contraindicated secondary to risk of uncontrollable hemorrhage

What is the treatment?
Surgery via lateral rhinotomy with bleeding controlled by internal maxillary artery ligation or preoperative embolization, in the setting of hypotensive anesthesia; preoperative irradiation has also been used to shrink the tumor

ORAL CAVITY AND PHARYNX

PHARYNGOTONSILLITIS

What is it?
Acute or chronic infection of the naso- or oropharynx and/or Waldeyer's ring of lymphoid tissue (consisting of palatine, lingual, pharyngeal tonsils, and the adenoids)

What is the etiology?
Acute attacks can be viral (adenovirus, enterovirus, coxsackievirus; Epstein-Barr virus in infectious mononucleosis) or bacterial (group A β-hemolytic streptococci are the leading bacterial agent); chronic tonsillitis often with mixed population, including streptococci, staphylococci, and *M. catarrhalis*

What are the symptoms?
Acute—Sore throat, fever, local lymphadenopathy, chills, headache, malaise
Chronic—Noisy mouth breathing, speech and swallowing difficulties, apnea, halitosis

What are the signs?
Viral—Injected tonsils and pharyngeal mucosa; exudate may occur, but less often than with bacterial tonsillitis
Bacterial—Swollen, inflamed tonsils with white-yellow exudate in crypts and on surface; cervical adenopathy

How is the diagnosis made?
CBC, throat culture, monospot test

What are the possible complications?
Peritonsillar abscess (quinsy), retropharyngeal abscess (causing airway compromise), rheumatic fever, poststreptococcal glomerulonephritis (with β-hemolytic streptococci)

What is the treatment?
Viral—Symptomatic → acetaminophen, warm saline gargles, anesthetic throat spray
Bacterial—10 days PCN (erythromycin if PCN-allergic)

What are the indications for tonsillectomy?
Sleep apnea/cor pulmonale secondary to airway obstruction, suspicion of malignancy, hypertrophy causing malocclusion, peritonsillar abscess, recurrent acute or chronic tonsillitis

What are the possible complications?
Acute or delayed hemorrhage

PERITONSILLAR ABSCESS

What is the clinical setting?
Inadequately treated recurrent acute or chronic tonsillitis

What is the associated microbiology?
Mixed aerobes and anaerobes (which may be PCN-resistant)

What is the site of formation?
Begins at the superior pole of the tonsil

What are the symptoms?
Severe throat pain, dysphagia, odynophagia, trismus, cervical adenopathy, fever, chills, malaise

What are the signs?
Bulging, erythematous, edematous tonsillar pillar; swelling of uvula and displacement to contralateral side

What is the treatment?
IV antibiotics and surgical evacuation by incision and drainage; most experts recommend tonsillectomy after resolution of inflammatory changes

CANCER OF THE ORAL CAVITY

What is the usual cell type?
Squamous cell (in more than 90% of cases)

What are the most common sites?
LIP, tongue, floor of the mouth, gingiva, cheek, and palate

What is the etiology?
Linked to smoking, alcohol, and smokeless tobacco products (alcohol and tobacco together greatly increase the risk)

What is the frequency of the following conditions:

Regional metastasis?
About 30%

Second primary?
About 25%

Nodal metastasis?
Depends on size of tumor and ranges from 10% to 60%, usually to jugular and **jugulodigastric nodes, submandibular nodes**

Distant metastasis?
Infrequent

How is the diagnosis made?
Full history and physical exam, dental assessment, panorex or bone scan if mandible is thought to be involved, CT/MRI for extent of tumor and nodal disease

What is the treatment?
Radiation and/or surgery for small lesions; localized lesions can usually be treated surgically; larger lesions require combination therapy, possible mandibulectomy and neck dissection

What is the prognosis?
Depends on stage and site:
- Tongue: 20% to 70% survival
- Floor of mouth: 30% to 80% survival

Most common cause of death in successfully treated head and neck cancer is development of a second primary (occurs in 20%–40% of cases)

SALIVARY GLAND TUMORS

What is the frequency of gland involvement?	Parotid gland (80%) Submandibular gland (15%) Minor salivary glands (5%)
What is the potential for malignancy?	Greatest in **minor salivary gland** tumors (80% are malignant) and least in parotid gland tumors (80% are benign); the smaller the gland, the greater the likelihood of malignancy
How do benign and malignant tumors differ in terms of history and physical exam?	Benign—mobile, nontender, no node involvement or facial weakness Malignant—painful, fixed mass with evidence of local metastasis, and facial paresis/paralysis
What is the diagnostic procedure?	FNA; never perform excisional biopsy of a parotid mass. Superficial parotidectomy is the procedure of choice for benign lesions of the lateral lobe.
What is the treatment?	Involves adequate surgical resection, sparing facial nerve if possible, neck dissection for node-positive necks Postoperative radiation therapy if high-grade cancer, recurrent cancer, residual disease, invasion of adjacent structures, any T3 or T4 parotid tumors
What is the most common benign salivary tumor?	**Pleomorphic adenoma** (benign mixed tumor) accounts for two-thirds of total (think: **P**leomorphic = **P**opular)
What is the usual location?	Parotid gland
What is the clinical course?	They are well-delineated and slow growing.
What is the second most common benign salivary gland tumor?	Warthin's tumor (1% of all salivary gland tumors)
What is the usual location?	Ninety-five percent are found in parotid, 3% are bilateral

Describe the lesion.

Slow-growing, cystic mass usually located in the tail of the superficial portion of the parotid; rarely becomes malignant

What is the most common malignant salivary tumor?

Mucoepidermoid carcinoma (10% of all salivary gland neoplasms) Think: **M**ucoepidermoid = **M**alignant
Most common parotid malignancy
Second most common submandibular gland malignancy

What is the second most common malignant salivary tumor in adults?

Adenoid cystic carcinoma
- Less than 10% of all salivary gland neoplasms
- Most common malignancy in submandibular and minor salivary glands
- Second most common malignancy in parotid
- Tends to have perineural invasion

LARYNX

ANATOMY

Define the three parts.

1. Glottis: begins halfway between the true and false cords (in the ventricle) and extends inferiorly 1.0 cm below the edge of the vocal folds
2. Supraglottis: extends from superior glottis to superior border of hyoid and tip of epiglottis
3. Subglottis: extends from lower border of glottis to inferior edge of cricoid cartilage

Innervation?

Via the vagus nerve: superior laryngeal and recurrent laryngeal nerves; superior laryngeal supplies sensory to supraglottis and motor to inferior constrictor and cricothyroid muscle; recurrent laryngeal supplies sensory to glottis and subglottis and motor to all remaining intrinsic laryngeal muscles

CROUP (LARYNGOTRACHEOBRONCHITIS)

What is it?

A viral infection of the larynx and trachea, generally affecting children (boys > girls)

What is the usual cause?	Parainfluenza virus (think: crou**P** = **P**arainfluenza)
What age group is affected most?	Ages 6 months to 3 years
Is the condition considered seasonal?	Yes; outbreaks most often occur in autumn
What are the precipitating events?	Usually preceded by URI
What is the classic symptom?	Barking (seal-like), nonproductive cough
What are the other symptoms?	Respiratory distress, low-grade fever
What are the signs?	Tachypnea, inspiratory retractions, prolonged inspiration, inspiratory stridor, expiratory rhonchi/wheezes
What is the differential diagnosis?	Epiglottitis, bacterial tracheitis, foreign body, diphtheria, retropharyngeal abscess, peritonsillar abscess, asthma
How is the diagnosis made?	A-P neck x-ray shows classic "steeple sign," indicating subglottic narrowing; ABG may show hypoxemia plus hypercapnia
What is the treatment?	**Keep child calm** (agitation only worsens obstruction), cool mist, steroids, aerosolized racemic EPI may be administered to reduce edema/airway obstruction
What are the indications for intubation?	If airway obstruction is severe or child becomes exhausted
What is the usual course?	Resolves in 3 to 4 days; secondary bacterial infection (streptococcal, staphylococcal) may require antibiotics

EPIGLOTTITIS

What is it?	Severe, rapidly progressive infection of the epiglottis

What is the usual causative agent?	*Haemophilus influenzae* type B
What age group is affected?	Children 2 to 5 years old
What are the signs/ symptoms?	Sudden onset, high fever (40°C); "hot potato" voice; dysphagia (→ drooling); no cough; patient prefers to sit upright, **lean forward;** patient appears toxic and stridulous
How is the diagnosis made?	Can usually be made clinically and does **not** involve direct observation of the epiglottis (which may worsen obstruction by causing laryngospasm)
What is the treatment?	Involves immediate airway support via OR intubation or possibly tracheotomy; medical treatment is comprised of steroids and IV antibiotics against *H. influenzae* (ampicillin + chloramphenicol)

MALIGNANT LESIONS OF THE LARYNX

What is the incidence?	Accounts for approximately 2% of all malignancies, more often in males
What is the most common site?	Glottis (two-thirds)
What is the second most common type?	Supraglottis (one-third)
Which type has the worst prognosis?	Subglottic tumors (infrequent)
What are the risk factors?	Tobacco, alcohol
What is the pathology?	Ninety percent are squamous cell carcinoma
What are the symptoms?	Hoarseness, throat pain, dysphagia, odynophagia, neck mass, (referred) ear pain

SUPRAGLOTTIC LESIONS

What is the usual location? Laryngeal surface of epiglottis

What area is often involved? Preepiglottic space

Extension? Tend to remain confined to supraglottic region, though may extend to vallecula or base of tongue

What is the associated type of metastasis? High propensity for nodal metastasis

GLOTTIC LESIONS

What is the usual location? Anterior part of true cords

Extension? May invade thyroid cartilage, cross midline to invade contralateral cord, or invade paraglottic space

What is the associated type of metastasis? Rare nodal metastasis

What is the treatment? Total or supraglottic laryngectomy, depending on location and extent of lesion; neck dissection if nodal involvement. Radiation therapy or surgery is given for early (T1 or T2) lesions. Combination therapy (surgery + radiation) is given for advanced (T3 and T4) disease.

What is the 5-year survival for:

T1 lesions? 90%

T2 lesions? 80%

T3 lesions? 75%

T4 lesions? 30%

NECK MASS

What is the usual etiology in infants? Congenital (branchial cleft cysts, thyroglossal duct cysts)

What is the usual etiology in adolescents?	Inflammatory (cervical adenitis is number one), with congenital also possible
What is the usual etiology in adults?	Malignancy (squamous is number one), especially if painless and immobile
What is the "80% rule"?	In general, 80% of neck masses are **benign** in children; 80% are **malignant** in adults over the age of 40
What are the seven cardinal symptoms of neck masses?	Dysphagia, odynophagia, hoarseness, stridor (signifies upper airway obstruction), globus, speech disorder, referred ear pain (via CN V, IX, or X)
Define dysphagia.	Difficulty swallowing
Define odynophagia.	Painful swallowing
Define globus.	Sensation of a "lump in the throat"
What comprises the workup?	Full head and neck exam, indirect laryngoscopy, CT and MRI to search for hidden primary; **FNA for tissue diagnosis;** biopsy is contraindicated because it has an adverse effect on survival if malignant
What is the differential diagnosis?	Inflammatory: cervical lymphadenitis, cat-scratch disease, infectious mononucleosis, infection in neck spaces Congenital: thyroglossal duct cyst (midline, elevates with tongue protrusion), branchial cleft cysts (lateral), dermoid cysts (midline submental), hemangioma, cystic hygroma Neoplastic: primary or metastatic
What is the treatment?	Surgical excision for congenital or neoplastic; two most important procedures for cancer treatment are radical and modified neck dissection

RADICAL NECK DISSECTION

What is involved?

Classically, removal of: **nodes** from clavicle to mandible, **sternocleidomastoid muscle, submaxillary gland,** tail of **parotid,** internal **jugular vein, digastric muscles, stylohyoid** and **omohyoid muscles, fascia** within the anterior and posterior triangles, **CN XI,** and cervical plexus sensory nerves

What are the indications?

1. Presence of clinically positive nodes that likely contain metastatic cancer
2. Clinically negative neck, but high probability of metastasis from a primary tumor elsewhere
3. A fixed cervical mass that is resectable

What are the contraindications?

1. Distant metastasis
2. Fixation to structure that cannot be removed (e.g., carotid artery)
3. Low neck masses

MODIFIED NECK DISSECTION

What are the types:

Type I?

Spinal accessory nerve preserved

Type II?

Spinal accessory and internal jugular preserved

Type III?

Spinal accessory, IJ, and sternocleidomastoid preserved

What are the advantages?

Increased postoperative function and decreased morbidity (especially if bilateral), most often used in N0 lesions; these modifications are usually intraoperative decisions based on the location and extent of tumor growth

What are the disadvantages?

May result in increased mortality from local recurrence

FACIAL FRACTURES

MANDIBLE FRACTURES

What are the symptoms?	Gross disfigurement, pain, **malocclusion,** drooling
What are the signs?	Trismus, fragment mobility and lacerations of gingiva, hematoma in floor of mouth
What are the possible complications?	Malunion, nonunion, osteomyelitis, TMJ ankylosis
What is the treatment?	Open or closed reduction MMF = maxillomandibular fixation (wiring jaw shut)

MIDFACE FRACTURES

How are they evaluated? Careful physical exam and CT

Classification

Le Fort I? Transverse maxillary fracture above the dental apices, which also traverses the pterygoid plate; palate is mobile, but nasal complex is stable

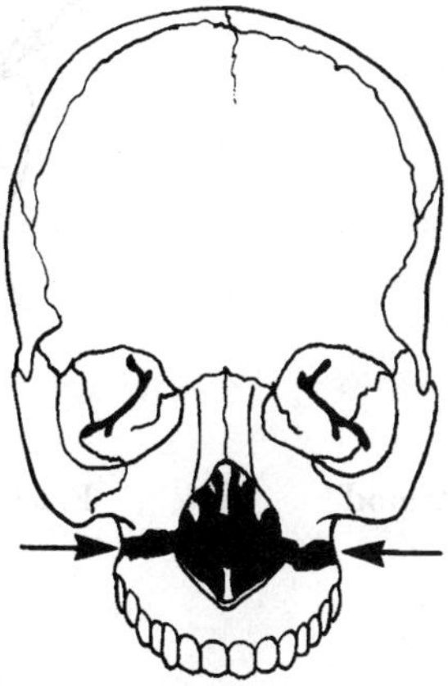

Le Fort I

Le Fort II? Fracture through the frontal process of the maxilla, through the orbital floor, and pterygoid plate; midface is mobile

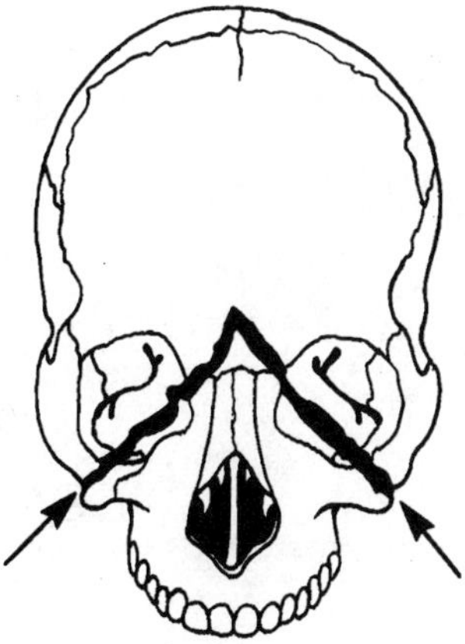

Le Fort II

Le Fort III?

Complete craniofacial separation, differs from II in that it extends through the nasofrontal suture and frontozygomatic sutures

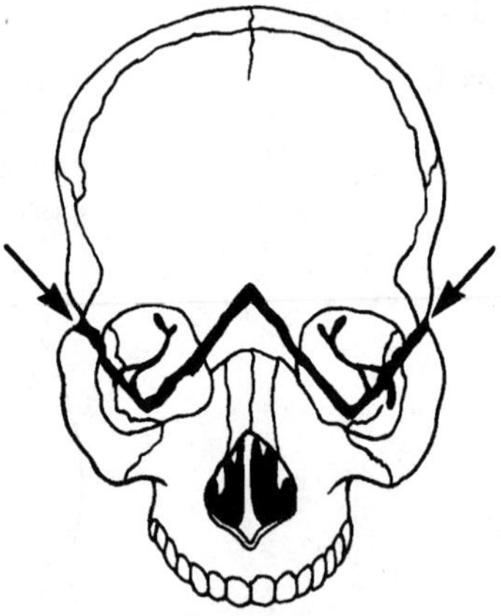

Le Fort III

What is a "tripod" fracture?

Fracture of the zygomatic complex

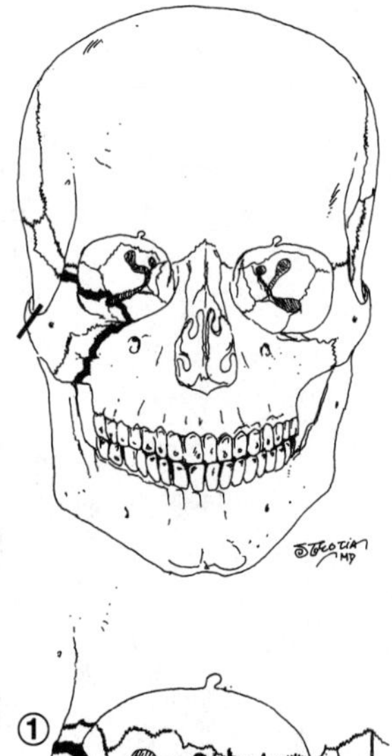

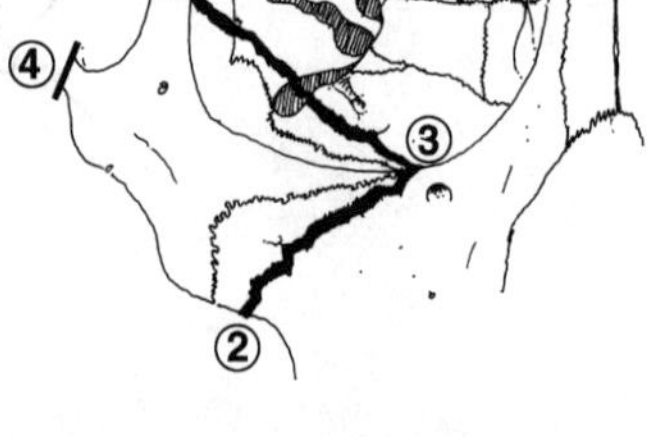

	Involves four fractures: 1. Frontozygomatic suture 2. Zygomaticomaxillary suture 3. Inferior orbital rim 4. Zygomaticotemporal suture
What is a "blowout" fracture?	Orbital fracture with "blowout" of supporting bony structural support of orbital floor; patient has enophthalmos (sunken-in eyeball)
What is "entrapment"?	Orbital fracture with "entrapment" of periorbital tissues within the fracture opening, including entrapment of extraocular muscles; loss of extraocular muscle mobility (e.g., lateral tracking) and diplopia (double vision).
What is a "step off"?	Fracture of the orbit with palpable "step off" of bony orbital rim (inferior or lateral)
Are mandibular fractures usually a single fracture?	No; because the mandible forms an anatomic ring, more than 95% of mandible fractures have more than one fracture site.
What is the best x-ray study for mandibular fractures?	Panorex
What must be ruled out and treated with a broken nose (nasal fracture)?	Septal hematoma; must drain to remove chance of a pressure-induced septal necrosis

ENT WARD QUESTIONS

How can otitis externa be distinguished from otitis media on exam?	Otitis externa is characterized by severe pain upon manipulation of the auricle
What causes otitis media?	The majority are caused by pneumococcus and *H. influenzae.*
What causes otitis externa?	*Pseudomonas aeruginosa*
What must be considered in unilateral serous otitis?	Nasopharyngeal carcinoma
What is most the common cause of facial paralysis?	**Bell's palsy,** which has an unidentified etiology

What is the single most important prognostic factor in Bell's palsy?	Whether or not the affected muscles are completely paralyzed (if not, prognosis is > 95% complete recovery)
What is the most common cause of parotid swelling?	Mumps
What is Heerfordt's syndrome?	Sarcoidosis with: parotid enlargement, facial nerve paralysis, and uveitis
Which systemic disease causes salivary gland stones?	Gout
What is the most common salivary gland site of stone formation?	Submandibular gland
What is Mikulicz's syndrome?	Any cause of bilateral enlargement of the parotid, lacrimal, and submandibular glands
What are the three major functions of the larynx?	1. Airway protection 2. Airway/respiration 3. Phonation
What is a cricothyroidotomy?	Emergent surgical airway by incising the cricothyroid membrane
Name the four major indications for a tracheostomy?	1. Prolonged mechanical ventilation (usually > 2 weeks) 2. Upper airway obstruction 3. Poor life-threatening pulmonary toilet 4. Severe obstructive sleep apnea
What is a Ranula?	Sublingual retention cyst
What is Frey's syndrome?	Flushing, pain, and diaphoresis in the auriculotemporal nerve distribution initiated by chewing; due to abnormal regeneration of the sympathetic/ parasympathetic nerves upon cutting the auriculotemporal nerve, usually during a parotidectomy. These parasympathetic fibers, once destined for the parotid gland, find new targets in skin sweat glands. Thus, people sweat when eating.
What is the classic triad of Meniere's disease?	Hearing loss, tinnitus, vertigo

What is the most common posterior fossa tumor and where is it located?	Acoustic neuromas, usually occurring at the cerebellopontine angle
What is the most common site of sinus cancer?	Maxillary sinus
What tumor arises from olfactory epithelium?	Esthesioneuroblastoma
What cell type is most common in head and neck cancer?	Squamous cell
What are the most important predisposing factors to head and neck cancer?	Excessive alcohol use and **tobacco** abuse of any form
What is the most frequent site of salivary gland tumor?	Parotid gland
What is the most common salivary gland neoplasm:	Minor salivary glands (> 75% malignant)
Benign?	Pleomorphic adenoma
Malignant?	Mucoepidermoid carcinoma
What is the classic feature of croup?	Barking, seal-like cough
What are the classic features of epiglottitis?	"Hot potato" voice, sitting up, **drooling,** toxic appearance, high fever, **leaning forward**
What comprises the workup of neck mass?	Do NOT biopsy; obtain tissue **via FNA** and complete head and neck exam
What is Ramsay Hunt's syndrome?	Painful facial nerve paralysis due to herpes zoster of the ear
What is the most common malignant neck mass in children, adolescents, and young adults?	Lymphoma
What is the most common primary malignant solid tumor of the head and neck in children?	Rhabdomyosarcoma

63

Thoracic Surgery

THORACIC OUTLET SYNDROME

What is it?

Compression of the:
Subclavian artery
Subclavian vein or
Brachial plexus at the superior outlet of the thorax

What are the causes? (2)

1. Various congenital anomalies, including cervical rib or abnormal fascial bands to the first rib, or abnormal anterior scalene muscle
2. Trauma:
   Fracture of clavicle or first rib
   Dislocation of humeral head
   Crush injuries

What are the symptoms?

Paresthesias (neck, shoulder, arm, hand); 90% in ulnar nerve distribution
Weakness (neural/arterial)
Coolness of involved extremity (arterial)
Edema, venous distension, discoloration (venous)

What is the most common problem seen with TOS?

Neurologic symptoms

Which nerve is most often involved?

Ulnar nerve

What are the signs?

Paget-von Schroetter syndrome—venous thrombosis leading to edema, arm discoloration, and distension of the superficial veins
Weak brachial and radial pulses in the involved arm
Hypesthesia/anesthesia
Occasionally, atrophy in the distribution of the ulnar nerve
Positive Adson maneuver/Tinel's sign
Edema

What is the Adson maneuver?

Evaluates for arterial compromise
Patient:
1. Extends neck (lifts head)
2. Takes a deep breath
3. Turns head toward examined side

Physician:
- Monitors radial pulse on examined side
- Test is positive if the radial pulse decreases or disappears during maneuver

What is Tinel's test?

Tapping of the supraclavicular fossa producing paresthesias

What is the differential diagnosis?

Cervical spine
- Ruptured intervertebral disk
- Osteoarthritis
- Spinal cord tumors

Peripheral neuropathy
Brachial plexus palsy
Arterial
- Aneurysm
- Embolism
- Occlusive disease
- Thromboangiitis obliterans
- Raynaud's disease

Venous
- Thrombophlebitis
- Vasculitis, collagen disease

What is the treatment?

Physical therapy (vast majority of cases)
Decompression of the thoracic outlet by resecting the first rib and cervical rib (if present) if physical therapy fails and as a last resort

CHEST WALL TUMORS

Benign

What are the most common types?

1. Fibrous rib dysplasia
2. Chondroma
3. Osteochondroma

What is the treatment?

Wide excision and reconstruction with autologous or prosthetic grafts

MALIGNANT TUMORS

What are the most common types?
1. Fibrosarcoma
2. Chondrosarcoma
3. Osteogenic sarcoma
4. Rhabdomyosarcoma
5. Myeloma
6. Ewing's sarcoma

What is the treatment?
Excision with or without radiation

DISEASES OF THE PLEURA

PLEURAL EFFUSION

What is it?
Fluid in the pleural space

What are the causes?
1. Pulmonary infections (pneumonia)
2. Congestive heart failure
3. SLE or rheumatoid arthritis
4. Pancreatitis (sympathetic effusion)
5. Trauma
6. Pulmonary embolism
7. Renal disease
8. Cirrhosis
9. Malignancy (mesothelioma/ lymphoma/metastasis)
10. Postpericardiotomy syndrome

What are the symptoms?
Dyspnea, pleuritic chest pain

What are the signs?
Decreased breath sounds
Dullness to percussion
Egophony at the upper limit

What are the properties of a transudate?
Specific gravity < 1.016
Protein < 3 g/dl
Few cells

What are the properties of an exudate?
Specific gravity > 1.016
Protein > 3 g/dl
Many cells

What is the key diagnostic test?
Thoracentesis (needle drainage) with studies including cytology

What is the treatment?
1. Pigtail catheter or thoracostomy (chest tube)
2. Treat underlying condition
3. Consider sclerosis

What is an empyema?
Infected pleural effusion; must be drained, usually with chest tube(s)
Decortication may be necessary if the empyema is solid

What is a decortication?
Thoracotomy and removal of an infected fibrous rind from around the lung (think of it as taking off a fibrous "cortex" from the lung)

LUNG ABSCESS

What are the signs/symptoms?
Fever, sputum, sepsis, fatigue

What are the associated diagnostic studies?
CXR: air-fluid level
CT scan to define position and to differentiate from a empyema
Bronchoscopy (looking for cancer/culture)

What is the treatment?
Antibiotics and bronchoscopy for culture and toilet
With or without surgery

What are the indications for surgery?
Underlying cancer/tumor
Refractory to antibiotics

What are the surgical options?
Lobectomy of lobe with abscess
Tube drainage

HEMOPTYSIS

What is it?
Bleeding into the bronchial tree

What are the causes?
1. Bronchitis (50%)
2. Tumor mass (20%)
3. TB (8%)

Other causes: bronchiectasis, pulmonary catheters, trauma

Define MASSIVE hemoptysis.
More than 600 cc/24 hours

What comprises the workup?
CXR
Bronchoscopy
Bronchial A-gram

What is the treatment if massive?
Bronchoscopy, intubation of unaffected side, Fogarty catheter, occlusion of bleeding bronchus, bronchial A-gram with or without embolization, surgical resection of involved lung

What is the treatment of moderate to mild bleeding?
Laser coagulation

SPONTANEOUS PNEUMOTHORAX

What is it?
Atraumatic spontaneous development of a pneumothorax

What are the causes?
Idiopathic (primary), bleb disease-emphysema, etc. (secondary)

What body habitus is associated with spontaneous pneumothorax?
Thin and tall

How is the diagnosis made?
CXR

What is the treatment?
Chest tube

What are the options if refractory, recurrent, or bilateral?
Pleurodesis: scar from the lung to the parietal pleura with a sclerosant (talc) via chest tube/thoracoscopy or by thoracotomy and mechanical abrasion

Who might also need a pleurodesis after the first episode?
Those with lifestyles in which a pneumothorax may be at higher risk of occurrence (e.g., pilots, skin divers)

MESOTHELIOMA

Malignant Mesothelioma

What is it?
A primary pleural neoplasm

What are the two types?
1. Localized (benign or malignant)
2. Diffuse (highly malignant)

What are the risk factors?
Exposure to asbestos
Smoking

What are the symptoms?
Localized: pleuritic pain, joint pain and swelling, dyspnea
Diffuse: chest pain, malaise, weight loss, cough

What are the signs?
Pleural effusion (present in only 10% to 15% of patients with local disease, almost always in diffuse disease [> 75%])

What are the associated radiographic tests?
X-ray may reveal a peripheral mass, often forming an obtuse angle with the chest wall; **CT**

How is the diagnosis made?
Pleural biopsy, pleural fluid cytology

What is the treatment if localized?
Surgical excision

What is the treatment if diffuse?
Early stages may be resected, followed by radiation (brachytherapy); more advanced stages: radiation and/or chemotherapy

What is the prognosis?
Localized: poor if tumor is malignant
Diffuse: **dismal** (average life span after diagnosis is about 1 year)

Benign Mesothelioma

What is it?
Benign pleural mesothelioma

What pleura is usually involved?
Visceral pleura

What is the gross appearance?
Pedunculated "broccoli or cauliflower" tumor on a stalk coming off of the lung

What is the treatment?
Surgical resection with at least 1 cm clear margin

What is the prognosis?	In contrast to malignant mesothelioma, the benign mesothelioma has an excellent prognosis with cure in the vast majority of cases (possibility of transformation into a malignant mesothelioma if inadequate resection).

DISEASES OF THE LUNGS

BRONCHOGENIC CARCINOMA

What is the annual incidence of lung cancer in the United States?	150,000 new cases
What is the number of annual deaths from lung cancer?	100,000 (increasing in women); most common cancer death in the United States
What is the number one risk factor?	Smoking (surprise!)
Does asbestos exposure increase the risk in patients who smoke?	Yes
What type of lung cancer arises in nonsmoking patients?	Adenocarcinoma
What are the signs/ symptoms?	Change in a chronic cough Hemoptysis, chest pain, dyspnea Pleural effusion (suggests chest wall involvement) Hoarseness (recurrent laryngeal nerve involvement) Superior vena cava syndrome Diaphragmatic paralysis (phrenic nerve involvement) Symptoms of metastasis/paraneoplastic syndrome Finger clubbing
What is Pancoast's tumor?	Tumor at the apex of the lung or superior sulcus that may involve the brachial plexus, sympathetic ganglia, and vertebral bodies, leading to pain, upper extremity weakness, and Horner's syndrome

What is Horner's syndrome?

Injury to the cervical sympathetic chain:
1. Miosis (small pupil)
2. Ptosis
3. Enophthalmos
4. Decreased sweating on affected side

What are the four most common sites of extrathoracic metastases?

1. Bone
2. Liver
3. Adrenals
4. Kidney

What are paraneoplastic syndromes?

Syndromes that are associated with tumors, but which may affect distant parts of the body; they may be caused by hormones released from endocrinologically active tumors or may be of uncertain etiology

Name five general types of paraneoplastic syndromes.

1. Metabolic: Cushing's, SIADH, hypercalcemia
2. Neuromuscular: Eaton-Lambert syndrome, cerebellar ataxia
3. Skeletal: hypertrophic osteoarthropathy
4. Dermatologic: acanthosis nigricans
5. Vascular: thrombophlebitis

What are the associated radiographic tests?

Chest x-ray and CT scan

How is the tumor diagnosed?

1. Sputum cytology
2. Needle biopsy (CT or fluoro guidance)
3. Bronchoscopy with brushings and/or biopsies
4. With or without mediastinoscopy, mediastinotomy, scalene node biopsy, or open lung biopsy for definitive diagnosis

For each tumor listed, recall its usual site in the lung and its natural course:

Squamous cell?

Two-thirds occur centrally in lung hilus; may also be a Pancoast's tumor; slow growth, late metastasis; associated with smoking (**think:** **S**quamous = **S**entral)

Adenocarcinoma?	Peripheral; rapid growth with hematogenous/nodal metastasis; associated with lung scarring
Small (oat) cell?	Central, highly malignant, usually not operable
Large cell?	Usually peripheral; very malignant
What are the stages of NON-small cell carcinoma of the lungs:	
Stage I?	Any tumor size without extension to chest wall, mediastinum, pericardium, or diaphragm, no nodes, no mets (> 2 cm from carina)
Stage II?	Stage I tumor with positive nodes in ipsilateral hilum and/or peribronchial nodes; no distant metastases
Stage IIIa?	Any tumor size with extension to pericardium, diaphragm, or chest wall, but not involving the heart, aorta, pulmonary artery, trachea, or esophagus, with or without positive ipsilateral hilar/peribronchial nodes **or** Positive subcarinal nodes, positive ipsilateral mediastinal nodes (no distant metastasis)
Stage IIIb?	Nodal metastasis: scalene nodes, supraclavicular nodes, contralateral hilar nodes, contralateral mediastinal nodes Tumor: extension to mediastinal structures including heart, great vessels, esophagus, trachea, malignant pleural effusion (no distant metastasis)
Stage IV?	Distant metastasis
What are the surgical contraindications by stage for NON-small cell carcinoma?	Stage IV, Stage IIIb

What is the treatment by stage for NON-small cell lung carcinoma:

Stage I? Surgical resection

Stage II? Surgical resection

Stage IIIa? Surgical resection, chemotherapy with or without radiation

Stage IIIb? Chemotherapy and radiation

Stage IV? Chemotherapy

What is the prognosis (5-year survival) after treatment of NON-small cell lung carcinoma by stage:

Stage I? Approximately 65%

Stage II? Approximately 45%

Stage IIIa? Approximately 30%

Stage IV? Basically 0%

How is small cell carcinoma treated? Chemotherapy with or without x-ray therapy

What are the six contraindications to surgery for lung cancer?

1. **S**uperior vena cava syndrome, **S**upraclavicular node mets, **S**calene node mets
2. **T**racheal carina involvement
3. **O**at cell carcinoma (treat with chemotherapy with or without radiation)
4. **P**ulmonary function tests shows FEV1 < 1
5. Myocardial **I**nfarction, (or cardiac cripple)
6. **T**umor elsewhere (metastatic disease)

Acronym: **STOP IT**

What postop FEV1 must you have?

FEV1 of more than 800 cc; thus, a preop FEV1 of more than 2 is usually needed for a pneumonectomy
If FEV1 is less than 2, a ventilation perfusion scan should be performed

What is hypertrophic pulmonary osteoarthropathy?

Periosteal proliferation and new bone formation at the end of long bones and in the bones of the hand (seen in 10% of patients with lung cancer)

SOLITARY PULMONARY NODULES (COIN LESIONS)

What are they?

Peripheral circumscribed pulmonary lesions

What is the differential diagnosis?

Granulomatous disease, benign neoplasms, malignancy

What percentage are malignant?

Overall, 5% to 10% (but > 50% malignant in smokers over 50 years old)

Is there a gender risk?

Yes; the incidence of coin lesions is 3 to 9 times higher in men, and malignancy is nearly twice as common.

What are the symptoms?

Usually asymptomatic with solitary nodules, but may include coughing, weight loss, chest pain, and hemoptysis

What are the signs?

Physical findings are uncommon; clubbing is rare; hypertrophic osteoarthropathy implies more than an 80% chance of malignancy.

How is the diagnosis made?

Chest x-ray, chest CT

What is the significance of "popcorn" calcification?

Most likely benign (i.e., hamartoma)

What are the risk factors for malignancy?

1. Size: lesions more than 1 cm have a significant chance of malignancy and those more than 4 cm are very likely to be malignant.
2. Indistinct margins (corona radiata)
3. Documented growth on follow-up x-ray (if no change in 2 years, most likely benign)
4. Increasing age

What are the associated lab tests?	1. TB skin tests, etc. 2. Sputum cultures 3. Sputum cytology is diagnostic in 5% to 20% of cases
Which method of tissue diagnosis is used?	Chest CT with needle biopsy, bronchoscopy (+/- transtracheal biopsy), excisional biopsy (open or thoracoscopic)
What is the treatment?	Surgical excision is the mainstay of treatment. Excisional biopsy is therapeutic for benign lesions, solitary metastasis, and for primary cancer in patients who are poor risks for more extensive surgery. Lobectomy for centrally placed lesions Lobectomy with node dissection for primary cancer (if resectable by preop evaluations)
Which solitary nodule can be followed without a tissue diagnosis?	Popcorn calcifications Mass unchanged for 2 years on previous CXR
What is the prognosis?	For malignant coin lesions less than 2 cm, 5-year survival is approximately 70%
What if the patient has an SPN and pulmonary hypertrophic osteoarthropathy?	The patient has more than a 75% chance of having a carcinoma.
What is hypertrophic pulmonary osteoarthropathy?	Periosteal proliferation and new bone formation at the end of long bones and in bones of the hand
What is the incidence?	Seen in 2% to 12% of patients with lung cancer
What are the signs?	Associated with clubbing of the fingers; diagnosed by x-ray of long bones revealing periosteal bone hypertrophy

CARCINOID TUMOR

What is it?	An APUD cell (amine-precursor uptake and decarboxylation) tumor of the bronchus
What is its natural course in the lung?	Slow growing (but may be malignant)
What are the primary local findings?	Wheezing and atelectasis caused by bronchial obstruction/stenosis
What condition may it be confused with?	Asthma
What is the incidence of carcinoid syndrome?	Very rare with bronchial carcinoid
How is the diagnosis made?	Bronchoscopy reveals round red-yellow-purple mass covered by epithelium that protrudes into bronchial lumen
What is the treatment?	Surgical resection (lobectomy with lymph node dissection) Sleeve resection is also an option for proximal bronchial lesions
What is a sleeve resection?	Resection of a ring segment of bronchus (with tumor inside) and then end-to-end anastomosis of the remaining ends, allowing salvage of lower lobe
What is the prognosis (5-year survival) after complete surgical resection of carcinoid:	
Negative nodes?	More than 90% alive at 5 years
Positive nodes?	Two-thirds alive at 5 years
What are the types of bronchial adenomas?	Carcinoid, mucoepidermoid carcinoma, mucous gland adenoma, adenoid cystic carcinoma
What is the most common bronchial adenoma?	Carcinoid (85%)

Are bronchial adenomas benign?
No, it is a misconception. Most can be malignant.

What is the most common benign lung tumor?
Hamartoma (normal cells in a weird configuration)

PULMONARY SEQUESTRATION

What is it?
Abnormal benign lung tissue with separate blood supply that **DOES NOT** communicate with the normal tracheobronchial airway

Define the following terms:

Interlobar
Sequestration in normal lung tissue covered by normal visceral pleura

Extralobar
Sequestration not in normal lung covered by its own pleura

What are the signs/ symptoms?
Asymptomatic, recurrent pneumonia

How is the diagnosis made?
CXR, chest CT, A-gram, U/S with Doppler flow to ascertain blood supply

What is the treatment in the following cases:

Extralobar?
Surgical resection

Intralobar?
Lobectomy

What is the major danger during surgery for sequestration?
Anomalous blood supply from below the diaphragm (these can be cut and retract into the abdomen and result in exsanguination!)
Always document blood supply by A-gram or U/S with Doppler flow.

DISEASES OF THE MEDIASTINUM

MEDIASTINAL ANATOMY

What structures lie in the following locations:

Anterior mediastinum?
Thymus, ascending aorta, aortic arch, great vessels, lymph nodes

Middle mediastinum?	Heart, trachea and bifurcation, lung hila, phrenic nerves, lymph nodes
Posterior mediastinum?	Esophagus, descending aorta, thoracic duct, vagus and intercostal nerves, sympathetic trunks, azygous and hemizygous veins, lymph nodes
What is the major differential diagnosis for tumors of the mediastinum:	
Anterior mediastinum?	The classic **"four Ts": T**hyroid tumor, **T**hymoma, **T**errible lymphoma, **T**eratoma; also parathyroid tumor, lipoma, vascular aneurysms
Middle mediastinum?	Lymphadenopathy (e.g., lymphoma, sarcoid), teratoma, fat pad, cysts, hernias, extension of esophageal mass, bronchogenic cancer
Posterior mediastinum?	Neurogenic tumors, lymphoma, aortic aneurysm, vertebral lesions, hernias
What is the differential diagnosis for a neurogenic tumor?	Schwannoma (A.K.A. neurolemmoma), neurofibroma, neuroblastoma, ganglioneuroma, ganglioneuroblastoma, pheochromocytoma

PRIMARY MEDIASTINAL TUMORS

Thymona

Where are they found in the mediastinum?	Anterior
How is the diagnosis made?	CT
What is the treatment?	All thymomas should be surgically resected via midline sternotomy and, if malignant, treated with postop radiation therapy (33% ten-year survival rate for malignant thymoma treated with surgery and radiation).

What percentage of thymomas are malignant?
Approximately 25%

How is a malignant thymoma diagnosed?
At surgery with invasion into surrounding structures (not by histology!)

What is myasthenia gravis?
Autoimmune disease with antibodies against the muscle acetylcholine receptors

What percentage of patients with myasthenia gravis have a thymoma?
Approximately 15%

What percentage of patients with thymoma have or will have Myasthenia gravis?
Approximately 75%!

Teratomas

What are they?
Tumors of branchial cleft cells; the tumors contain ectoderm, endoderm, and mesoderm

What is a dermoid cyst?
A teratoma made up of ectodermal derivatives (e.g., teeth, skin, hair)

Which age-group is affected?
Usually adolescents, but can occur at any age

Where in the mediastinum do they occur?
Anterior

What are the characteristic x-ray findings?
Calcifications or teeth; tumors may be cystic

What percentage are malignant?
Approximately 15%

What is the treatment of benign dermoid cysts?
Surgical excision

What is the treatment of malignant teratoma?
Preoperative chemotherapy until tumor markers are normal, then surgical resection

Which tumor markers are associated with malignant teratomas?

AFP, CEA

Neurogenic Tumors

What is the incidence?

Most common mediastinal tumors in all age-groups

Where in the mediastinum do they occur?

Posterior, in the paravertebral gutters

What percentage are malignant?

50% in children
10% in adults

What are the histologic types (5)? (note cells of origin and whether benign or malignant)

Neurilemmoma or schwannoma (benign)—arise from Schwann cell sheaths of intercostal nerves
Neurofibroma (benign)—arise from intercostal nerves; can degenerate into:
- Neurosarcoma (malignant)
- Ganglioneuroma (benign)—from sympathetic chain
- Neuroblastoma (malignant)—also from sympathetic chain

LYMPHOMA

Where in the mediastinum do they occur?

Anywhere, but most often in the anterior mediastinum

What percentage of lymphomas involve mediastinal nodes?

Approximately 50%

What are the symptoms?

Cough, fever, chest pain, weight loss, SVC syndrome, chylothorax

How is the diagnosis made?

1. Chest x-ray, CT
2. Mediastinoscopy or mediastinotomy with node biopsy

What is the treatment?

Nonsurgical (chemotherapy and/or radiation)

MEDIASTINITIS

Acute Mediastinitis

What is it?
Acute suppurative mediastinal infection

Name the six etiologies:
1. Esophageal perforation (Boerhaave's syndrome)
2. Postop wound infection
3. Head and neck infections
4. Lung or pleural infections
5. Rib or vertebral osteomyelitis
6. Distant infections

What are the clinical features?
Fever, chest pain, dysphagia (especially with esophageal perforation), respiratory distress, leukocytosis

What is the treatment?
1. **A**irway, **B**reathing, and **C**irculation (always first!)
2. Wide drainage
3. Treatment of primary cause
4. Antibiotics

CHRONIC MEDIASTINITIS

What is it?
Mediastinal fibrosis secondary to chronic granulomatous infection

What is the most common etiology?
Histoplasma capsulatum

What are the clinical features?
Fifty percent are asymptomatic; symptoms are related to compression of adjacent structures: SVC syndrome, bronchial and esophageal strictures, constrictive pericarditis

How is the diagnosis made?
CXR or CT may be helpful, but surgery/biopsy often makes the diagnosis

What is the treatment?
Antibiotics; surgical removal of the granulomas is rarely helpful

SUPERIOR VENA CAVA SYNDROME

What is it?
Obstruction of the superior vena cava, usually by extrinsic compression

What is the number one cause?

Malignant tumors cause approximately 90% of the cases; lung cancer is by far the most common; other tumors include thymoma, lymphoma, and Hodgkin's disease.

Name three other causes.

1. Chronic mediastinitis
2. Benign tumors
3. Thrombosis (often due to long-term central line)

What are the clinical manifestations?

1. Blue discoloration and puffiness of the face, arms, and shoulders
2. CNS manifestations may include headache, nausea, vomiting, visual distortion, stupor, and convulsions
3. Cough, hoarseness, and dyspnea

What may aggravate the symptoms?

Lying flat or bending over

What is the clinical course?

Depends on the rapidity of onset; rapid onset of severe obstruction with no time to develop collateral circulation leads to severe symptoms and possibly fatal cerebral edema; chronic onset, as in fibrosing mediastinitis, may be very insidious and mild as collateral drainage develops

How is the diagnosis made?

1. Measure upper extremity venous pressure.
2. Venography localizes the obstruction.
3. CT scan evaluates for tumor.

What is the treatment?

1. Diuretics and fluid restriction
2. Prompt radiation therapy with or without chemotherapy for any causative cancer
3. With or without surgery to bypass SVC, replace it, or recanalize the lumen (rarely for tumor causation)
4. In chronic total obstruction, patients may gradually improve without treatment.

What is the prognosis? SVC obstruction itself is fatal in less than 5% of cases; mean survival time in patients with malignant obstruction is about 7 months.

DISEASES OF THE ESOPHAGUS

ANATOMIC CONSIDERATIONS

What is the primary function of the UES? Swallowing

What is the primary function of the LES? Prevention of reflux

The esophageal venous plexus drains inferiorly into the gastric veins. Why is this important? The gastric veins are part of the portal venous system; portal hypertension can thus be referred to the esophageal veins, leading to varices.

Identify the esophageal muscle type:

Proximal third Skeletal muscle

Mid third Smooth muscle >> skeletal muscle

Distal third? Smooth muscle

What is the length of the esophagus? Approximately 25 cm in the adult (40 cm from teeth to LES)

Why is the esophagus notorious for anastomotic leaks? The esophagus has no serosa (same as the distal rectum)

What nerve runs with the esophagus? The vagus nerves

OROPHARYNGEAL DYSPHAGIA

What is it? Improper relaxation of the upper esophageal sphincter

Describe the pathophysiology and the resulting complication.

Incoordination between relaxation of the upper esophageal sphincter and contraction of the pharynx leads to eventual formation of **Zenker's diverticulum,** which is a false diverticulum (mucosa only) above the cricopharyngeus muscle.

What are the symptoms?

Dysphagia, reflux of undigested food, left-sided neck mass, halitosis

What are the diagnostic tests?

History and physical exam; endoscopy to rule out other esophageal disorders (must be taken with caution as not to rupture through the diverticulum)

What is the treatment?

1. Myotomy of cricopharyngeus muscle
2. Excision of diverticulum

What muscle is involved with a Zenker's diverticulum?

Cricopharyngeus muscle

ACHALASIA

What is it?

1. **Failure of the lower esophageal sphincter to relax** during swallowing
2. Loss of esophageal peristalsis

What are the proposed etiologies?

1. **Neurologic** (ganglionic degeneration of Auerbach's plexus and/or vagus nerve); possibly infectious in nature
2. Chagas' disease in South America

What are the associated long-term conditions?

Esophageal carcinoma secondary to Barrett's esophagus due to food stasis

What are the symptoms?

Dysphagia for both solids and liquids, followed by regurgitation; dysphagia for liquids is worse

What are the diagnostic findings?

Radiographic contrast studies reveal dilated esophageal body with narrowing inferiorly

Manometry: motility studies reveal increased pressure in the LES and failure of the LES to relax during swallowing

What is the treatment?

1. Balloon dilation of LES
2. Medical treatment of reflux versus Belsey Mark IV 270 degree fundoplication (do not perform 360 Nissen)
3. Myotomy of the lower esophagus and LES

DIFFUSE ESOPHAGEAL SPASM

What is it?

Strong, nonperistaltic contractions of the esophageal body; sphincter function is usually **normal**

What is the associated condition?

Gastroesophageal reflux

What are the symptoms?

Spontaneous chest pain that radiates to the back, ears, neck, jaw, or arms

What is the differential diagnosis?

Angina pectoris
Psychoneurosis
Nutcracker esophagus

What are the associated diagnostic tests?

Esophageal manometry: Motility studies reveal repetitive, high-amplitude contractions with normal sphincter response
Upper GI may be normal, but 50% show segmented spasms or corkscrew esophagus
Endoscopy

What is the classic finding on esophageal contrast study (UGI)?

"Corkscrew esophagus"

What is the treatment?

Medical (antireflux measures, Ca blockers, nitrates)
Long esophagomyotomy in refractory cases

NUTCRACKER ESOPHAGUS

What is it also known as?

Hypertensive peristalsis

What is it?
Very strong **peristaltic** waves

What are the symptoms?
Spontaneous chest pain that radiates to the back, ears, neck, jaw, or arms

What is the differential diagnosis?
Angina pectoris
Psychoneurosis
Diffuse esophageal spasm

What are the associated diagnostic tests?
1. **Esophageal manometry:** Motility studies reveal repetitive, high-amplitude contractions with normal sphincter response
2. Upper GI may be normal (rule out mass)
3. Endoscopy

What is the treatment?
Medical (antireflux measures, Ca blockers, nitrates)
Long esophagomyotomy in refractory cases

ESOPHAGEAL REFLUX

What is it?
Reflux of gastric contents into the lower esophagus due to the decreased function of the LES

What are the causes?
1. Decreased LES tone
2. Decreased esophageal motility
3. Hiatal hernia
4. Gastric outlet obstruction

Name four associated conditions/factors.
1. Sliding hiatal hernia
2. Tobacco and alcohol
3. Scleroderma
4. Decreased endogenous gastrin production

What are the symptoms?
Substernal pain, heartburn, regurgitation; symptoms are worse when patient is supine and after meals

How is the diagnosis made?
1. pH probe in the lower esophagus reveals acid reflux
2. EGD shows esophagitis
3. Manometry reveals decreased LES pressure
4. Barium swallow

What is the treatment?

Usually medical: cisapride, H_2 blockers; antacids; metoclopramide, omeprazole
Elevation of the head of the bed; small, multiple meals

Which four complications require surgery?

1. Failure of medical therapy
2. Esophageal strictures
3. Progressive pulmonary insufficiency secondary to documented nocturnal aspiration
4. Barrett's esophagus

Describe each of the following types of surgery:

Nissen

360° fundoplication: wrap fundus of stomach all the way around the esophagus

Belsey Mark IV

270° fundoplication: wrap fundus of stomach, but not all the way around

Hill

Tighten arcuate ligament around esophagus and tack stomach to diaphragm

Lap Nissen

Nissen via laparoscope

What is Barrett's esophagus?

Replacement of the lower esophageal squamous epithelium with columnar epithelium secondary to reflux

Why is it significant?

This lesion is premalignant.

What is the treatment?

People with significant reflux should be followed with regular EGDs with biopsies, H_2-blockers, and antireflux precautions; many experts believe that patients with severe dysplasia should undergo esophagectomy.

ESOPHAGEAL STRICTURES

Caustic Strictures

Which agents may cause strictures if ingested?

Lye, oven cleaners, drain cleaners, batteries, sodium hydroxide tablets (Clinitest)

How is the diagnosis made?

History; EGD is clearly indicated early on to assess the extent of damage (< 24 hrs); scope to level of severe injury (deep ulcer) only, water soluble contrast study for deep ulcers to rule out perforation

What is the initial treatment?

1. NPO/IVF/H_2-blocker
2. **Do NOT induce emesis**
3. Corticosteroids (controversial—probably best for shallow/moderate ulcers), antibiotics (penicillin/gentamicin) for moderate ulcers
4. Antibiotic for deep ulcers
5. Upper GI at 10 to 14 days

What is the treatment if stricture develops?

Dilation with Maloney dilator/balloon catheter
In severe refractory cases, esophagectomy with colon interposition or gastric pull-up

What is the long-term follow-up?

Because of increased risk of esophageal squamous cancer (especially with ulceration), patients need endoscopies every other year.

What is a Maloney dilator?

Mercury-filled rubber dilator

ESOPHAGEAL CARCINOMA

What are the two main types?

1. **Squamous cell carcinoma** in most of the esophagus
2. **Adenocarcinoma** at the GE junction

What is the age and gender distribution?

Most common in the sixth decade of life; men predominate

What are the etiologic factors (4)?

1. Tobacco
2. Alcohol
3. GE reflux
4. Barrett's esophagus

What are the symptoms?

Dysphagia, weight loss
Others symptoms include: chest pain, back pain, hoarseness, symptoms of metastasis

What comprises the workup?

1. UGI
2. EGD
3. Transesophageal ultrasound (TEU)
4. CT scan of chest/abdomen

What is the differential diagnosis?

Leiomyoma, metastatic tumor, lymphomas, benign stricture, achalasia, diffuse esophageal spasm, GERD

How is the diagnosis made?

1. Upper GI localizes tumor
2. EGD obtains biopsy and assesses resectability
3. Full metastatic workup (CXR, bone scan, CT, LFTs)

Describe the stages of esophageal cancer:

Stage I

Tumor: invades **lamina propria or submucosa**
Nodes: negative

Stage IIa

Tumor: invades muscularis propria or adventitia
Nodes: negative

Stage IIb

Tumor: ANY TUMOR that invades up to the muscularis propria
Nodes: positive regional nodes

Stage III

Tumor: invades adventia
Nodes: positive regional nodes **OR**
Tumor: invades adjacent structures
Nodes: positive or negative nodes

Stage IV

Distant metastasis

What is the treatment?

Total thoracic esophagectomy with gastric pull-up or colon interposition (± chemotherapy/radiation, usually in a clinical trial)

What is the operative mortality rate?

About 5%

What is the prognosis (5-year survival) by stage:

I?

80%

II?	33%
III?	15%
IV?	Basically 0%

MISCELLANEOUS

Name four tumors of the anterior mediastinum

"Four **Ts**":
1. **T**hymomas
2. **T**eratomas
3. **T**hyroid tumor
4. **T**errible lymphomas

What are the classic locations of aspiration pneumonia?

RUL—posterior segment
RLL—superior segment

What bronchus is inadvertently intubated most often?

The right main stem (less of angle from the trachea than the left)

What is Tietze's syndrome?

Nonsuppurative inflammation of the costochondral cartilage—painful and of unknown etiology

64

Cardiovascular Surgery

What do the following abbreviations stand for:

IABP?	**I**ntra-**A**ortic **B**alloon **P**ump
VAD?	**V**entricular **A**ssist **D**evice
CABG?	**C**oronary **A**rtery **B**ypass **G**rafting
AI?	**A**ortic **I**nsufficiency
CAD?	**C**oronary **A**rtery **D**isease
CPB?	**C**ardio**P**ulmonary **B**ypass
MR?	**M**itral **R**egurgitation
VSD?	**V**entricular **S**eptal **D**efect
AS?	**A**ortic **S**tenosis
LAD?	**L**eft **A**nterior **D**escending coronary artery
IMA?	**I**nternal **M**ammary **A**rtery
PTCA?	**P**ercutaneous **T**ransluminal **C**oronary **A**ngioplasty (balloon angioplasty)

Define the following terms:

Stroke volume (SV)	ml of blood pumped per heart beat
Cardiac output (CO)	Amount of blood pumped by the heart/min: heart rate × stroke volume
Cardiac Index (CI)	CO/BSA (body surface area)

Ejection fraction — Percentage of blood pumped out of the left ventricle: SV ÷ end diastolic volume (nl 55%–70%)

Compliance — Change in volume/change in pressure

SVR — **S**ystemic **V**ascular **R**esistance

$$\frac{\text{MAP} - \text{CVP}}{\text{CO}} \times 80$$

Preload — Left ventricular end diastolic pressure or volume

Afterload — Arterial resistance the heart pumps against

PVR — **P**ulmonary **V**ascular **R**esistance
$PA_{(mean)} - PCWP / CO \times 80$

MAP — **M**ean **A**rterial **P**ressure = Diastolic BP + 1/3 (Systolic BP – Diastolic BP)

What are the ways to increase cardiac output?

Increase inotropes (increase contractility)
Increase chronotropes: increase heart rate (until SV decreases due to decreased "filling time")
Decrease afterload (decrease SVR)
Increase preload (Frank-Starling curve)

When does most of the coronary blood flow take place?

During **diastole (66%)**

Name the three major coronary arteries.

1. **L**eft **a**nterior **d**escending (LAD)
2. Circumflex
3. Right coronary

What are the three main "cardiac electrolytes"?

1. Calcium (inotropic)
2. Potassium (arrhythmias)
3. Magnesium (arrhythmias)

ACQUIRED HEART DISEASE

CORONARY ARTERY DISEASE (CAD)

What is it?

Atherosclerotic occlusive lesions of the coronary arteries; segmental nature makes coronary artery bypass grafting possible

What is the incidence?

Number one killer in the western world; more than 50% are triple vessel diseases involving the LAD, circumflex, and right coronary arteries

What are the symptoms?

If ischemia occurs (low flow, vasospasm, thrombus formation, plaque rupture, or a combination), patient may experience: chest pain; crushing, substernal shortness of breath; nausea/upper abdominal pain; sudden death; or may be asymptomatic, fatigue

Who classically gets "silent" MIs?

Patients with diabetes (autonomic dysfunction)

What are the risk factors?

HTN
Smoking
High (> 240) cholesterol/lipids
Obesity
Diabetes mellitus
Family history

Which diagnostic tests should be performed?

Exercise stress testing (± thallium)
Echocardiography
  Localize dyskinetic wall segments
  Valvular dysfunction
  Estimate ejection fraction
Cardiac catheterization with coronary angiography and left ventriculography (definitive test)

What is the treatment?

Medical therapy (β-blockers, aspirin, nitrates, HTN medications), angioplasty (PTCA), surgical therapy: CABG

CABG

What is it?

Coronary **A**rtery **B**ypass **G**raft

What are the indications?

Left main disease
Three-vessel disease (main arteries—not branches)
Unstable angina or disabling angina unresponsive to medical therapy
Postinfarct angina
Coronary artery rupture, dissection, thrombosis after PTCA

What procedures are most often used in the treatment?	Coronary arteries grafted (usually 3–6): internal mammary pedicle graft and saphenous vein free graft are most often used (IMA 95% ten-year patency vs. 60%–70% with saphenous); procedure is performed under CPB
What other vessels are occasionally used for grafting?	Gastroepiploic and inferior epigastric veins
What are the possible complications?	MI, arrhythmias Infection Hemorrhage Graft thrombosis Sternal dehiscence Postpericardiotomy syndrome, stroke
What is the operative mortality?	Between 1% and 3% for elective CABG (vs. 5%–10% for acute MI)
What medication should every patient be given after a CABG?	Aspirin

POSTPERICARDIOTOMY SYNDROME

What is it?	Pericarditis after pericardiotomy (unknown etiology), occurs weeks to 3 months postoperatively
What are the signs/ symptoms?	Fever Chest pain, atrial fibrillation Malaise Pericardial friction rub Pericardial effusion/pleural effusion
What is the treatment?	NSAIDs, with or without steroids
What is pericarditis after an MI called?	Dressler's syndrome

CARDIOPULMONARY BYPASS (CPB)

What is it?	Pump and oxygenation apparatus remove blood from SVC and IVC and return it to the aorta, bypassing the heart and lungs and allowing cardiac arrest for open heart procedures, heart transplant,

lung transplant, or heart–lung transplant, as well as procedures on the proximal great vessels.

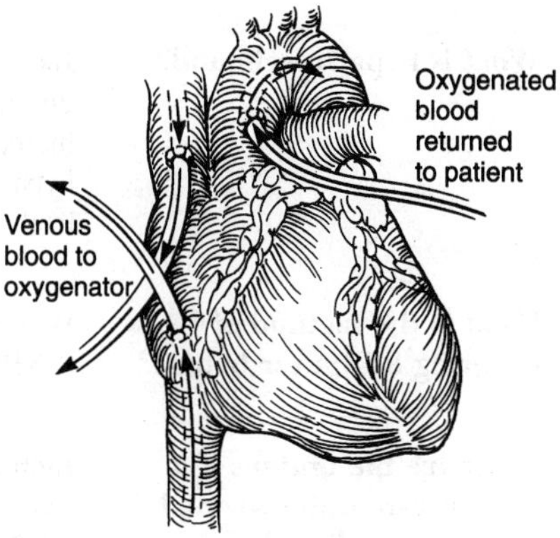

What is the proper procedure?

Roller pump provides nonpulsatile flow (pulse pressure < 20 mm Hg)

Is anticoagulation necessary?

Yes, just before and during the procedure, with heparin

How is anticoagulation reversed?

Protamine

What are the five ways to manipulate cardiac output after bypass?

1. Preload—fluids
2. Inotropic state—calcium, dobutamine/epinephrine, and VAD as a last resort
3. Afterload—vasodilators, heat, IABP
4. Rate, rhythm—pacer, antiarrhythmics

What mechanical problems can decrease CO after a cardiopulmonary bypass procedure?

Cardiac tamponade, pneumothorax

What are the possible complications?

Trauma to formed blood elements (especially thrombocytopenia and platelet dysfunction)
Pancreatitis (low flow)
Heparin rebound
CVA
Failure to wean from bypass

	Technical complications (operative technique) MI
What is heparin rebound?	Increased anticoagulation after bypass due to increased heparin levels, as increase in peripheral blood flow after bypass returns heparin residual that was in the peripheral tissues
What is the method of lowering SVR after bypass?	Warm the patient, sodium nitroprusside (SNP), dobutamine
What are the options if a patient cannot be weaned from the cardiopulmonary bypass?	Inotropes (e.g., epinephrine) IABP VAD
What percentage of patients go into AFib after CPB?	Up to one-third
What is the workup of a postoperative patient with AFib?	Rule out PTX (CXR), rule out acidosis (ABG), rule out electrolyte abnormality (chem 10), rule out ischemia (EKG)
What is the treatment of AFib?	
± Cardioversion	Correction of electrolytes and underlying problem
± Procainamide	Digitalis and β-blocker or Ca^{+}-channel blocker for rate control

AORTIC STENOSIS (AS)

What is it?	Destruction and calcification of valve leaflets, resulting in obstruction of left ventricular outflow
What are the causes?	Calcification of bicuspid aortic valve Rheumatic fever Acquired calcific aortic stenosis (7th–8th decades)

What are the symptoms?

Angina (5 years life expectancy if untreated)
Syncope (3 years life expectancy if untreated)
CHF (2 years life expectancy if untreated)
Often asymptomatic until late

Mnemonic:
Aortic **S**tenosis **C**omplications
(**A**ngina **S**yncope **C**HF)—5,3,2

What are the signs?

Murmur: crescendo–decrescendo systolic second right intercostal space with radiation to the carotids
Left ventricular heave or lift due to left ventricular hypertrophy

What lab tests should be performed?

Echocardiography
Cardiac catheterization—needed to plan operation

What is the treatment?

Valve replacement with tissue or mechanical prosthesis, if patient is symptomatic or valve cross-sectional area is less than 0.7 cm^2 (normal 2.5–3.5 cm^2) and gradiant > 50 mm Hg

What are the pros/cons of mechanical valve?

Mechanical valve is more durable, but requires lifetime anticoagulation.

AORTIC INSUFFICIENCY (AI)

What is it?

Incompetency of the aortic valve

What are the causes?

Bacterial endocarditis (*Staphylococcus aureus, Streptococcus viridans*)
Rheumatic fever
Annular ectasia due to collagen vascular disease (especially Marfan's syndrome)

What are the predisposing conditions?

Bicuspid aortic valve

What are the symptoms?

Palpitations due to arrhythmias and dilated left ventricle
Dyspnea/orthopnea due to left ventricular failure
Angina due to decreased diastolic BP and coronary flow (*Note:* most coronary blood flow occurs during diastole and aorta rebound)

What are the signs?

Murmur: blowing, decrescendo diastolic at left sternal border
Austin-Flint murmur: reverberation of regurgitant flow
Increased pulse pressure: "pistol shots," "water-hammer" pulse palpated over peripheral arteries

Which diagnostic tests should be performed?

1. CXR: increasing heart size can be used to follow progression
2. Echocardiogram
3. Catheterization (definitive)

What is the treatment?

Aortic valve replacement is indicated with the onset of CHF and significant left-ventricular dysfunction

What is the prognosis?

Low operative risk; surgery gives symptomatic improvement and may improve longevity

MITRAL STENOSIS (MS)

What is it?

Calcific degeneration and narrowing of the mitral valve due to rheumatic fever in most cases

What are the symptoms?

1. Dyspnea due to increased left atrial pressure causing pulmonary edema (i.e., CHF)
2. Hemoptysis (rarely life-threatening)
3. Hoarseness due to dilated left atrium impinging on the recurrent laryngeal nerve

What are the signs?

Murmur: crescendo diastolic rumble at apex
Irregular pulse from AFib due to dilated left atrium

	Stroke due to systemic emboli from left atrium (AFib and obstructed valve allows blood to pool in the left atrium and can lead to thrombus formation)
Which diagnostic tests should be performed?	Echocardiogram Catheterization
What is the treatment?	1. Open commissurotomy: open heart operation with cardiopulmonary bypass in which the valve is cut 2. Balloon valvuloplasty: percutaneous, if unsuccessful, surgery is required 3. Valve replacement
What is the prognosis?	More than 80% of patients are well at 10 years with successful operation

MITRAL REGURGITATION (MR)

What is it?	Incompetence of the mitral valve
What are the causes?	Severe mitral valve prolapse (some prolapse is present in 5% of the population, with women ≥ men) Rheumatic fever Post-MI due to papillary mm dysfunction/rupture Ruptured chordae
What is the most common cause?	Ruptured chordae/papillary muscle dysfunction
What are the symptoms?	Often insidious and late: dyspnea, palpitations, fatigue
What are the signs?	Murmur: holosystolic, apical radiating to the axilla
What are the indications for treatment?	Indications for surgery differ from those for MS; in MR, catheter and echocardiogram findings are more revealing than symptoms (e.g., increasing regurgitation, decreasing EF). *Note:* EF first increases in MR; therefore, normal EF may actually indicate decompensation.

What is the treatment?
1. Valve replacement
2. Annuloplasty: suture a prosthetic ring to the dilated valve annulus

What is a normal ejection fraction?
From 55% to 70%

ARTIFICIAL VALVE PLACEMENT

What is it?
Replacement of damaged valves with tissue or mechanical prosthesis

What are the types of valves?
Tissue: glutaraldehyde-fixed porcine valves deteriorate over time (about 20% require replacement in 10 years); however, they do not require long-term anticoagulation
Contraindicated in children because of calcification
Mechanical: can last for the life of the patient, but require lifelong anticoagulation
Contraindicated in those with bleeding tendency (e.g., PUD, ETOH abuse)

What is the operative mortality?
From 1% to 5% in most series

What are the possible postoperative complications?
Valve failure
Valve deterioration, especially rapid calcification of tissue valves in children
Hemorrhagic complications in anticoagulated patients (1% per year)
Thromboembolic—2% to 5% per patient-year, even with adequate anticoagulation
Conduction abnormalities due to the proximity of valvular suture lines to the conduction system (especially mitral valve and bundle of His)

INFECTIOUS ENDOCARDITIS

What is it?
Microbial infection of heart valves

What are the predisposing conditions?
Pre-existing valvular lesion, procedures that lead to bacteremia/IV drug use

What are the common causative agents?
Streptococcus viridans: associated with abnormal valves
Staphylococcus aureus: associated with IV drug use
Staphylococcus epidermidis: associated with prosthetic valves

What are the signs/ symptoms?
Murmur (new or changing)
Petechiae
Splinter hemorrhage (fingernails)
Roth spots (on retina)
Osler nodes (raised, **painful** on soles and palms; Osler = Ouch!)
Janeway lesions (similar to Osler nodes, but flat and **painless)**
(Janeway = pain **away**)

Which diagnostic tests should be performed?
Echocardiogram
Serial blood cultures (definitive)

What is the treatment?
Prolonged IV therapy with bactericidal antibiotics, to which infecting organisms are sensitive

What is the prognosis?
Infection can progress, requiring valve replacement

CONGENITAL HEART DISEASE

VENTRICULAR SEPTAL DEFECT (VSD)

What is its claim to fame?
Most common congenital heart defect

What is it?
Failure of ventricular septum to completely close; **80% involve the membranous portion of the septum,** resulting in left-to-right shunt, increased pulmonary blood flow, and CHF if pulmonary:systemic flow is more than 2:1

What is Eisenmenger's syndrome?
Irreversible pulmonary HTN due to chronic changes in pulmonary arterioles and increased right heart pressures; cyanosis develops when the shunt reverses (becomes right to left across the VSD)

What is the treatment of Eisenmenger's syndrome?
The only option is heart–lung transplant; otherwise, the disease is untreatable

What is the incidence of VSD?
Thirty percent of heart defects (most common defect)

PATENT DUCTUS ARTERIOSUS (PDA)

What is it?
Physiologic right-to-left shunt in fetal circulation connecting the pulmonary artery to the aorta bypassing fetal lungs; often, this shunt persists in the neonate

What are the factors preventing closure?
Hypoxia
Increased prostaglandins

What are the symptoms?
Often asymptomatic
Poor feeding
Respiratory distress
CHF with respiratory infections

What are the signs?
Acyanotic, unless other cardiac lesions are present; continuous "machinery" murmur

Which diagnostic tests should be performed?
Physical exam
Echocardiogram (to rule out associated defects)
Catheter (seldom required)

What is the medical treatment?
Indomethacin is an NSAID: prostaglandin (PG) inhibitor (PG keeps PDA open)

What is the surgical treatment?
Ligation electively at 1 to 2 years, but if CHF occurs, operate acutely

What is the prognosis?
Surgically curable lesion

TETRALOGY OF FALLOT (TOF)

What is it?

Malalignment of the infundibular septum in early development, leading to the characteristic tetrad:

1. Pulmonary stenosis/obstruction of right ventricular outflow
2. Overriding aorta
3. Right ventricular hypertrophy
4. VSD

What are the symptoms?

Hypoxic spells (squatting behavior increases SVR and increases pulmonary blood flow)

What are the signs?

Cyanosis
Clubbing
Murmur: SEM at left third intercostal space

Which diagnostic tests should be performed?

CXR: small, "boot-shaped" heart and decreased pulmonary blood flow
Cardiac catheterization (definitive)

What is the prognosis?

Ninety percent success rate for surgical correction

What is IHSS?

Idiopathic **h**ypertrophic **s**ubaortic **s**tenosis

What is the usual presentation?

Can present with sudden death due to:

1. Arrhythmias
2. Syncope
3. CHF

COARCTATION OF THE AORTA

What is it?

Narrowing of the thoracic aorta, with or without intraluminal "shelf" (infolding of the media); usually found near ductus/ligamentum arteriosum

What are the three types?

1. Preductal (fatal in infancy if untreated)
2. Juxtaductal
3. Postductal

What percentage are associated with other cardiac defects?
Sixty percent (bicuspid aortic valve is most common)

What is the major route of collateral circulation?
Subclavian artery to the IMA to the intercostals to the descending aorta

What is the incidence?
From 10% to 15% of defects

What are the symptoms?
Headache
Epistaxis
Lower extremity fatigue→ claudication

What are the signs?
Pulses: decreased lower extremity pulses
Murmurs:
1. Systolic—due to turbulence across coarctation, often radiating to infrascapular region
2. Continuous—due to dilated collaterals

Other signs that can be associated with fatal consequences:
1. CHF
2. Aortic dissection
3. Intracranial aneurysmal rupture (due to HTN)
4. Bacterial endocarditis

Which diagnostic tests should be performed?
CXR
  "3" sign is aortic knob, coarctation, and dilated poststenotic aorta
  Rib notching is bony erosion due to dilated intercostal collaterals
Catheterization with aortography
Echocardiogram

What is the treatment?
Surgery
  Resection with end-to-end anastomosis
  Patch graft (rare)
  Subclavian artery flap (favored in infants)
  Interposition graft

What are the indications for surgery?
Symptomatic patient
Asymptomatic patient more than 3 to 4 years old

What are the possible postoperative complications?	Paraplegia "Paradoxic" HTN (postop) Mesenteric necrotizing panarteritis (GI bleeding)
What is the prognosis?	Untreated life expectancy: 30 to 40 years
What are the long-term concerns?	Aortic dissection, HTN

TRANSPOSITION OF THE GREAT VESSELS

What is it?	Aorta originates from the right ventricle and the pulmonary artery from the left ventricle; fatal without PDA, ASD, or VSD to allow communication between the left and right circulations
What is the incidence?	From 5% to 8% of defects
What are the signs/ symptoms?	Most common lesion that presents with cyanosis and CHF in neonatal period (> 90% by day 1)
Which diagnostic tests should be performed?	CXR: "egg-shaped" heart contour Catheterization (definitive)
What is the treatment?	Arterial switch operation

EBSTEIN'S ANOMALY

What is it?	Tricuspid valve is placed abnormally low in the right atrium, forming a large right atrium and a small right ventricle, leading to tricuspid regurgitation and decreased right ventricular output
What are the risk factors?	Four hundred times the risk if the mother has taken lithium

VASCULAR RINGS

What are they?	Many types; represent an anomalous development of the aorta/pulmonary artery from the embryonic aortic arch that surrounds and obstructs the trachea/ esophagus

What are the signs/ symptoms?

Most prominent is stridor due to tracheal compression

CYANOTIC HEART DISEASE

What are the causes?

The five "Ts" of cyanotic heart disease:
- **T**etralogy of Fallot
- **T**runcus arteriosus
- **T**otally anomalous pulmonary venous return (TAPVR)
- **T**ricuspid atresia
- **T**ransposition of the great vessels

CARDIAC TUMORS

What is the most common benign lesion?

Myxoma in adults, commonly found in the left atrium with pedunculated morphology (60%–80% of primary cardiac tumors)

What is the most common malignant tumor in children?

Rhabdomyosarcoma

DISEASES OF THE GREAT VESSELS

THORACIC AORTIC ANEURYSM

What is it?

Aneurysm of the thoracic aorta

What is the cause?

Vast majority are due to atherosclerosis

What is the major differential diagnosis?

Aortic dissection

What percentage of patients have aneurysms of the aorta at a distant site?

About one-third! (rule out AAA)

What are the signs/ symptoms?

Most are asymptomatic
Chest pain, stridor, hemoptysis (rare), recurrent laryngeal nerve compression

What is the most common way to diagnose?

Routine CXR

Which diagnostic tests should be performed?
CXR, CT, MRI

What are the indications for surgical treatment?
More than 6 cm in diameter
More than 2.5 times contiguous normal aortic diameter
Symptoms
Rapid increase in diameter

What is the treatment?
Replace with graft

What are the dreaded complications after treatment of a thoracic aortic aneurysm?
Paraplegia (up to 20%)
Anterior spinal syndrome

What is anterior spinal syndrome?
Syndrome characterized by:
- Paraplegia
- Incontinence (bowel/bladder)
- Pain and temperature sensation loss

What is the cause?
Occlusion of the great radicular artery of **Adamkiewicz,** which is one of the intercostal/lumbar arteries from T8 to L4

AORTIC DISSECTION

What is it?
Separation of the walls of the aorta due to an intimal tear and disease of the tunica media; a false lumen is formed and a "reentry" tear may occur, resulting in "double-barrel" aorta

What are the aortic dissection classifications?
DeBakey classification
Stanford classification

Define the DeBakey classifications:

DeBakey type I — Involves ascending **and** descending aorta

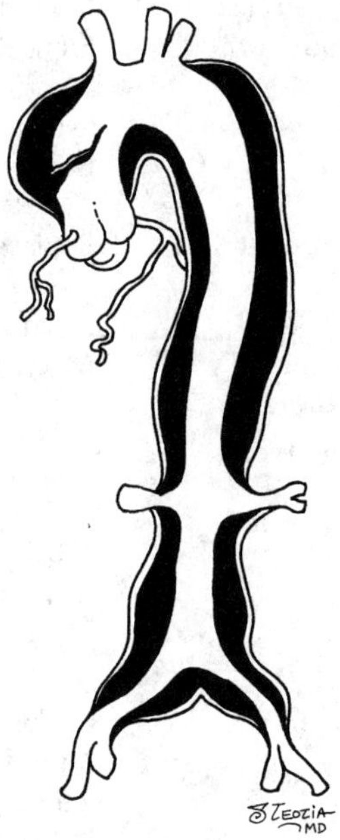

DeBakey type II — Involves ascending aorta only

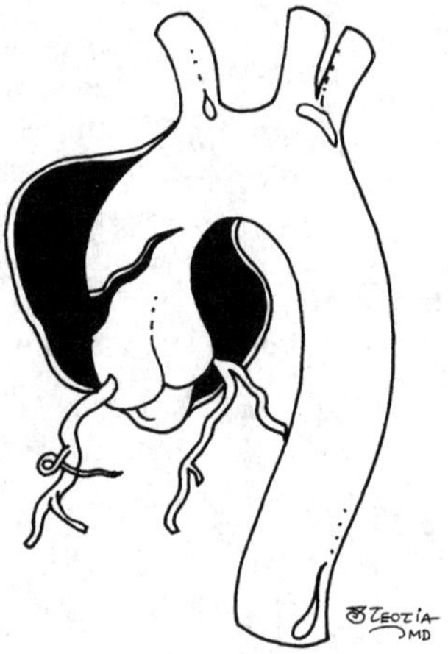

DeBakey type III Descending aorta only

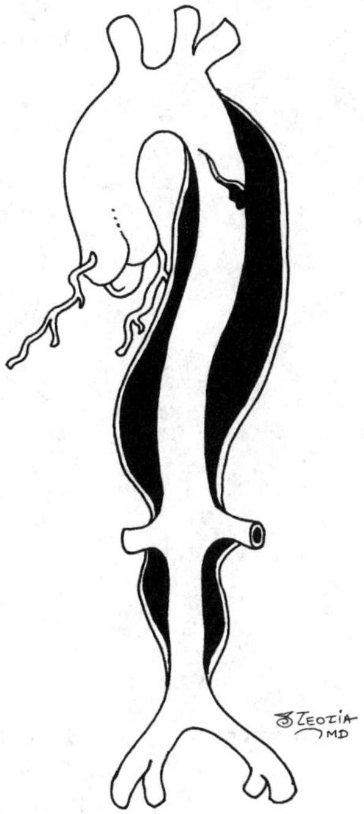

Define the Stanford classifications:

Type A Ascending aorta (requires surgery) ± Descending aorta (includes DeBakey Types I and II)

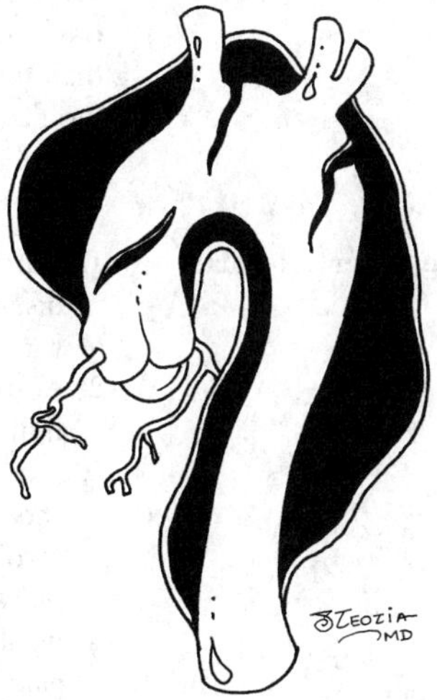

Type B

Descending aorta only (nonoperative, except for complications) (same as DeBakey Type III)

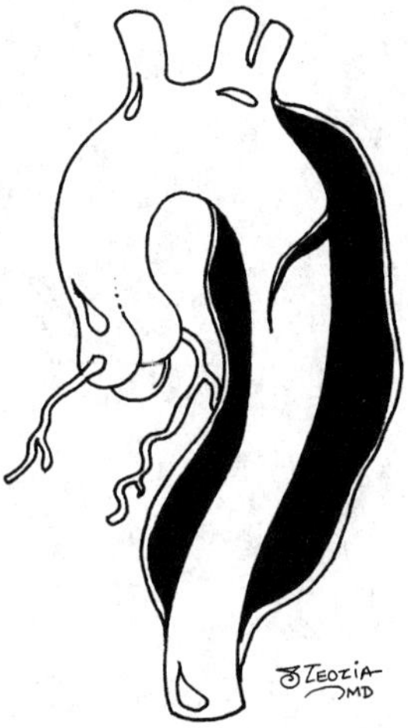

What is the etiology?

HTN (most important)
Marfan's syndrome
Bicuspid aortic valve
Coarctation of the aorta
Cystic medial necrosis
Proximal aortic aneurysm

What are the signs/ symptoms?

Abrupt onset of severe chest pain, most often radiating/tearing to the back; onset is typically more abrupt than that of MI; the pain can migrate as the dissection progresses; patient describes a **"tearing pain"**

Note three other sequelae.

1. Cardiac tamponade; Beck's triad—distant heart sounds, increased CVP with JVD, decreased blood pressure
2. Aortic insufficiency—diastolic murmur
3. Aortic arterial branch occlusion/ shearing, leading to ischemia in the involved circulation (i.e., unequal pulses, CVA, paraplegia, renal insufficiency, bowel ischemia, claudication)

Which diagnostic tests are indicated?

CXR
1. Widened mediastinum
2. Pleural effusion

TEE (transesophageal echo)
CT
Aortography (definitive gold standard!)

What is a dissecting aortic aneurysm?

A misnomer! Not an aneurysm!

What is the treatment of the various types:

Types I and II (Stanford type A)?

Surgical because of risk of:
1. Aortic insufficiency
2. Compromise of cerebral and coronary circulation
3. Tamponade
4. Rupture

Type III (Stanford type B)?

Medical (control BP), unless complicated by rupture or significant occlusions

Describe the surgery for an aortic dissection.

Open the aorta at the proximal extent of dissection, and then sew—graft to—intimal flap and adventia circumferentially.

What is the preoperative treatment?

Control BP with sodium nitroprusside **and β-blockers** (e.g., esmolol; β-blockers decrease shear stress)

What is the postoperative treatment?

Lifetime control of BP and monitoring of aortic size

What is the Edwards' procedure?

Replace the ascending aorta with a graft and replace the aortic valve; reimplantation of coronaries

What is the possible cause of MI in a patient with aortic dissection?

Dissection involves the coronary arteries or underlying LAD.

What are the EKG signs of the following disorders:

Atrial fibrillation? Irregularly irregular

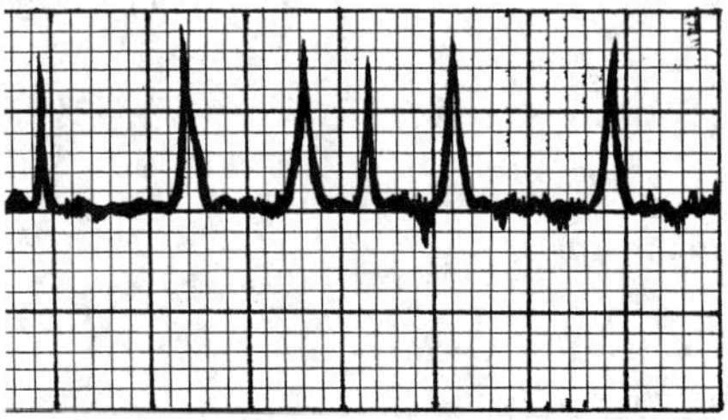

PVC? **P**remature **v**entricular **c**omplex: Wide QRS

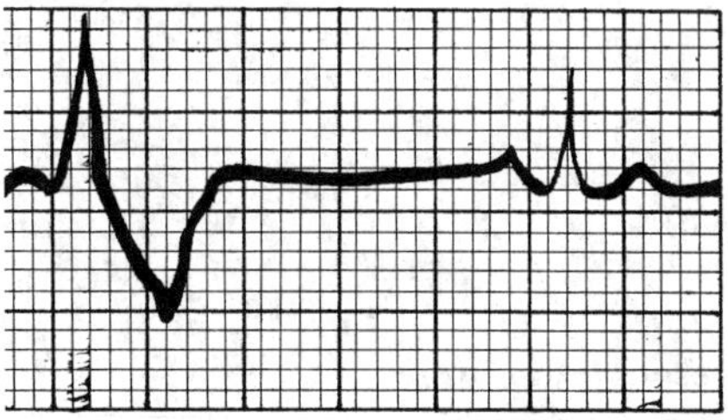

Ventricular aneurysm? ST elevation

Ischemia? ST elevation/ST depression/flipped T waves

Infarction? Q waves

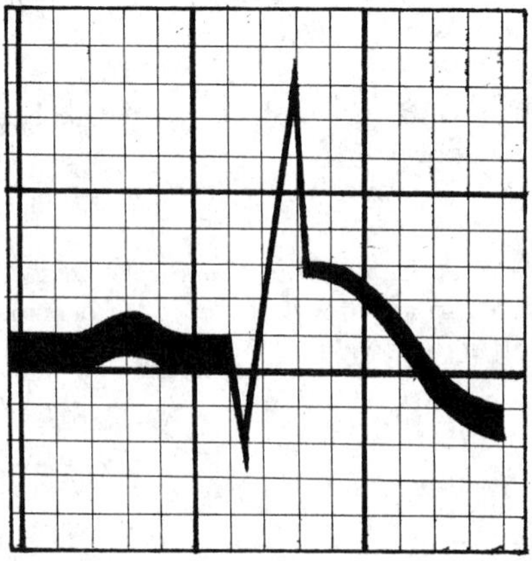

Pericarditis?	ST elevation throughout leads
RBBB?	**R**ight **b**undle **b**ranch **b**lock: wide QRS and "rabbit ears" or R-R in V1 or V2
LBBB?	**L**eft **b**undle **b**ranch **b**lock: wide QRS and "rabbit ears" or R-R in V5 or V6
Wolff-Parkinson-White	Delta wave = slurred upswing on QRS
First degree A-V block?	Prolonged P-R interval (≥ 0.2 second)
Second degree A-V block?	Dropped QRS; not all P waves transmit to produce ventricular contraction
Wenckebach phenomenon?	Second-degree block with progressive delay in P-R interval prior to dropped beat
Third-degree A-V block?	Complete A-V dissociation; random P wave and QRS

MISCELLANEOUS

What is Mondor's disease?	Thrombophlebitis of the thoracoepigastric veins
What is a VAD?	**V**entricular **A**ssist **D**evice
How does an IABP work?	The **i**ntra-**a**ortic **b**alloon **p**ump has a balloon tip resting in the aorta. The balloon inflates in diastole, increasing diastolic blood pressure and coronary blood flow. In systole the balloon deflates, creating a negative pressure, lowering afterload, and increasing systolic blood pressure.
What electrolyte must be monitored during diuresis after cardiopulmonary bypass?	K^+
How is extent/progress of postbypass diuresis followed?	Daily weight, I's and O's, CXR, JVD, edema, etc.

During a CABG, what can be used in place of the saphenous vein?

IMA, inferior epigastric vessels, radial artery, gastroepiploic vessels (*Note:* prosthetic material cannot be used)

What are the indications for CABG?

Left main coronary disease
Triple vessel disease
Unstable/disabling angina not responsive to medical treatment
Postinfarct angina
Damage to coronary during cardiac catheterization
Disabling/refractory angina

What are the five ways of increasing cardiac output?

1. Inotropes
2. Chronotropes
3. Increase preload
4. Decrease afterload
5. Improve heart compliance

What side effect is associated with protamine?

Hypotension

What is an Austin Flint murmur?

Diastolic murmur of AI secondary to regurgitant turbulent flow

Where is the least-oxygenated blood in the body?

Coronary sinus

What is the most common cause of a cardiac tumor?

Metastasis

65

Transplant Surgery

Define the following terms:	
Autograft	Same individual is donor and recipient
Isograft	Donor and recipient are genetically identical (identical twins)
Allograft	Donor and recipient are genetically dissimilar, but of the same species
Xenograft	Donor and recipient belong to different species
Orthotopic	Donor organ placed in anatomic position (liver, heart)
Heterotopic	Donor organ placed in different anatomic position (kidney, pancreas)
Paratopic	Donor organ is placed close to original organ

BASIC IMMUNOLOGY

What are histocompatibility antigens?	Distinct (genetically inherited) cell surface proteins of the human leukocyte antigen system (HLA)
Why are they important?	They are targets (class I antigens) and initiators (class II antigens) of immune response to donor tissue (i.e., distinguishing **self from nonself)**
Which cells have class I antigens?	All nucleated cells (think: type 1 = all cells and thus: "one for all")
Class II antigens?	Macrophages, monocytes, B cells, activated T cells, endothelial cells

What is the MHC called in humans? HLA—human leukocyte antigen

What is the location? Short arm of chromosome 6

What is the code? Class I, II, and III antigens

CELLS

T CELLS

What is the source? Thymus

What is the function? Cell-mediated immunity/rejection

What are the types?
Th (CD4): helper T—help B cells become plasma cells
Ts (CD8): suppressor T—regulate immune response
Tc (CD8): cytotoxic T—kill cell by direct contact

B CELLS

What is the function? Humoral immunity

What is the cell type that produces antibodies? B cells differentiate into **plasma cells**

MACROPHAGE

What is it? A monocyte in parenchymal tissue

What is its function? Processes foreign protein and **presents** it to lymphocytes

What is it also known as? Antigen presenting cell (APC)

Briefly describe the events leading to antibody production.

1. Macrophage engulfs antigen and presents it to Th cells and the macrophage produces IL-1.
2. The Th cells then produce IL-2 and the Th cells proliferate.
3. The Th cells then activate (via IL-4) B cells that differentiate into plasma cells, which produce antibodies against the antigen presented.

IMMUNOSUPPRESSION

Who needs to be immunosuppressed?	All recipients (except auto- or isograft)
What are the three major drugs used for immunosuppression?	Corticosteroids, azathioprine, cyclosporine
What are the other drugs?	ALG, OKT3, ATG
What are the new drugs?	FK-506, mycophenolate
What is the advantage of "triple therapy"?	Uses three immunosuppressive drugs and thereby can use lower doses of each and decrease the toxic side effects of each

CORTICOSTEROIDS

Which is most commonly used in transplants?	Prednisone
How does it function?	Primarily **blocks production of IL-1 by macrophage** and stabilizes lysosomal membrane of macrophage
What is the associated toxicity?	"Cushingoid," alopecia, striae, HTN, diabetes, pancreatitis, ulcer disease, osteomalacia, aseptic necrosis (especially of the femoral head)
What is the relative potency of the following corticosteriods:	
Cortisol?	1
Prednisone?	4
Methylprednisolone?	5
Dexamethasone?	25

AZATHIOPRINE (AZA [IMURAN])

How does it function?	Prodrug that is cleaved into mercaptopurine; inhibits synthesis of DNA and RNA, leading to decreased cellular (T/B cells) production

What is the associated toxicity?
Toxic to bone marrow (leukopenia + thrombocytopenia), hepatotoxic, associated with pancreatitis

When should a lower dose of AZA be administered?
When WBC is less than 4

What is the associated drug interaction?
Decrease dose if the patient is also on allopurinol, because allopurinol inhibits the enzyme xanthine oxidase, which is necessary for the breakdown of azathioprine.

CYCLOSPORINE (CSA)

What is its function?
Inhibits the production of IL-2 by Th cells

What is the associated toxicity?
1. Nephrotoxicity (dose-dependent, reversible)
2. Elevated LFTs (50%)
3. Neurotoxic tremor (50%), seizures (5%)
4. HTN
5. Gum hypertrophy
6. Hirsutism
7. Hyperkalemia

What drugs increase CSA levels?
Diltiazem
Ketoconazole
Erythromycin, fluconazole

What are the drugs of choice for HTN due to CSA?
Clonidine, calcium channel blockers

ATG/ANTITHYMOCYTE GLOBULIN

How does it function?
An antibody against thymocytes

How is it made?
Injection of human lymphoblasts and lymphocytes into a horse or rabbit and retrieval of antibodies

What is the associated toxicity?
Thrombocytopenia, leukopenia, serum sickness, rigors, fever, anaphylaxis, increased risk of viral infection

OKT3

How does it function?	Antibody that binds to CD3 receptor (a specific antigen on T cells)
What problem is it associated with?	Because it is monoclonal, blocking antibodies develop; therefore, it may be less effective each time it is used

What drug acts at the following sites:

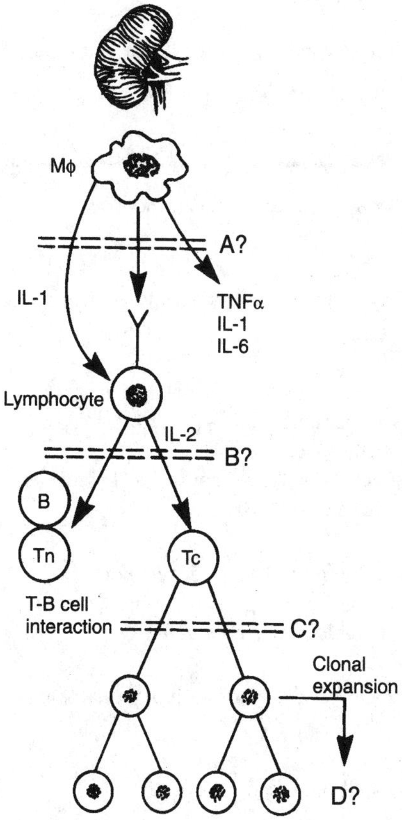

A?	Corticosteroids
B?	Cyclosporine
C?	Azathioprine
D?	OKT3/ATG

MATCHING OF DONOR AND RECIPIENT

How is ABO crossmatching performed?	Same procedure as in blood typing
What is the purpose of lymphocytotoxic crossmatching?	Test for HLA antibodies in serum; most important in kidney and pancreas transplants
How is the test performed?	Mix recipient serum with donor lymphocyte and rabbit complement
Is HLA crossmatching important?	Yes, for kidney and pancreas transplants

REJECTION

How many methods of rejection are there?	Two—humoral and cell-mediated
Name the types of rejection.	Hyperacute, accelerated acute, acute, chronic
What are the associated time courses by type?	Hyperacute—immediate in OR Accelerated acute—7 to 10 days post-transplant Acute—weeks to months post transplant Chronic—months to years
What happens in hyperacute rejection?	Antigraft antibodies in recipient recognize foreign antigen immediately after blood perfuses organ
What causes accelerated acute rejection?	T-cell mediated or antibody rejection
What happens in acute rejection?	T-cell mediated rejection
What type of rejection is responsible for chronic rejection?	Cellular and/or antibody (humoral)
What is the treatment of hyperacute rejection?	Remove transplanted organ

What is the treatment of acute rejection?	High-dose steroids/OKT3
What is the treatment of chronic rejection?	Not much (irreversible) Or retransplant

REVIEW OF MECHANISMS OF REJECTION

Hyperacute?	Secondary to recipient preformed antibodies to donor ABO or HLA antigen
Accelerated acute?	Humoral or cell mediated
Acute?	Cellular immunity
Chronic?	Humoral and/or cellular immunity

ORGAN PRESERVATION

What is the storage temperature of an organ?	4°C—keep on ice in a cooler
Why should it be kept cold?	Cold decreases the rate of chemical reactions; decreased energy use minimizes effects of hypoxia and ischemia.
What is U-W solution?	University of Wisconsin solution; used to perfuse an organ prior to removal from the donor
What is in it?	Potassium phosphate, buffers, starch, steroids, insulin, electrolytes, adenosine
Why should it be used?	Lengthens organ preservation time

MAXIMUM TIME BETWEEN HARVEST AND TRANSPLANT OF ORGAN

Heart?	4 hours
Lungs?	6 hours
Pancreas?	24 hours
Liver?	24 hours

Kidney? Up to 48 hours

KIDNEY TRANSPLANT

HISTORY

In what year was the first transplant performed in man?
1954

By whom?
J.E. Murray—1990 Nobel Prize winner in medicine

What are the indications for transplant?
Irreversible renal failure due to:
1. Glomerulonephritis (leading cause)
2. Pyelonephritis
3. Polycystic kidney disease
4. Malignant HTN
5. Reflux pyelonephritis
6. Goodpasture's syndrome (antibasement membrane)
7. Congenital renal hyperplasia
8. Fabry's disease
9. Alport's syndrome
10. Renal cortical necrosis
11. Damage due to IDDM

Define renal failure.
GFR less than 20% to 25% of normal; as GFR drops to 5% to 10% of normal, uremic symptoms begin (e.g., lethargy, seizures, neuropathy, electrolyte disorders)

STATISTICS

What are the sources of donor kidneys?
Cadaveric (70%)
Living related donor (LRD; 30%)

What survival rate is associated with cadaveric source?
Eighty-five percent at 1 year if HLA matched; 80% at 1 year if not HLA matched; 75% graft survival at 3 years

What survival rate is associated with LRD?
Between 90% and 95% patient survival at 3 years; 75% to 85% graft survival at 3 years

What are the tests for compatibility?

ABO, HLA typing

If a choice of left or right donor kidney is available, which is preferred?

Left—longer renal vein allows for easier anastomosis

Should the placement of the kidney be hetero- or orthotopic?

Heterotopic—retroperitoneal in the right lower quadrant or left lower quadrant above the inguinal ligament

Why?

Preserves native kidneys, allows easy access to iliac vessels, places ureter close to the bladder, easy to biopsy kidney

Define anastomoses of a heterotopic kidney transplant.

1. Renal artery to iliac artery
2. Renal vein to iliac vein
3. Ureter to bladder

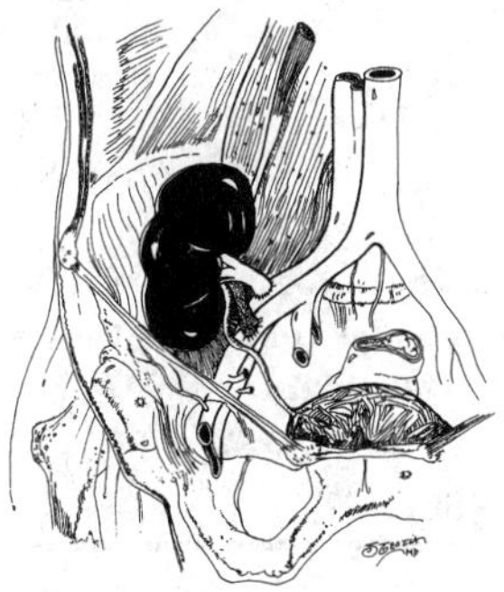

What is the correct placement of the ureter?

Submucosally through the bladder wall—decreases reflux

Why keep native kidneys?

Increased morbidity if they are removed

What is the indication for removal of native kidneys?

Uncontrollable HTN, ongoing renal sepsis

IMMUNOSUPPRESSION

For cadaveric transplant?

Cyclosporine, azathioprine (Imuran), steroids, ATG, OKT3

For LRD transplant?

Cyclosporine, azathioprine (Imuran), steroids

REJECTION

What is the red flag that indicates rejection?	Increasing creatinine
What is the differential diagnosis of increased creatinine?	(Remember: "**-tion**") obstruc**tion,** dehydra**tion,** infec**tion,** intoxica**tion** (CSA); plus lymphocele, ATN
What are the signs/ symptoms?	Fever, malaise, HTN, ipsilateral leg edema, pain at transplant site, oliguria
What is the workup for the following tests:	
US/Doppler?	Look for fluid collection around the kidney, hydronephrosis, flow in vessels
Radionuclide scan?	Look at flow and function
Biopsy?	Distinguish between rejection and cyclosporine toxicity
What is the time course for return of normal renal function after transplant?	LRD—3 to 5 days Cadaveric—7 to 15 days

LIVER TRANSPLANT

What are the indications?

Liver failure due to:

1. Cirrhosis (leading indication in adults)
2. Budd-Chiari
3. Biliary atresia (leading indication in children)
4. Neonatal hepatitis
5. Chronic active hepatitis
6. Fulminant hepatitis with drug toxicity—acetaminophen
7. Sclerosing cholangitis
8. Caroli's disease
9. Subacute hepatic necrosis
10. Congenital hepatic fibrosis
11. Inborn errors of metabolism
12. Fibrolamellar hepatocellular carcinoma

Define the following terms:

Liver failure — Stage III or IV encephalopathy in patients with liver disease; also, abnormal synthetic function

Stage III encephalopathy — Deep somnolence, incoherent speech

Stage IV encephalopathy — Coma

What is the test for compatibility? — ABO typing

What is the placement? — Orthotopic

What are the options for biliary drainage?

1. Donor common bile to recipient common bile duct end to end
2. Roux-en-Y choledochojejunostomy

What is the correct proportionate size? — Donor body weight should be approximately 50% greater than or 50% less than recipient

Immunosuppression? — Cyclosporine, azathioprine (Imuran), steroids

REJECTION

What are the red flags indicating rejection? — Decreased bile drainage, increased serum bilirubin, increased LFTs

What is the site of rejection? — Rejection involves the biliary epithelium first and later the vascular endothelium.

What is the workup with the following tests:

U/S with Doppler? — Look at flow in portal vein, hepatic artery; rule out thrombosis, leaky anastomosis, infection (abscess)

Cholangiogram? — Look at bile ducts (easy to do; patients usually have a T-tube if they have first-degree biliary anastomosis)

Biopsy? — Especially important 3 to 6 weeks postop, when CMV is of greatest concern

Does hepatorenal syndrome renal function improve after liver transplant?	Yes

SURVIVAL STATISTICS

What is the 1-year survival rate?	Approximately 80%–85%
What percentage of patients require retransplant?	Approximately 20%
Why?	Usually due to primary graft dysfunction, rejection, infection, vascular thrombosis, or recurrence of primary disease

PANCREAS TRANSPLANT

What are the indications?	Type I (juvenile diabetes mellitus) associated with severe complications (renal failure, blindness, neuropathy) or very poor glucose control
What are the tests for compatibility?	ABO, Dr matching (class II)
What is the placement?	Heterotopic, in iliac fossa or paratopic
Anastomosis of the exocrine duct (in heterotopic placement)?	To the bladder
Why?	Measures the amount of amylase in urine, gives an indication of pancreatic function (i.e., high urine amylase indicates good pancreatic function)
What is the associated electrolyte complication?	Loss of bicarbonate
Anastomosis of exocrine duct (in paratopic placement)?	To the jejunum
Why?	It is close by and physiologic

What is the advantage of paratopic placement?	Endocrine function drains to the portal vein directly to the liver, and pancreatic contents stay within the GI tract (no need to replace bicarbonate)
Immunosuppression?	Cyclosporine, azathioprine (Imuran), steroids
What are the red flags indicating rejection?	Hyperamylasemia, hyperglycemia, hypoamylasuria, graft tenderness
Why should the kidney and pancreas be transplanted together?	Kidney function is a better indicator of rejection; also better survival of graft is associated with kidney–pancreas transplant than pancreas alone.
Why is hyperglycemia not a good indicator for rejection surveillance?	Hyperglycemia appears relatively late with pancreatic rejection

HEART TRANSPLANT

What are the indications?	Age birth to 65 years with terminal acquired heart disease—class IV of New York Heart Association classification (inability to do any physical activity without discomfort = 10% chance of surviving 6 months)
What are the contraindications?	Over age 65 (variable) Active infection Poor pulmonary function Increased pulmonary artery resistance
What are the tests for compatibility?	ABO, size
What is the placement?	Orthotopic anastomosis of atria, aorta, pulmonary artery
Immunosuppression?	Cyclosporine, azathioprine (Imuran), steroids

REJECTION

What are the red flags of rejection?	Fever, hypo- or hypertension, increased T4/T8 ratio

What are the tests?	Endomyocardial biopsy—much more important than clinical signs/symptoms; patient undergoes routine biopsy

SURVIVAL STATISTICS

What is the 1-year graft survival rate?	Between 85% and 95%

LUNG TRANSPLANT

What are the indications?	Generally, disease that substantially limits activities of daily living and is likely to result in death within 12 to 18 months: Pulmonary fibrosis COPD Eosinophilic granuloma Primary pulmonary HTN Eisenmenger's syndrome Cystic fibrosis
What are the contraindications?	Current smoking Active infection
What tests comprise the pretransplant assessment of recipient?	1. Pulmonary—PFTs, V/Q scan 2. Cardiac—Echo, cath, angiogram 3. Exercise tolerance test
What are the donor requirements?	1. Age less than 55 2. Clear chest film 3. PA oxygen tension of 300 on 100% oxygen and 5 cm PEEP 4. No purulent secretions on bronchoscopy
Necessary anastomoses?	Bronchi, PA, pulmonary veins Bronchial artery is not necessary
What are the red flags of rejection?	Decreased arterial O_2 tension Fever Increased fatigability Infiltrate on x-ray
What are the survival rates associated with the following conditions:	
Single lung, 1 year?	Approximately 65%

Double lung, 1 year?	Approximately 70%

TRANSPLANT COMPLICATIONS

Note four major complications.	1. Infection 2. Rejection 3. Post-transplant lymphoproliferative disease 4. Complications of steroids

INFECTION

What are the usual agents?	DNA viruses, especially CMV, HSV, VZV
When should CMV infection be suspected?	More than 21 days post-transplant
What is the time of peak incidence of CMV infections?	Four to six weeks post-transplant
What are the signs/ symptoms of CMV?	Fever, neutropenia, signs of rejection of transplant; also can present as viral pneumonitis, hepatitis, colitis
How is CMV diagnosed?	Biopsy of transplant to differentiate rejection, cultures of blood, urine
What is the treatment of CMV?	Ganciclovir, with or without immunoglobin; foscarnet
What are the complications of Ganciclovir?	Bone marrow suppression
What are the signs/ symptoms of HSV?	Herpetic lesions, shingles, fever, neutropenia, rejection of transplant
What is the treatment of HSV?	Acyclovir until patient is asymptomatic

MALIGNANCY

What are the most common types?	1. Skin/lip cancer (40%) 2. B-cell cancer (15%) 3. Cervical cancer [three-fourths in situ] in women (20%), other types: T-cell lymphoma, Kaposi's sarcoma

Which epithelial cancers are important after transplant?	Skin/lip cancer, especially basal cell and squamous cell
What is the treatment of malignancy?	Epithelial—standard operative procedure; lymphomas are difficult to treat
What is post-transplant lymphoma associated with?	Multiple doses of OKT3 EBV Young > elderly
What is the treatment for post-transplant lymphoproliferative disease?	1. Drastically reduce immunosuppression 2. ± Radiation 3. ± Chemotherapy

66

Orthopaedic Surgery

What do the following abbreviations stand for:

ORIF?	**O**pen **R**eduction **I**nternal **F**ixation
ROM?	**R**ange **O**f **M**otion
FROM?	**F**ull **R**ange **O**f **M**otion
ACL?	**A**nterior **C**ruciate **L**igament
PCL?	**P**osterior **C**ruciate **L**igament
MCL?	**M**edial **C**ollateral **L**igament
PWB?	**P**artial **W**eight **B**earing
FWB?	**F**ull **W**eight **B**earing
WBAT?	**W**eight **B**earing **A**s **T**olerated
THR?	**T**otal **H**ip **R**eplacement
TKR?	**T**otal **K**nee **R**eplacement
TJR?	**T**otal **J**oint **R**eplacement

Define the following terms:

Supination	Palm up
Pronation	Palm down
Plantarflexion	Foot down at ankle joint (plant foot in ground)
Foot dorsiflexion	Foot up at ankle joint
Adduction	Movement toward the body (**ADD**uction = **ADD** to the body)

Abduction	Movement away from the body
Inversion	Foot sole faces midline
Eversion	Foot sole faces laterally
Volarflexion	Hand flexes at wrist joint toward flexor tendons
Wrist dorsiflexion	Hand flexes at wrist joint toward extensor tendons
Allograft bone	Bone from human donor other than patient
Reduction	Maneuver to restore proper alignment to fracture or joint
Closed reduction	Reduction done without surgery (e.g., casts, splints)
Open reduction	Surgical reduction
Fixation	Stabilization of a fracture after reduction by means of surgical placement of hardware (e.g., pins, plates, screws); can be external or internal
Unstable fracture or dislocation	Fracture or dislocation in which further deformation will occur if reduction is **not** performed

Varus

Extremity abnormality with apex of defect pointed away from midline (e.g., genu varum = bowlegged; with valgus, this term can also be used to describe fracture displacement)
Think, knees are very VARIED apart

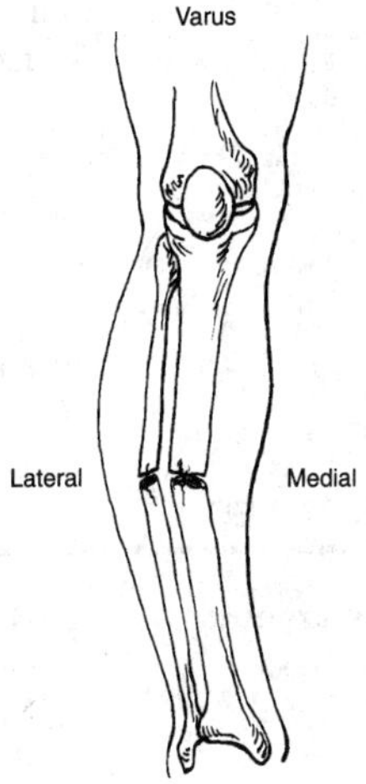

Valgus

Extremity abnormality with apex of defect pointed toward the midline (e.g., genu valgus = knock-kneed)

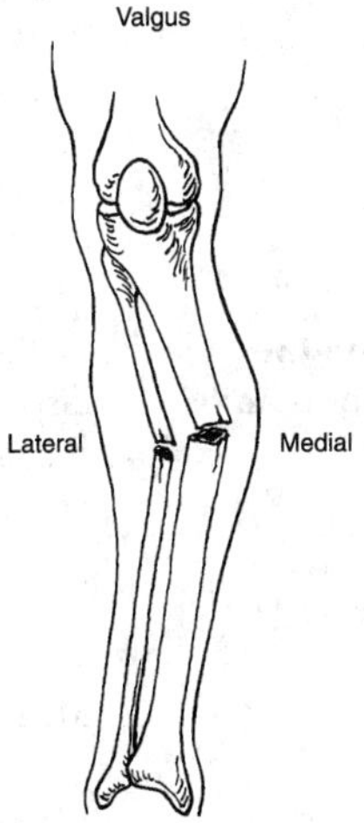

Dislocation

Total loss of congruity between articular surfaces of a joint

Subluxation — Loss of congruity between articular surfaces

Arthroplasty — Total joint replacement (most last 10–15 years)

Arthrodesis — Joint fusion with removal of articular surfaces

Osteotomy — Cutting bone (usually wedge resection) to help realigning of joint surfaces

Non-union? — Failure of a fracture to heal (failure to fuse and thus no union of the fractured bone ends)

GENERAL PRINCIPLES

Define extremity exam in fractured extremities.

1. Observe entire extremity (e.g., open, angulation)
2. Neurologic (sensation, movement)
3. Vascular (e.g., pulses, cap refill)

Which x-rays should be obtained? — Two views (also joint above and below fracture)

How are fractures described?

1. Skin status (open or closed)
2. Bone (by thirds: proximal/middle/distal)
3. Pattern of fracture (e.g., comminuted)
4. Degree of angulation

How do you define the degree of angulation and/or displacement? — Define lateral/medial/anterior/posterior displacement and angulation of the distal fragment(s) in relation to the proximal bone.

Define the following terms:

Diaphysis — Main shaft of long bone

Metaphysis — Flared end of long bone

Physis — Growth plate, found only in immature bone

Define:

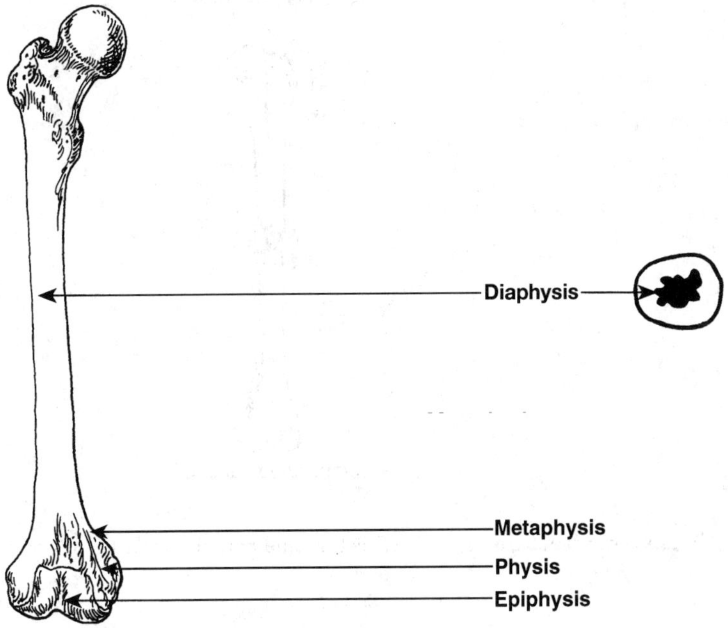

FRACTURES

Define the following patterns of fracture:

Closed fracture — Intact skin over fracture/hematoma

Open fracture — Wound overlying fracture, through which fracture fragments are in continuity with outside environment; high risk of infection
Note: Called compound fracture in the past

Simple fracture — One fracture line, two bone fragments

Comminuted fracture

Results in more than two bone fragments; also known as fragmentation

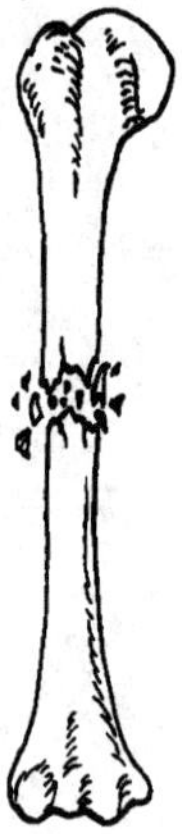

Comminuted fracture

Transverse fracture

Fracture line perpendicular to long axis of bone

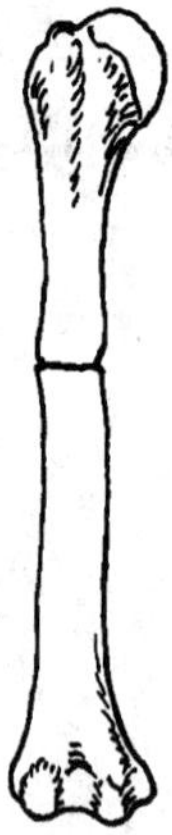

Transverse fracture

Oblique fracture

Fracture line creates an oblique angle with long axis of bone

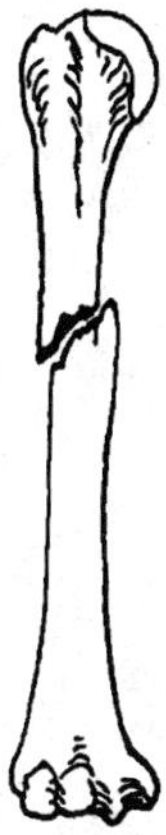

Oblique fracture

Spiral fracture

Severe oblique fracture in which fracture plane rotates along the long axis of bone; caused by a twisting injury

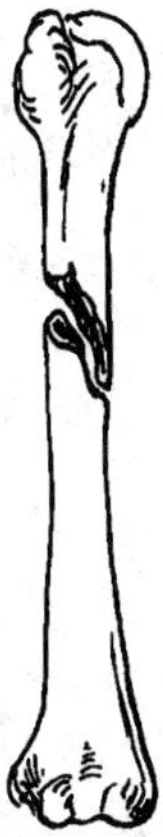

Spiral fracture

Impaction fracture

Due to "end on" stress/force

Longitudinal fracture

Fracture line parallel to long axis of bone

Impacted fracture

Fracture due to compressive force; end of bone is driven into contiguous metaphyseal region without displacement

Pathologic fracture

Fracture through abnormal bone (e.g., tumor-laden or osteoporotic bone)

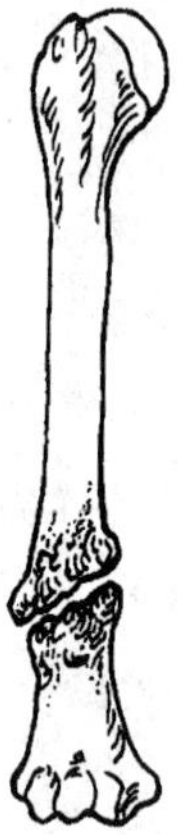

Pathologic fracture

Stress fracture

Fracture in normal bone due to cyclic loading on bone

Greenstick fracture

Incomplete fracture in which cortex on only one side is disrupted; seen in children

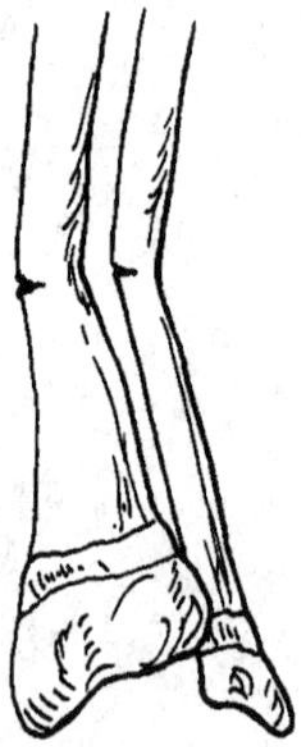

Greenstick fracture

Torus fracture

Impaction injury in children in which cortex is buckled but not disrupted (A.K.A. buckle fracture)

Displaced fracture

Occurs when cortices of fractured bone are knocked out of alignment without angulation; the **displacement** is measured and noted

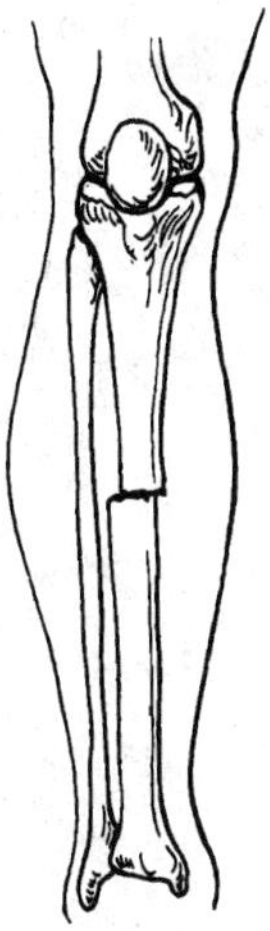

Displaced fracture

Angulated fracture

Occurs when an angle is created between the long axes of the two main bone fragments; the angulation is measured and noted

Rotated fracture

Occurs when one bone fragment rotates in relation to the other along the longitudinal axis; the rotation is usually difficult to see on x-ray and is usually noted clinically

Avulsion fracture

Fracture in which tendon is pulled from bone, carrying with it a bone chip

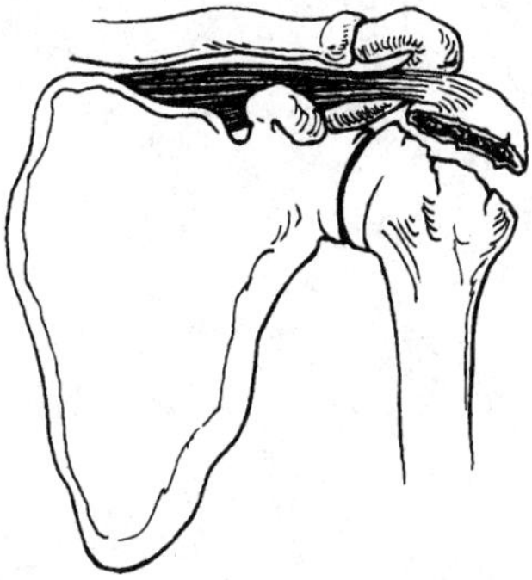

Avulsion fracture

Periarticular fracture

Fracture close to but not involving the joint

Intraarticular fracture

Fracture through the articular surface of a bone

Define the following specific fractures:

Colles' fracture

Fracture of the distal end of the radius, usually from falling on an outstretched hand

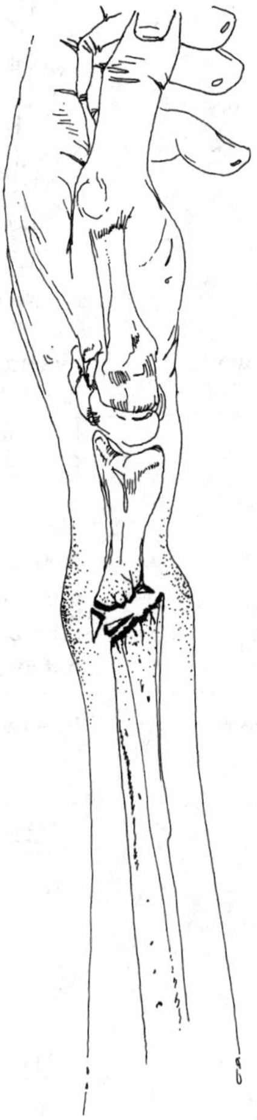

Jones' fracture

Fracture at the base of the fifth metatarsal diaphysis

Bennett's fracture — Fracture of the base of the first metacarpal with involvement of carpometacarpal joint

Smith's fracture — Opposite of Colles' fracture; fracture of the distal radius, but from falling on the dorsum of the hand

Boxer's fracture — Fracture of the metacarpal neck, "classically" of the small finger

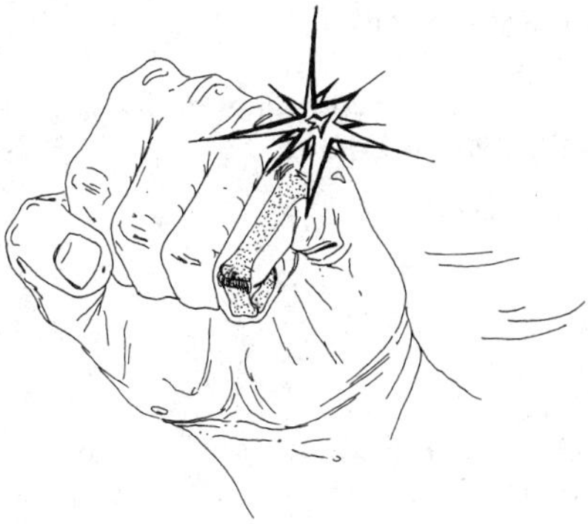

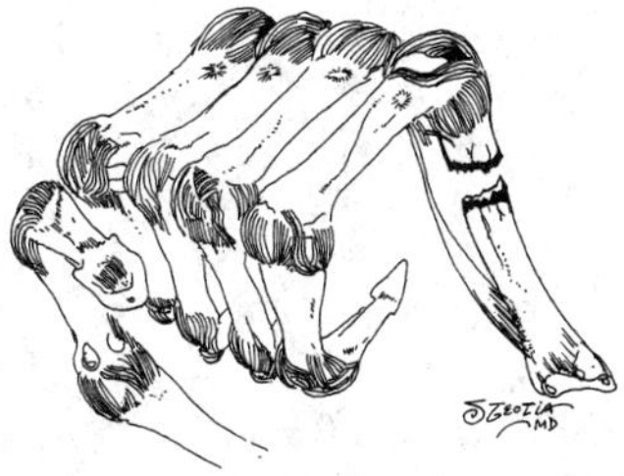

Clay shoveler's fracture — Fracture of spinous process of C7

Hangman's fracture — Fracture of the pedicles of C2

Transcervical fracture — Fracture through the neck of the femur

Tibial plateau fracture — Fracture in the proximal tibia (the plateau is the flared proximal end)

Monteggia fracture — Fracture of the proximal third of the ulna with a dislocation of the radial head

Galeazzi fracture — Fracture of the radius at the junction of the middle and distal thirds accompanied by disruption of the distal radioulnar joint

Pott's fracture — Fracture of distal fibula

Pott's disease — Tuberculosis of the spine

ORTHOPAEDIC TRAUMA

Which fracture has the highest mortality?

Pelvic fracture

What factors determine the extent of injury?

1. Age: suggests susceptible point in musculoskeletal system:
   Child—growth plate
   Adolescent—ligaments
   Elderly—metaphyseal bone
2. Direction of forces
3. Magnitude of forces

What are indications for open reduction?

1. Intraarticular fractures
2. Extremity function requiring perfect reduction
3. Failed closed reduction
4. Multiple trauma; to allow mobilization at earliest possible date
5. Elderly patients in cases in which a long period without ambulation carries a risk of compromised cardiopulmonary function

What is the acronym for indications for OPEN reduction?

"NO CAST":
N: **N**onunion
O: **O**pen fracture

C: **C**ompromise of blood supply
A: **A**rticular surface malalignment
S: **S**alter Harris grade III, IV, V fracture
T: **T**rauma patients who need early ambulation

What are the major orthopaedic emergencies?

1. Open fractures/dislocations
2. Vascular injuries (e.g., knee dislocation)
3. Compartment syndromes

4. Neural compromise, especially spinal injury
5. Osteomyelitis/septic arthritis; acute, i.e., when aspiration is indicated
6. Hip dislocations—require immediate reduction or patient will develop avascular necrosis; "reduce on the x-ray table"
7. Exsanguinating pelvic fracture (M.A.S.T., external fixator)

What is the main risk when dealing with an open fracture?

Infection

How are open fractures classified:

Grade I?

Less than 1-cm laceration

Grade II?

More than 1 and less than 10-cm laceration

Grade IIIA?:

Open fracture with massive tissue devitalization/loss

Grade IIIB?

Open fracture with massive tissue devitalization/loss *and* extensive periosteal stripping or extensive gross contamination

Grade IIIC?

Open fracture with massive tissue devitalization/loss *and* major vascular injury

What is the initial treatment of an open fracture?

1. Prophylactic antibiotics to include IV gram-positive ± anaerobic coverage
   Grade I—cefazolin (Ancef)
   Grade II or III—cefoxitin/gentamicin
2. Surgical debridement
3. Inoculation against tetanus
4. Lavage wound less than 6 hours postincident with high-pressure sterile irrigation
5. Open reduction of fracture and stabilization (e.g., use of external fixation)

What is acute compartment syndrome?

Increased pressure within an osseofascial compartment that leads to compromised circulation and function

What are the causes?

Fractures, vascular compromise, reperfusion injury, but can occur after any musculoskeletal injury

What is the most common site?

Calf (four compartments: anterior, lateral, deep posterior, superficial posterior compartments)

What situations should immediately alert one to be on the lookout for a developing compartment syndrome?

1. Supracondylar elbow fractures in children
2. Proximal/midshaft tibial fractures
3. Electrical burns
4. Arterial/venous disruption

What are the symptoms of compartment syndrome?

Pain, paresthesias, paralysis

What are the signs of compartment syndrome?

Pain on passive movement (out of proportion to injury), cyanotic or pallor, hypoesthesia (decreased sensation, decreased two point discrimination), firm compartment

How is the diagnosis made?

Clinically or by placing needle in extremity compartment and measuring pressure: positive if pressures **are more than 40 mm Hg**; pressure between 30 and 40 mm Hg—gray area, depends on clinical exam

Can a patient have a compartment syndrome with a palpable or Doppler-detectable distal pulse?

YES!

What are the possible complications of compartment syndrome?

Muscle necrosis, nerve damage

What is the treatment of compartment syndrome?

Fasciotomy within 4 hours if at all possible (6–8 hours max)

Name the classic associated orthopedic injury distant from the following:

Clavicle fracture due to a fall

Scaphoid fracture—due to outstretched hand (pain in snuff-box)

Calcaneus fracture	L-spine fracture
Knee pain	Hip dislocation/fracture—hip pain can be referred to the knee
Seizures/electrical shock	Posterior shoulder dislocation (remember, 90% of shoulder dislocations are **anterior)**

Name the nerves of the brachial plexus.

Think: morning rum or **A.M. RUM** = **A**xillary, **M**edian, then **R**adial, **U**lnar, **M**usculocutaneous nerves

Give the motor function and sensory domain of the following:

	MOTOR; DERMATOME
Radial	Wrist extension; back of forearm/hand
Ulnar	Finger abduction; pinkie side of hand
Median	Thumb opposition; hand
Axillary	Arm abduction; shoulder
Musculocutaneous	Elbow flexion lateral; forearm

Name the structure at risk with the following fracture:

Shoulder dislocation	Axillary nerve
Humerus fracture	Radial nerve, brachial artery
Elbow dislocation	Ulnar nerve, median nerve, brachial artery
Hip dislocation	Sciatic nerve, artery to the femoral head
Knee dislocation	Peroneal nerve, popliteal artery

How is a peripheral nerve injury treated?

Follow for 6 to 8 weeks, then EMG

What are the indications for operative exploration with a peripheral nerve injury?

1. Loss of nerve function *after* reduction of fracture
2. No EMG signs of nerve regeneration after 8 weeks (nerve graft)

DISLOCATIONS

SHOULDER

What is the most common type?	Ninety-five percent are anterior (posterior are often seen with epilepsy or electrocution)
Which structures are at risk?	Axillary nerve and axillary artery
How is it diagnosed?	Indentation of soft tissue beneath acromion
What is the treatment?	1. Reduction via gradual traction 2. Immobilization for 3 weeks in internal rotation 3. ROM exercises

ELBOW

What is the most common type?	Posterior
Which structures are at risk?	Brachial artery
What is the treatment?	Reduce and splint for 7 to 10 days

HIP

What is the most common type?	Posterior—"dashboard dislocation"—often involves fracture of posterior lip of acetabulum
Which structures are at risk?	Sciatic nerve; blood supply to femoral head—AVN
What is the treatment?	Closed or open reduction

KNEE

What are the common types?	Anterior or posterior

Which structures are at risk?

Popliteal artery and vein, peroneal nerve—especially with posterior dislocation (*Note:* need arteriogram)

What is the treatment?

Often requires ligament repair for reconstruction

COMMON FRACTURES AND DISLOCATIONS IN ADULTS

What is the most common cause of a "pathologic" fracture in adults?

Osteoporosis

THE KNEE

What are the ligaments of the knee?

Anterior cruciate ligament (ACL), posterior cruciate ligament (PCL), medial collateral ligament (MCL), lateral collateral ligament (LCL), patellar ligament

What is a "drawer test" of the knee?

Test to ascertain the anterior stability of the knee and integrity of the ACL. Knee is placed in 90° flexion and pulled forward (like opening a drawer). If the tibia is pulled forward, the test is positive and is consistent with an ACL tear.

What is the meniscus of the knee?

The cartilage surface of the tibia plateau (lateral and medial meniscus); tears are repaired usually by arthroscopy with removal of torn cartilage fragments

What is the "unhappy triad"?

Lateral knee injury resulting in ACL tear, MCL tear, and a medial meniscus injury

What is a chief concern in humeral shaft fractures?

Radial nerve palsy

What are the signs of an Achilles tendon rupture?

Severe calf pain, also bruised swollen calf, two ends of ruptured tendon may be felt, patient will have weak plantar flexion due to great toe flexors that should be intact

Name the test for an intact Achilles tendon.	Thompson's test: a squeeze of the gastrocnemius muscle results in plantar flexion of the foot
What must be done when both forearm bones are broken?	Because precise movements are needed, open reduction and internal fixation are a must.
How have femoral fractures been repaired traditionally?	Traction for 4 to 6 weeks
What is the newer technique?	Intramedullary rod placement
What are the advantages?	Nearly immediate mobility with decreased morbidity/mortality
What is the chief concern following tibial fractures?	Recognition of associated compartment syndrome
When do hip dislocations usually occur?	High-velocity injuries (e.g., MVA)
What is suggested by pain in the anatomic snuff-box?	Fracture of scaphoid bone (A.K.A. navicular fracture)

ROTATOR CUFF

What muscles form the rotator cuff?	1. Supraspinatus (acronym = **"SITS"**) 2. Infraspinatus 3. Teres minor 4. Subscapularis
When do tears usually occur?	Fifth decade
What is the usual history?	Intermittent shoulder pain followed by an episode of acute pain corresponding to a tendon tear; weakness of abduction
What is the treatment?	Most tears: symptomatic pain relief Later: if poor muscular function persists, surgical repair is indicated
What is Volkmann's contracture?	Contracture of forearm flexors secondary to **forearm compartment syndrome**

What is the usual cause of Volkmann's contracture?	Brachial artery injury, **supracondylar humerus fracture,** radius/ulnar fracture, crush injury, etc.
Define the following terms:	
Dupuytren's contracture	Thickening and contracture of palmar fascia; incidence increases with age
Charcot's joint	Joint arthritis due to **peripheral neuropathy**
Tennis elbow	Tendinitis of the lateral epicondyle of the humerus (classically seen in tennis players)
Turf toe	Hyperextension of the great toe (tear of the tendon of the flexor hallucis brevis); classically seen in football players.
Shin splints	Excercise-induced anterior compartment hypertension (compartment syndrome); seen in runners
Heel spur	Plantar fasciitis with abnormal bone growth in the plantar fascia Classically seen in runners and walkers
What is traumatic myositis ossificans?	Abnormal bone deposit in a muscle after blunt trauma deep muscle contusion

ORTHOPAEDIC INFECTIONS

OSTEOMYELITIS

What is osteomyelitis?	Inflammation/infection of bone marrow and adjacent bone
What are the most likely causative organisms?	Neonates: *Staphylococcus aureus,* gram-negative Children: *Staphylococcus aureus*, *H. influenzae* Adults: *Staphylococcus aureus* Immunocompromised/drug addicts: gram-negative Sickle cell: *Salmonella, Staphylococcus*

What is the most common organism isolated in osteomyelitis in the general adult population?	*Staphylococcus aureus*
What is the most common isolated organism in patients with sickle cell disease?	*Salmonella*
What is seen on physical exam?	Tenderness, decreased movement, swelling
What are diagnostic steps?	History and physical exam, needle aspirate, CBC, ESR, bone scan
What are the treatment options?	Antibiotics with or without surgical drainage
What is a Marjolin's ulcer?	Squamous cell carcinoma that arises in a chronic sinus due to osteomylitis

SEPTIC ARTHRITIS

What is septic arthritis?	Inflammation of a joint beginning as synovitis and ending with destruction of articular cartilage if left untreated
What are the causative agents?	Same as in osteomyelitis, except that *Gonococcus* is a common agent in the adult population
What are the findings on physical exam?	Joint pain, decreased motion, joint swelling, joint warm to the touch
What are the diagnostic steps?	Needle aspirate (look for pus; culture plus Gram stain), x-ray
What is the treatment?	Decompression of the joint via needle aspiration and IV antibiotics; hip, shoulder, and spine must be surgically incised, debrided, and drained

ORTHOPAEDIC TUMORS

What is the most common type in adults?	Metastatic!

What are the common sources?
Breast, lung, prostate, kidney, and multiple myeloma

What is the usual presentation?
May present as bone pain or as a pathologic fracture

What is the most common primary malignant bone tumor?
Multiple myeloma

What is the differential diagnosis of a possible bone tumor?
1. Metastatic disease
2. Primary bone tumors
3. Metabolic disorders (e.g., hyperparathyroidism)
4. Infection

What are the benign bone tumors?
1. Osteochondroma
2. Enchondroma
3. Unicameral bone cyst
4. Osteoid osteoma
5. Chondroblastoma
6. Fibroxanthoma
7. Fibrous dysplasia

What are the malignant bone tumors?
1. Osteosarcoma
2. Chondrosarcoma
3. Ewing's sarcoma
4. Giant cell tumor (locally malignant)
5. Malignant melanoma
6. Metastatic

Compare benign and malignant bone tumors in terms of:

Size
Benign—small; < 1 cm
Malignant— > 1 cm

Bone reaction
Benign—sclerotic bone reaction
Malignant—little reaction

Margins
Benign—sharp
Malignant—poorly defined

Invasive
Benign—confined to bone
Malignant—often extends to surrounding tissues

Are most pediatric tumors benign or malignant?
Eighty percent are benign (most common is osteochondroma)

Are most adult bone tumors benign or malignant?
Sixty-six percent are malignant (most commonly metastatic)

What are the diagnostic steps?
1. PE/lab tests
2. Radiographs
3. CT and/or technetium scan
4. Biopsy

What are radiographic signs of malignant tumors?
Large size
Aggressive bone destruction
Ineffective bone rxn to tumor
Extension to soft tissues

What are the radiographic signs of benign tumor?
Small
Well circumscribed
Lytic lesion with sclerotic rim
No extension

What are some specific radiographic findings of the following:

Osteosarcoma?
"Sunburst pattern"

Fibrous dysplasia
Radiolucent, "ground glass"

Ewing's sarcoma
"Onion skinning"

What is the mainstay of treatment?
Surgery (excision plus debridement) for both malignant and benign lesions; x-ray therapy and chemotherapy as adjuvant for many malignant tumors

OSTEOSARCOMA

What is the usual age at presentation?
Between 10 and 20 years

What is the gender distribution?
Men > women

What is the most common location?
Approximately two-thirds in the distal femur, proximal tibia

What is the radiographic sine qua non? Bone formation somewhere within tumor

What is the treatment? Resection plus chemotherapy

What is the 5-year survival rate? Approximately 15%

What is the most common site of metastasis? Lungs

What is the most common benign bone tumor? **Osteochondroma;** it is cartilaginous in origin and may undergo malignant degeneration

What is a chondrosarcoma? Malignant tumor of cartilaginous origin; presents in middle-aged and older patients and is unresponsive to chemotherapy and radiotherapy

EWING'S SARCOMA

What is the usual presentation? Pain, swelling in involved area

What is the most common location? Around the knee (distal femur, proximal tibia)

What is the usual age at presentation? Evenly spread among those less than 20 years of age

What are the associated radiographic findings? Lytic lesion with periosteal reaction termed "onion skinning," which is calcified layering

What is a unicameral bone cyst? Fluid-filled cyst most commonly found in the proximal humerus in children ages 5 to 15 years

What is the usual presentation? Pain, pathologic fracture

What is the treatment? Steroid injections

ARTHRITIS

Which arthritides are classified as degenerative? Osteoarthritis
Posttraumatic arthritis

What signs characterize osteoarthritis?	Heberden's nodes/Bouchard's nodes **Symmetry,** usually of the hip, knee, or spine
What are Bouchard's nodes?	Enlarged PIP joints of the hand due to cartilage/bone growth; seen in osteoarthritis
What are Heberden's nodes?	Enlarged DIP joints of the hand due to cartilage/bone growth; seen in osteoarthritis
What is posttraumatic arthritis?	Usually involves **one joint** of past trauma
What are the treatment options for degenerative arthritis?	1. NSAIDS for acute flare-ups, **not** for long-term management 2. Local corticosteroid injections 3. Surgery
What are the characteristics of rheumatoid arthritis?	Autoimmune reaction in which hyaline articular cartilage is attacked by invasive pannus, rheumatoid factor (anti-IgG/IgM) in 80% of patients, three times more common in women versus men, skin nodules (e.g., rheumatoid nodule)
What is pannus?	Inflammatory exudate overlying synovial cells inside the joint
What are the classic hand findings with rheumatoid arthritis?	Wrist: radial deviation Fingers: ulnar deviation
What are the surgical management options for joint/bone diseases?	1. Arthroplasty 2. Arthrodesis (fusion) 3. Osteotomy
What is the major difference between gout and pseudogout?	Gout: caused by urate deposition Pseudogout: caused by calcium pyrophosphate positive birefringent square crystals (think: **P**ositive **S**quare crystals = **PS**eudogout)
What is a Charcot's joint?	Arthritic joint due to peripheral neuropathy

PEDIATRIC ORTHOPAEDICS

What are the major differences between pediatric and adult bones?	Children: increased bone flexibility, increased bone healing (and thus many fractures are treated closed whereas in an adult, O.R.I.F. should be required), fractures through physis (weak point)
What type of fractures are specific for children?	Greenstick fracture Torus fracture Fracture through physis

CONGENITAL HIP DISLOCATION

What is the epidemiology?	Women > men, firstborn children, breech presentation
% Bilateral?	Bilateral 10% of the time
How is the diagnosis made?	Barlow's maneuver Ortolani's sign Radiographic confirmation is required
What is Barlow's maneuver?	Patient is placed in the supine position and attempt is made to push femurs posteriorly with knees at 90°/hip flexed and hip will dislocate (think: push **B**ack = **B**arlow)
What is Ortolani's sign?	Rotate the hip with patient in the supine position and hip abducted; a "clunk" or "click" represents congenitally dislocated hip (think: legs **O**ut = **O**rtolani's)
What is the treatment?	Pavlik harness—maintains hip reduction with hips flexed at 100° to 110°

SCOLIOSIS

What is the definition?	Lateral curvature of a portion of the spine Nonstructural: corrects with positional change Structural: does not correct

What is the cause?
Most cases are termed idiopathic, but causes may include neuromuscular paralysis, painful lesion, radiation, thoracic surgery, and congenital anomalies.

What is the most common cause of scoliosis?
Idiopathic

What is the classic presentation?
Right thoracic curve, though thoracolumbar, lumbar, and double curves are seen; look for chest rotation and rib hump

What is the epidemiology?
Usually affects prepubertal females

What are the treatment options?
1. Braces (Milwaukee brace)
2. Surgery
3. Electrical stimulation

What are the indications for surgery for scoliosis?
Respiratory compromise
Rapid progressive
Curves more than 40°
Failure of brace

Define the following terms:

Legg-Calvé-Perthes disease
Idiopathic avascular necrosis of femoral head in children

Slipped capital femoral epiphysis
Migration of proximal femoral epiphysis of child on the metaphysis in children
Note: Hip pain in children often presents as knee pain

Blount's disease
Idiopathic varus bowing of tibia

Osgood-Schlatter's disease
Epiphysitis of the tibial tubercle resulting from repeated powerful contractions of the quadriceps seen in adolescents with an open physis
Treatment of mild cases: activity restriction
Treatment of severe cases: cast

SALTER CLASSIFICATION

What does it describe? Fractures in children involving physis

What does it indicate high risk of? Growth arrest potential

Define the following terms:

Salter I Through physeal plate only

Salter II Involves physis and metaphysis

Salter III Involves physis and epiphysis

Salter IV Fracture extends from metaphysis through physis, into epiphysis

Salter V Axial force crushes physeal plate

Define the following fractures by Salter-Harris grade:

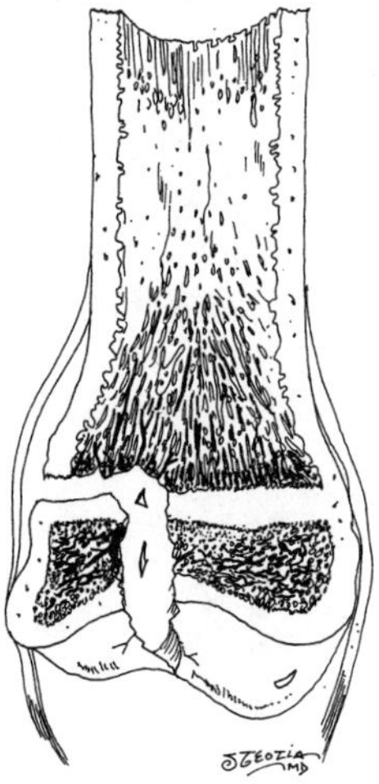

Salter III

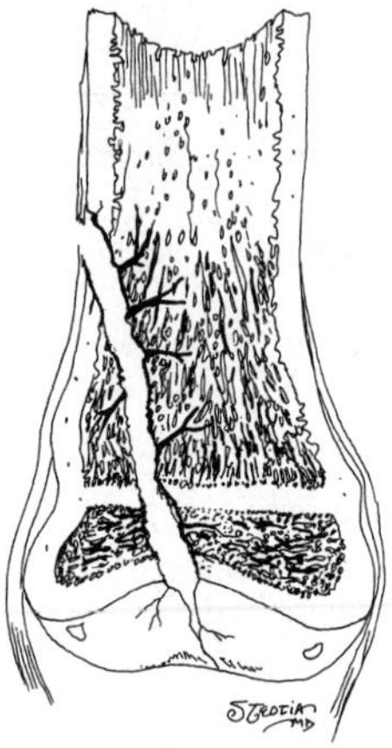

Salter IV

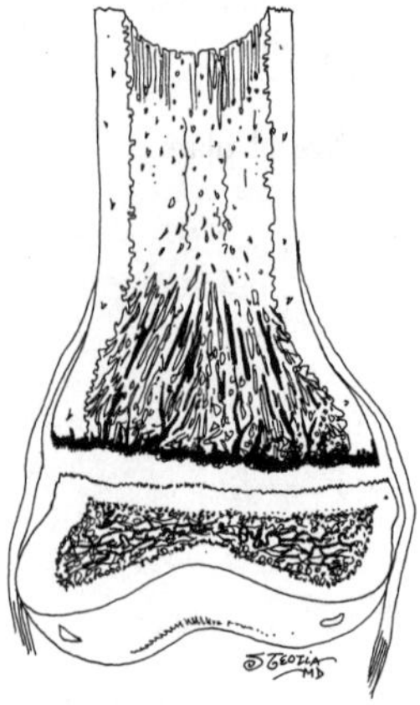

Salter I

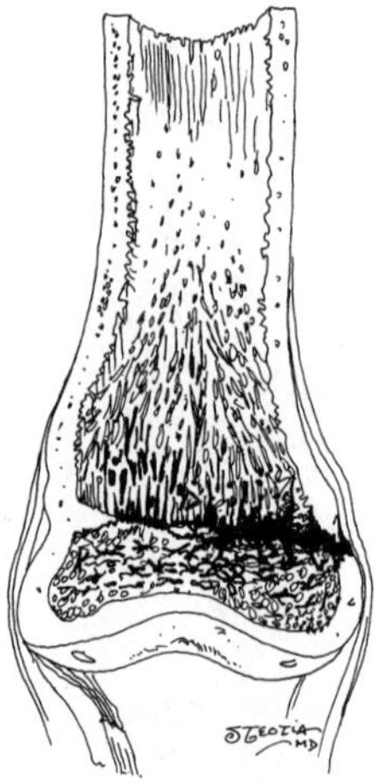

Salter V

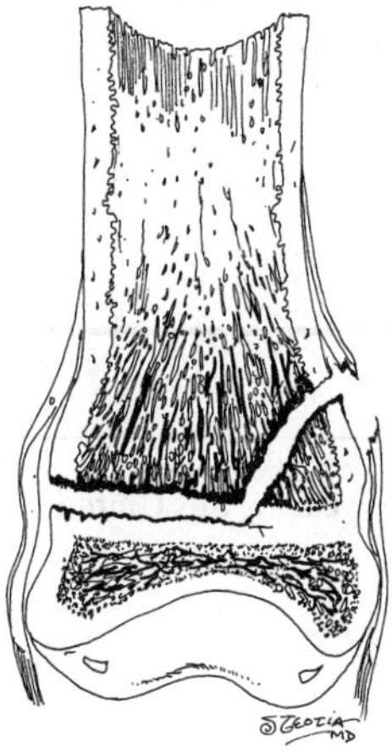

Salter II

SELECTED PEDIATRIC FRACTURES

Why is the growth plate of concern in childhood fractures?

The growth plate represents the "weak link" in the musculoskeletal system of the child. Fractures involving the growth plate of long bones may compromise normal growth, so special attention should be given to them.

What is a chief concern when oblique/spiral fractures of long bones are seen in children?

Child abuse is a possibility and other signs of abuse should be investigated

What is usually done during reduction of a femoral fracture?

A small amount of overlap is allowed because increased vascularity due to injury may make the affected limb **longer** if overlap is not present. Treatment after reduction is a spica cast.

What is unique about ligamentous injury in children?

Most "ligamentous" injuries are actually fractures involving the growth plate!

What two fractures have a high incidence of associated compartment syndrome?

1. Tibial fractures
2. Supracondylar fractures of humerus (Volkmann's contracture)

What is the most common pediatric bone tumor?

Osteochondroma (remember, 80% of bone tumors are benign in children)

67 Neurosurgery

TRAUMA

HEAD TRAUMA

What is the incidence?

70,000 fatal injuries/year in the United States

What percentage of trauma deaths are due to head trauma?

50% (MVA = 60%)

What is the Glasgow Coma Scale (GCS) and why is it important?

The GCS is a measure of brain dysfunction and is used as a predictor of prognosis in head-injured patients. Responses are graded for verbal, motor, and ocular responses. Patients with a GCS score of 3 to 8 are defined as comatose. Patients with an initial score of 3 to 4 have a more than 95% incidence of death or persistent vegetative state.

GCS scoring system

Eyes?

Eye Opening (E)
4—opens spontaneously
3—opens to voice (command)
2—opens to painful stimulus
1—does not open eyes
(Think = "4 eyes")

Motor?

Motor Response (M)
6—obeys commands
5—localizes painful stimulus
4—withdraws from pain
3—decorticate posture
2—decerebrate posture
1—no movement
(Think = 6-cylinder motor)

Verbal?	**Verbal Response (V)** 5—appropriate and oriented 4—confused 3—inappropriate words 2—incomprehensible sounds 1—no sounds **(Think = Jackson 5 = verbal 5)**
Coma by GCS score?	8
What does unilateral, dilated, nonreactive pupil suggest?	Focal mass lesion/herniation with compression of CN III
What does bilateral fixed and dilated pupil suggest?	Diffusely increased ICP
What are the four signs of basilar skull fracture?	1. **Raccoon eyes—**periorbital ecchymoses 2. **Battle's sign—**postauricular ecchymoses 3. **Hemotympanum** 4. **CSF** rhinorrhea/otorrhea
What is the initial radiographic imaging in trauma?	1. Plain films of C-spine (C1-C7/T1): AP, LAt, Odontoid 2. Head CT (if LOC or GCS < 15) 3. T/L spine AP and Lateral
Should the trauma head CT be with or without IV contrast?	Without!
What is normal ICP?	Between 5 and 15 mm H_2O
What is the worrisome ICP?	More than 20 mm H_2O
What determines ICP (Monroe-Kelly hypothesis)?	1. Volume of brain 2. Volume of blood 3. Volume of CSF
What is the CPP?	**C**erebral **P**erfusion **P**ressure = Mean arterial pressure − ICP (normal CPP is > 50)

What is Cushing's triad?

Physiologic response to increased ICP (A.K.A. Cushing's response)

1. Increased vascular resistance (increasing BP)
2. Bradycardia
3. Respiratory irregularity

What are the general indications to monitor ICP after trauma?

1. GCS less than 11 to 12
2. Altered level of consciousness or unconsciousness with multiple system trauma
3. Decreased consciousness with focal neuro exam abnormality

What nonoperative techniques are used to decrease ICP?

1. Reverse Trendelenburg position (if spine cleared)
2. Diuresis-Mannitol (osmotic diuretic), Lasix, limit fluids
3. Intubation plus hyperventilation
4. Reversible sedation
5. Pharmacologic paralysis
6. Pentobarbital coma (last resort)

What is a Kjellberg?

Decompressive bifrontal craniectomy (pronounced "shellberg") with removal of frontal bone placed in freezer for possible later replacement

How does cranial nerve exam localize the injury in a comatose patient?

The CNs proceed caudally in the brain stem as numbered. Presence of corneal reflex (CN 5 + 7) indicates intact pons. Intact gag reflex (CN 9 + 10) shows functioning upper medulla. Be aware that CN 6 palsy is often a false localizing sign.

EPIDURAL HEMATOMA

What is an epidural hematoma?

Collection of blood between the skull and dura

What causes it?

Usually occurs in association with a skull fracture as bone fragments lacerate meningeal arteries

What artery is associated with epidural hematomas?

Middle meningeal artery

What is the most common sign of an epidural hematoma?

More than 50% have ipsilateral blown pupil

What is the classic history with an epidural hematoma?

LOC followed by a "lucid interval" followed by neurologic deterioration

What are the classic CT findings with an epidural hematoma?

Lenticular-shaped hematoma

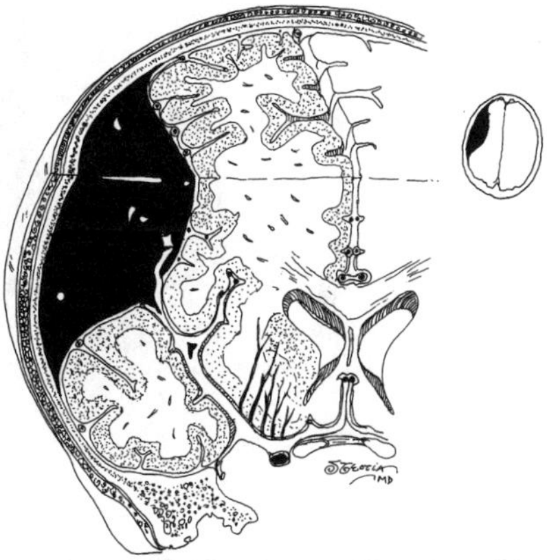

SUBDURAL HEMATOMA

What is it?

Blood collection under the dura

What causes it?

Tearing of veins that pass through the space between the cortical surface and the dural venous sinuses or injury to the brain surface with resultant bleeding from cortical vessels

What are the three types of subdurals?

1. Acute—symptoms within 72 hours of injury
2. Subacute—symptoms within 3 to 20 days
3. Chronic—symptoms after 3 weeks or longer

What is the treatment of epidural and subdural hematomas?

The mass effect (pressure) must be reduced. Whereas the previously mentioned medical measures can be employed to delay additional neurologic damage, craniotomy with the removal of clot is required. The surgeon must address any remaining bleeding to prevent reaccumulation of the hematoma.

What classic CT findings appear on head CT for a subdural hematoma?

Crescent-shaped hematoma

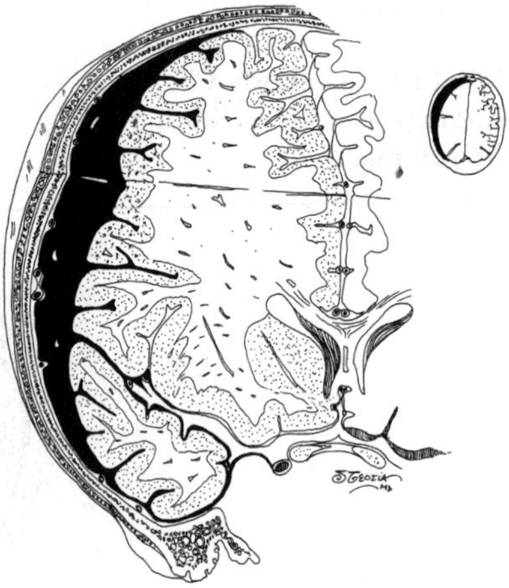

TRAUMATIC SUBARACHNOID HEMORRHAGE

What is it?

Head trauma resulting in blood below the arachnoid membrane and above the pia

What is the treatment?

Anticonvulsants and observation

CEREBRAL CONTUSION

What is it?

Hemorrhagic contusion of brain parenchyma

What is a coup and contrecoup injury?

Coup—injury at the site of impact
Contrecoup—injury at the site opposite the point of impact

What is DAI?

Diffuse **A**xonal **I**njury (shear injury to brain parenchyma) due to rapid deceleration injury; 33% mortality; long-term coma

SKULL FRACTURE

What is a depressed skull fracture?

A fracture in which one or more fragments of the skull are forced below the inner table of the skull.

What are the surgical indications?

1. Contaminated wound requiring cleaning and debridement
2. Severe deformity
3. Impingement on cortex
4. Open fracture
5. CSF leak

SPINAL CORD TRAUMA

What are the two general types of injury?

1. Complete—no motor/sensory function below the level of injury
2. Incomplete—residual function below the level of injury

Define "spinal shock"?

Loss of all reflexes and motor function
Hypotension

Define "sacral sparing"?

Sparing of sacral nerve level: anal sphincter intact, toe flexion, perianal sensation

What initial labs/ intervention are important?

1. ABCs—obtain airway and vent if needed
2. Maintain BP (IVF, pressors if refractory to fluids)
3. NG tube—prevents aspiration
4. Foley
5. High-dose steroids—proven to improve outcome
6. Complete cervical x-rays and those of lower levels as indicated by exam

What are the associated diagnostic studies?

Plain films, CT, MRI

What are the indications for emergent surgery with spinal cord injury?

Incomplete injury with extrinsic compression (e.g., bone chip, subluxation)

What is the indication for IV high-dose steroids with spinal cord injury?

Spinal cord injury with neurologic deficit (methylprednisolone: high-dose bolus [30 mg/kg] followed by continuous infusion [5.4 mg/kg] for 23 hours)

Describe the following conditions:

Anterior cord syndrome

Affects corticospinal and lateral spinothalamic tracts, paraplegia, loss of pain/temp sensation

Central cord syndrome

Preservaton of some lower extremity motor and sensory ability

Brown-Séquard syndrome

Hemisection of cord resulting in ipsilateral motor weakness and touch/ proprioception loss with contralateral pain/temperature loss

How can the findings associated with Brown-Séquard syndrome be remembered?

Think: Captain Brown Séquard = **CPT**
Brown Séquard = **CPT** = **C**ontralateral **P**ain **T**emperature loss

Posterior cord syndrome

Injury to posterior spinal cord with loss of proprioception distally

Define the following terms:

Jefferson's fracture

Fracture through **C1** arches due to axial loading (unstable fracture)

Hangman's fracture

Fracture through the pedicles of **C2** due to hyperextension; usually stable
Think: hangman (C2) is below stature of President T. Jefferson (C1)

Odontoid fracture

Fracture of the odontoid process of C2 (view with open-mouth odontoid x-ray)

Priapism

Penile erection seen with spinal cord injury

Chance fracture

Transverse vertebral fracture

Clay shoveler's fracture

Fracture of spinous process of C7

Odontoid fractures

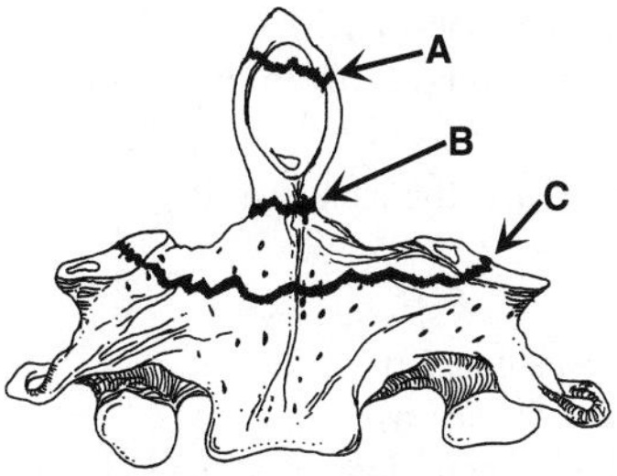

A: Type I—fracture through tip of dens
B: Type II—fracture through base of dens
C: Type III—fracture through body of C2

TUMORS

GENERAL

What is the incidence of CNS tumors?

Approximately 1% of all cancer; third leading cause of cancer deaths in people aged 15 to 34; second leading cause of cancer deaths in children

Define benign versus malignant in the setting of CNS tumors.

Malignant tumors are highly aggressive/proliferative tumors of poorly differentiated cells. Benign refers to a less aggressive, more differentiated cell line. However, a benign tumor can be as lethal as a malignant variety because of the continued ability to grow within the confines of the skull.

What is the usual location of primary tumors in adults/children?

In adults, roughly two-thirds of tumors are supratentorial, one-third are infratentorial; the reverse is true in children.

What is the differential diagnosis of a ring-enhancing brain lesion?

Metastatic carcinoma, abscess, GBM, lymphoma

What are the adverse effects of tumors on the brain?

1. Increased ICP
2. Mass effect on cranial nerves
3. Invasion of brain parenchyma, disrupting nuclei/tracts
4. Seizure foci
5. Hemorrhage into/around the tumor mass

What are the signs/ symptoms of brain tumors?

1. Neurologic deficit (two-thirds)
2. Headache (one-half)
3. Seizures (one-fourth)
4. Vomiting (classically in the morning)

How is the diagnosis made?

CT or MRI is the standard diagnostic study.

What are the surgical indications?

1. Establishing a tissue diagnosis
2. Relief of increased ICP
3. Relief of neurologic dysfunction due to tissue compression
4. Attempt to cure in the setting of localized tumor

What are the most common intracranial tumors in adults?

Metastatic neoplasms are most common; among primaries, gliomas are number 1 (one-half) and meningiomas number 2 (one-fourth).

What are the most common in children?

1. Medulloblastomas (one-third)
2. Astrocytomas (one-third)
3. Ependymomas (10%)

GLIOMAS

What is a glioma?

A general name for a number of tumors of neural origin (e.g., astrocytes, oligodendrocytes) that show a wide range of presentations

What is the most common glioma?

Astrocytoma (half of all gliomas)

What are the characteristics of a LOW-grade astrocytoma?

Nuclear atypia, high mitotic rate

What is the most common primary brain tumor in adults?

Glioblastoma multiforme (GBM)

What are its characteristics?

Poorly defined, highly aggressive tumors occurring in the white matter of the cerebral hemispheres; spread extremely rapidly

What is the average age of onset?	Fifth decade
What is the treatment?	Surgical debulking followed by radiation therapy
What is the prognosis?	Without treatment, more than 90% of patients die within 3 months of diagnosis. With treatment, 90% die within 2 years.

MENINGIOMAS

What is the layer of origination?	Arachnoid cap cells
What are the associated histologic findings?	Psammoma bodies (concentric calcifications), Whorl formations (onion skin pattern)
What is the histologic malignancy determination?	Brain parenchymal invasion
What is the peak age of occurrence?	Between 40 and 50
What is the gender ratio?	Females predominate almost 2:1
What is the clinical presentation?	Variable depending on location; lateral cerebral convexity tumors can cause focal deficits or headache; sphenoid tumors can present with seizures; posterior fossa tumors with CN deficits; olfactory groove tumors with anosmia
What is the treatment?	Preop embolization and surgical resection are the treatment of choice and is usually aimed at complete removal of the tumor.

CEREBELLAR ASTROCYTOMAS

What is the peak age of occurrence?	Between 5 and 9 years
What is the usual location?	Usually in the cerebellar hemispheres; less frequently in the vermis

What are the signs/ symptoms?
Usually lateral cerebellar signs occur: ipsilateral incoordination or dysmetria (patient tends to fall to side of tumor), as well as nystagmus and ataxia; CN deficits are also frequently present, especially CNs VI and VII

What are the treatment and prognosis?
Completely resectable in 75% of cases, which usually results in a cure; overall 5-year survival rate exceeds 90%

MEDULLOBLASTOMA

What is the peak age of occurrence?
First decade (3–7 years)

What is the cell of origin?
External granular cells of cerebellum

What is the most common location?
Cerebellar vermis in children; cerebellar hemispheres of adolescents and adults

What are the signs/ symptoms?
Headache, vomiting, and other signs of increased ICP; also usually truncal ataxia

What are the treatment and prognosis?
Best current treatment includes surgery to debulk the tumor, cranial and spinal radiation, and chemotherapy; 5-year survival rate is more than 50%

METASTATIC TUMORS

What are the three main patterns of intracranial metastasis and what are the most common primary tumors involved?
Metastases to
1. Skull/dura: breast, prostate, multiple myeloma
2. Brain parenchyma: lung, breast, skin, kidney, GI tract
3. Meningeal carcinomatosis: lung, leukemia, lymphoma, breast, GI

Where do cerebral metastases occur within the brain?
At the junction of gray and white matter

What are the signs/ symptoms?
Same as those of primary tumors

What are the treatment and prognosis?

Surgical resection if lesion is solitary and accessible; otherwise, radiation is most frequently used

Chemotherapy has been used with some success for lung, breast, and testicular primaries.

Average survival is approximately 6 months.

What are the signs/ symptoms of meningeal carcinomatosis?

Headache, backache, mental status changes, radiculopathy, and CN palsies are common.

How is the diagnosis of meningeal carcinomatosis made?

Head CT is usually normal, but may show a diffuse enhancement of the meninges. A demonstration of malignant cells in the CSF is required for diagnosis.

What are the treatment and prognosis?

Intrathecal chemotherapy and radiation; mean survival is about 6 months

VASCULAR NEUROSURGERY

OCCLUSIVE CEREBROVASCULAR DISEASE

What are the causes of cerebral infarction?

Thrombosis and embolism

What are the signs/ symptoms prior to infarction?

Most important are transient ischemic attacks (TIAs), i.e., temporary ischemic insults to the brain that usually signify cerebrovascular pathology; specific symptoms depend on what area of the brain is ischemic

Which artery is most often involved?

Middle cerebral artery

What is the treatment?

For severe stenosis (> 70%) of internal carotid artery, carotid endarterectomy is the most beneficial treatment. If stenosis is mild (< 70%) patients are given a trial of 1 g ASA per day. A patient who continues to have TIAs during treatment is a surgical candidate.

SUBARACHNOID HEMORRHAGE (SAH)

What are the usual causes?

Most cases are due to **trauma;** of nontraumatic SAH, the leading cause is ruptured **berry aneurysm,** followed by arteriovenous malformations

What is a berry aneurysm?

Saccular outpouching of vessels in the circle of Willis, usually at bifurcations

What is the usual location of a berry aneurysm?

Anterior communicating artery is number one (30%), followed by posterior communicating artery and middle cerebral artery

What medical disease increases the risk of berry aneurysms?

Polycystic kidney disease and connective tissue disorders (e.g., Marfan's syndrome)

What is an AVM?

A congenital abnormality of the vasculature with retainment of one or more primitive connections between the arterial and venous circulations; there is a failure to develop the connecting capillary network

Where do they occur?

More than 75% are supratentorial

What are the signs/symptoms of SAH?

Classic symptom is **"the worst headache of my life."** Meningismus is documented by neck pain and positive Kernig's and Brudzinski's signs. Occasionally LOC, vomiting, and CN deficits occur.

What comprises the workup of SAH?

If SAH is suspected, head CT should be the first test ordered to look for subarachnoid blood. LP may show xanthochromic CSF, but is not necessary if CT is definitive. This test should be followed by arteriogram to look for aneurysms or AVMs.

What are the possible complications of SAH?

1. Brain edema leading to increased ICP
2. Rebleeding (most common in the first 24–48 hours posthemorrhage)
3. Vasospasm (peaks 7–11 days after bleeding) of cerebral arteries is the

most common cause of morbidity and mortality

What is the treatment of aneurysm?

Surgical treatment by placing a metal clip on the aneurysm is the mainstay of therapy. Alternatives include balloon occlusion or coil embolization.

What is the treatment of AVM?

Many are on the brain surface and are accessible operatively. Preoperative embolization can reduce the size of the AVM. For surgically inaccessible lesions, radiosurgery (gamma knife) has been effective in treating AVMs less than 3 cm in diameter.

INTRACEREBRAL HEMORRHAGE

What is it?

Bleeding into the brain parenchyma

What is the etiology?

Number one is hypertensive/atherosclerotic disease giving rise to Charcot-Bouchard aneurysms (small tubular aneurysms along smaller terminal arteries); other causes include coagulopathies, AVMs, amyloid angiopathy, bleeding into a tumor, and trauma

Where does it occur?

Two-thirds occur in the basal ganglia; putamen is the structure most commonly affected

How often does blood spread to the ventricular system?

Two-thirds of cases

What is the usual presentation?

Two-thirds present with coma; large putamen bleeding classically presents with contralateral hemiplegia and hemisensory deficits, lateral gaze preference, aphasia, and homonymous hemianopsia

What is the associated diagnostic study?

CT

What are the surgical indications?

Cerebellar hemorrhages must be removed quickly to decrease the risk of tonsillar herniation and death. Large lobar lesions are also commonly removed.

What is the prognosis?

Poor, especially with ventricular or diencephalon involvement

EPILEPSY SURGERY

What are the indications for surgery?

Poorly controlled severe epilepsy of more than 1 year duration

What is the goal of surgery?

Resect seizure focus

How is seizure focus located?

CT, MRI, with or without surface electrodes (subdural grids)

SPINE

LUMBAR DISC HERNIATION

What is it?

Extrusion of the inner portion of the intervertebral disc (nucleus pulposus) through the outer annulus fibrosis, causing impingement on nerve roots exiting the spinal canal

Which nerve is affected?

The nerve exiting at the level below (e.g., an L4-L5 disc impinges on the L5 nerve exiting between L5-S1)

Who is affected?

Middle-aged and older individuals

What is the usual cause?

Loss of elasticity of the posterior longitudinal ligaments and annulus fibrosis due to aging

What are the most common sites?

L5-S1 (45%)
L4-L5 (40%)

What is the usual presenting symptom?

Low back pain

What are the signs:

L5-S1?

Decreased ankle jerk reflex
Weakness of plantar flexors in foot
Pain in back/midgluteal region to posterior calf to lateral foot
Ipsilateral radiculopathy on straight leg raise

L4-L5?

Decreased biceps femoris reflex
Weak extensors of foot
Pain in hip/groin region to posterolateral thigh, lateral leg, and medial toes

What is cauda equina syndrome?

Herniated disc compressing multiple S1, S2, S3, S4 nerve roots resulting in bowel/bladder incontinence, "saddle anesthesia" over buttocks/perineum, low back pain, sciatica

What is "sciatica"?

Radicular or nerve root pain

How is the diagnosis made?

CT, CT myelogram, or MRI

What is the treatment?

Conservative—bed rest and analgesics
Surgical—partial hemilaminectomy and discectomy (removal of herniated disc)

What are the indications for emergent surgery?

1. Cauda equina syndrome
2. Progressive motor deficits

CERVICAL DISC DISEASE

What is it?

Basically the same pathology as previously described, except in the cervical region; the disc impinges on the nerve exiting the canal at the same level of the disease (e.g., a C6-C7 disc impinges on the C7 nerve root exiting at the C6-C7 foramen)

What are the most common sites?

C6-C7 (70%)
C5-C6 (20%)
C7-T1 (10%)

What are the signs/ symptoms:

C7?

Decreased triceps reflex/strength, weakness of forearm extension
Pain from neck, through triceps and into index and middle finger

C6?

Decreased biceps and brachioradialis reflex
Weakness in forearm flexion
Pain in neck, radial forearm, and thumb

C8?

Weakness in intrinsic hand muscles, pain in fourth/fifth fingers

What is Spurling's sign?

Reproduction of radicular pain by having the patient turn his head to the affected side and applying axial pressure to the top of the head

How is the diagnosis made?

CT or MRI

What is the treatment?

Anterior or posterior discectomy with fusion PRN

What are the symptoms of central cervical cord compression from disc fragments?

Myelopathic syndrome with LMN signs at level of compression and UMN signs distally; e.g., C7 compression may cause bilateral loss of triceps reflex and bilateral hyperreflexia, clonus, and Babinski signs in lower extremities

SPINAL EPIDURAL ABSCESS

What is the etiology?

Hematogenous spread from skin infections is most common; also, distant abscesses/infections, UTIs, postoperative infections, and LPS, spine surgery

What is the commonly associated medical condition?

Diabetes mellitus

What are the most common sites?

1. Thoracic
2. Lumbar
3. Cervical

What is the most common organism?	*Staphylococcus aureus*
What are the signs/ symptoms?	Fever; severe pain over affected area and with flexion/extension of spine; weakness can develop, ultimately leading to paraplegia; 15% of patients have a back furuncle
How is the diagnosis made?	MRI is test of choice.
Which test is contraindicated?	LP, because of the risk of seeding CSF with bacteria, causing meningitis
What is the treatment?	Surgical drainage and appropriate antibiotic coverage
What is the prognosis?	Depends on preop condition; severe neurologic deficits (e.g., paraplegia) show little recovery; 15% to 20% of cases are fatal

SYRINGOMYELIA

What is it?	Central pathologic cavitation of the spinal cord
What is the etiology?	Unknown, but associated with cranial base malformations, intramedullary tumors, or traumatic necrosis of the cord
What is the anatomic location?	Most are in the cervical/upper thoracic region; they can extend either way (syringobulbia = extension into medulla)
What are the signs/ symptoms?	First, bilateral loss of pain and temperature sensation in "cape-like" distribution (lateral spinothalamic tract involvement); enlargement of syrinx will cause further motor and sensory loss
How is the diagnosis made?	MRI will show defect in cord
What is the treatment?	Surgical (syringosubarachnoid shunt)

PEDIATRIC NEUROSURGERY

HYDROCEPHALUS

What is it?
Abnormal condition consisting of an increase in the volume of CSF along with distension of CSF spaces

What are the three general causes?
1. Increased production of CSF
2. Decreased absorption of CSF
3. Obstruction of flow of normal CSF (90% of cases)

What is the normal daily CSF production?
Approximately 500 ml

What is the normal volume of CSF?
Approximately 150 ml in the average adult

Define "communicating" versus "noncommunicating" hydrocephalus.
Communicating—unimpaired connection of CSF pathway from lateral ventricle to subarachnoid space
Noncommunicating—complete or incomplete obstruction of CSF flow within or at the exit of the ventricular system

What are the specific causes of hydrocephalus?
1. Congenital malformation
   Aqueductal stenosis
   Myelomeningocele
2. Tumors obstructing CSF flow
3. Inflammation causing impaired absorption of fluid
   Subarachnoid hemorrhage
   Meningitis
4. Choroid plexus papilloma causing increased production of CSF

What are the signs/ symptoms?
Signs of increased ICP: HA, nausea, vomiting, ataxia, increasing head circumference exceeding norms for age-related children

What is Sheehan's syndrome?
1. Bulging fontanelle
2. Paralysis of upward gaze
3. Scalp vein engorgement

How is the diagnosis made?
CT, MRI, measurement of head circumference

What is the treatment?
1. Remove obvious offenders
2. Bypass obstruction with ventriculoperitoneal shunt or ventriculoatrial shunt

What is the prognosis if untreated?
50% mortality; survivors show decreased IQ (mean = 69); neurologic sequelae: ataxia, paraparesis, visual deficits

What are the possible complications of treatment?
1. Blockage/shunt malfunction
2. Infection

What is hydrocephalus ex vacuo?
Increased volume of CSF spaces due to brain atrophy, not due to any pathology in the amount of CSF absorbed or produced

What is a "shunt series"?
A series of x-rays covering the entire shunt length—looking for shunt disruption/kinking to explain malfunction of shunt

SPINAL DYSRAPHISM/NEURAL TUBE DEFECTS

What is the incidence?
Approximately 1/1000 live births in the United States

What are the race/gender demographics?
More common in white patients and female patients

Define spina bifida occulta.
Defect in the development of the posterior portion of the vertebrae

What are the signs/ symptoms?
Usually asymptomatic, though it may be associated with other spinal abnormalities; usually found incidentally on x-rays

What is the most common clinically significant defect?
Myelomeningocele: herniation of nerve roots and spinal cord through a defect in the posterior elements of the vertebra(e); the sac surrounding the neural tissue may be intact, but more commonly is ruptured and therefore exposes the CNS to the external environment

What is the most common anatomic site?	Lumbar region; next most common is the lower thoracic and upper sacral region
What are the signs/ symptoms?	Variable from mild skeletal deformities to a complete motor/sensory loss; bowel/ bladder function is difficult to evaluate, but often is affected and can adversely affect survival
What is the treatment?	With open myelomeningoceles, patients are operated on immediately to prevent infection.
What is the prognosis?	Approximately 95% survival for the first 2 years, compared with 25% in patients not undergoing surgical procedures
Which vitamin is thought to lower the rate of neural tube defects in utero?	Folic acid

CRANIOSYNOSTOSIS

What is it?	Premature closure of one or more of the sutures between the skull plates
What is the incidence?	1/200 live births in the United States
What are the types?	Named for the suture that is fused (e.g., sagittal, coronal, lambdoid); sagittal craniosynostosis accounts for more than 50% of all cases; more than one suture can be fused, and all or part of a suture may be affected
How is the diagnosis made?	Physical exam can reveal ridges along fused sutures and lessened suture mobility. Plain x-rays can show a lack of lucency along the fused suture, but are rarely required.
What are the indications for surgery?	Most often the reasons are cosmetic, as the cranial vault will continue to deform with growth. Occasionally, a child will present with increased ICP secondary to restricted brain growth.

What is the timing of surgery?

Usually 3 to 4 months of age; earlier surgery increases the risk of anesthesia; later surgeries are more difficult due to the worsening deformities and decreasing malleability of the skull

What is the operative mortality?

Less than 1%

MISCELLANEOUS

What anesthetic decreases the seizure threshold?

Enflurane, so **isoflurane** is preferred in neurosurgical cases

Which IV anesthetic causes an increase in ICP?

Ketamine; consequently, this medication should be avoided in head trauma patients

What is the most common cause of postneurosurgery meningitis?

Staphylococcus aureus (skin flora)

What classically presents as the "worst headache of my life"?

Spontaneous subarachnoid hemorrhage

What classically has a "lucid interval"?

Epidural hemorrhage

What is the most common location of a hypertensive intracerebral hemorrhage?

Putamen

What is Horner's syndrome?

Cervical sympathetic chain lesion:
1. Ptosis
2. Miosis
3. Decreased tearing and diaphoresis on ipsilateral face

What is a third-nerve palsy?

Think: the third nerve does three things:
1. Diplopia
2. Ptosis
3. Mydriasis

What is Millard-Gubler syndrome?

Pons infarction:
1. VI nerve palsy
2. VII nerve palsy
3. Contralateral hemiplegia

68 Urology

Define the following terms:

Cystogram	Contrast study of the bladder
Ureteral stents	Plastic tubes placed via cystoscope into the ureters for stenting, identification, etc.
Cystoscope	Scope placed into the urethra and into the bladder to visualize the bladder
Perc nephrostomy	Catheter placed through the skin into the kidney pelvis to drain urine with distal obstruction, etc.
Retrograde pyelogram	Dye injected into the ureter up into the kidney and films taken
RUG	**R**etrograde **U**rethro**G**ram (dye injected into the urethra and films taken; rules out urethral injury, usually in trauma patients)
Gomco clamp	Clamp used for circumcision; protects penis glans
Bell clapper's deformity	Condition of congenital absence of gubernaculum attachment to scrotum
Fournier's gangrene	Extensive tissue necrosis/infection of the perineum in patients with diabetes
Coudé's catheter	Basically, a Foley catheter with hook on the end to get around a large prostate
Foley catheter	Straight bladder catheter placed through the urethra

Suprapubic catheter	Bladder catheter placed through the skin above the pubic symphysis into the bladder
Posthitis	Foreskin infection
Hydrocele	Clear fluid in the processus vaginalis membrane
Communicating hydrocele	Hydrocele that communicates with peritoneal cavity and, thus, gets smaller and larger as fluid drains and then reaccumulates
Noncommunicating hydrocele	Hydrocele that does not communicate with the peritoneal cavity Hydrocele remains the same size
Varicocele	Abnormal dilation of the pampiniform plexus to the spermatic vein in the spermatic cord; described as a "sac of worms"
Epididymitis	Infection of the epididymis
Prehn's sign	Elevation of the painful testicle that reduces the pain of epididymitis
Orchitis	Inflammation/infection of the testicle
Pseudohermaphroditism	Genetically ONE sex; partial or complete opposite-sex genitalia
Urgency	Overwhelming sensation to void immediately
Dysuria	Painful urination (usually burning sensation)
Frequency	Urination more times than usual
Polyuria	Urination in larger amounts than usual
Nocturia	Awakening to urinate
Hesitancy	Delay in urination

Pneumoturia	Air passed with urine via the urethra
Pyuria	WBC in urine; usually more than 10 WBC/HPF
Cryptorchidism	Undescended testicle
IVP	**I**ntra**V**enous **P**yelogram (dye is injected into the vein, collects in the renal collecting system, and an x-ray is taken)
Hematuria	RBCs in urine
Space of Retzius	Anatomic extraperitoneal space in front of the bladder
Enuresis	Involuntary urination while asleep
Incontinence	Involuntary urination
TURP	**T**rans**U**rethral **R**esection of the **P**rostate
PVR	**P**ost**V**oid **R**esidual
Priapism	Prolonged, painful erection
Paraphimosis	Foreskin held (stuck) in the retracted position
Phimosis	Inability to retract the foreskin
Balanitis	Inflammation/infection of the glans penis
Balanoposthitis	Inflammation/infection of the glans and prepuce of the penis
UTI	**U**rinary **T**ract **I**nfection
Peyronie's disease	Abnormal fibrosis of the penis shaft resulting in a bend upon erection
BPH	**B**enign **P**rostatic **H**yperplasia
Epispadias	Abnormal urethral opening on the dorsal surface of the penis

Hypospadiasis	Abnormal urethral opening on the ventral surface of the penis
Impotence	Inability to achieve an erection
Sterility	Inability to reproduce
Appendix testis	Common redundant testicular tissue
VUR	**V**esico**U**reteral **R**eflux

UROLOGIC DIFFERENTIAL DIAGNOSIS

What is the differential diagnosis of scrotal mass?	Cancer, torsion, epididymitis, hydrocele, spermatocele, varicocele, inguinal hernia, testicular appendage, swollen testicle after trauma, nontesticular tumor (paratesticular tumor: e.g., rhabdomyosarcoma, leiomyosarcoma, liposarcoma)
What is the differential diagnosis of hematuria?	Bladder cancer, trauma, UTI, cystitis from chemotherapy or radiation, stones, kidney lesion, BPH
What is the most common cause of severe gross hematuria without trauma or chemotherapy/radiation?	Bladder cancer
What is the differential diagnosis of bladder outlet obstruction?	BPH, stone, foreign body, urethral stricture, urethral valve
What is the differential diagnosis of ureteral obstruction?	Stone, tumor, iatrogenic (suture), stricture, gravid uterus, radiation injury, retroperitoneal fibrosis
What is the differential diagnosis of kidney tumor?	Renal cell carcinoma, sarcoma, adenoma, angiomyolipoma, hemangiopericytoma, oncocytoma

RENAL CELL CARCINOMA

What is it?	Most common solid renal tumor (90%); originates from proximal renal tubular epithelium

What is the epidemiology?	Primarily a tumor of adults 40 to 60 years of age with a 2:1 male:female ratio; makes up less than 5% of cancer in adults; equal incidence in white and African-American patients
What are the symptoms?	Pain (40%), hematuria (35%), weight loss (35%), flank mass (25%), HTN (20%)
What is the classic triad of renal cell carcinoma?	Flank pain, hematuria, and palpable mass (occurs in 10% to 15% of cases)
Radiologic tests?	1. IVP 2. Abdominal CT with contrast
Define the stages:	
I	Intact renal capsule
II	Extends to perinephric fat
III	IVC or main renal vein Regional lymph nodes Vessels and nodes
IV	Distant metastasis, spread to adjacent organs
What is the metastatic workup?	CXR, IVP, CT, LFTs, calcium
What are the sites of metastases?	Lung, liver, brain, bone; tumor thrombus entering renal vein or IVC is not uncommon
What is the unique route of spread?	Tumor thrombus into **IVC lumen**
What is the treatment?	Radical nephrectomy (excision of the kidney and adrenal, including Gerota's fascia) for stages I through IV

BLADDER CANCER

What is the incidence?	Second most common urologic malignancy Male:female ratio of 3:1 White patients are more commonly affected than African-American patients
What is the histology?	Transitional cell carcinoma (TCC)—90%; remaining cases are squamous or adenocarcinomas
What are the risk factors?	Smoking, industrial carcinogens (aromatic amines), schistosomiasis, truck drivers, petroleum workers
What are the symptoms?	**Hematuria,** with or without irritative symptoms (e.g., dysuria)
What is the classic presentation of bladder cancer?	"Painless hematuria"
What tests are included in the workup?	Urinalysis and culture, IVP, cystoscopy with cytology and biopsy
Define the stages (according to the Jewett/Marshall system):	
O	Superficial, limited to mucosa; also known as carcinoma in situ (CIS)
A	Involves lamina propria
B	Muscle invasion
C	Extends to perivesicular fat
D	Abdominal organ metastasis, lymph node metastasis, distant metastasis
What is the treatment according to stage:	
Stage O?	Bladder chemotherapy (intravesical chemotherapy)

Stage A?	TURB
Stages B and C?	Radical cystectomy, lymph node dissection, removal of prostate/uterus/ovaries/anterior vaginal wall, and urinary diversion (e.g., ileal conduit)
Stage D?	+/- Cystectomy and **systemic chemotherapy**
What is TURB?	**T**rans-**U**rethral **R**esection of the **B**ladder
What is the recurrence rate?	Increased risk because of "field effect"; field effect refers to the uniform exposure of the urothelium as it is bathed in urinary carcinogens; therefore, requires surveillance with repeat cystoscopy and urinary cytology every 3 to 4 months

PROSTATE CANCER

What is the incidence?	Number one GU cancer (> 100,000 new cases per year in the U.S.); most common carcinoma in men in the United States; second most common cause of death in men in the United States
What is the epidemiology?	"A disease of elderly men" present in one-third of men aged 70 to 79 and two-thirds aged 80 to 89 at autopsy; African-American patients have a 50% higher incidence than white patients
What is the histology?	Adenocarcinoma (95%)
What are the symptoms?	Often asymptomatic; usually presents as a nodule found on routine rectal exam; in 70% of cases, cancer begins in the periphery of the gland and moves centrally; thus, obstructive symptoms occur late; 40% of patients have metastatic disease at presentation, with symptoms of bone pain and weight loss

What are the common sites of metastasis?
Osteoblastic bony lesions, lung, liver, adrenal

What provides lymphatic drainage?
Obturator and hypogastric nodes

What is the significance of Batson's plexus?
Spinal cord venous plexus; route of isolated skull/brain metastasis

What are the steps in early detection and surveillance?
1. Prostate-specific antigen (PSA)—most sensitive and specific marker
2. Acid phosphatase—often elevated in metastatic prostate cancer; used mostly to detect recurrences
3. Rectal exam

How is the diagnosis made?
Transrectal biopsy

What are the indications for transrectal biopsy with normal rectal exam?
PSA more than 10 or abnormal transrectal ultrasound

Gleason histologic grading system

Define the following Gleason scores:

2 to 4
Well-differentiated cancer

5 to 7
Moderately differentiated cancer

8 to 10
Poorly differentiated cancer

What are the steps in staging workup?
1. Digital rectal exam
2. Transrectal ultrasonography
3. CT for lymph node involvement
4. PSA
5. Bone scan

Define the stages:

A
Nonpalpable—confined to prostate

B
Palpable nodule, but confined to prostate

C
Extends beyond capsule without metastasis

D	Metastatic disease
What are the treatment options according to stage:	
Stage A?	Radical prostatectomy (10% to 50% are impotent and 1% to 10% are incontinent) External beam radiation
Stage B?	Radical prostatectomy, with or without radiation
Stage C?	Radiation therapy or hormonal therapy
Stage D?	Hormonal treatment, with or without radiation (some benefit from radical prostatectomy with better local control)
What is the hormonal treatment?	Hormonal therapy (palliative); androgen blockade with estrogen diethylstilbestrol (DES) or LH-RH agonists Surgical castration (orchiectomy; palliative)
What are the steps in follow-up?	Rectal exam and PSA every 6 months

BENIGN PROSTATIC HYPERPLASIA

What is it also known as?	BPH
What is it?	Disease of elderly men (average age is 60–65 years); prostate gradually enlarges, creating symptoms of urinary outflow obstruction due to benign hyperplasia
What is the size of a normal prostate?	Between 20 and 25 gm
Where does BPH occur?	Periurethrally (note: prostate cancer occurs in the periphery of the gland)
What are the symptoms?	Obstructive-type symptoms: hesitancy, weak stream, nocturia, intermittency, UTI, urinary retention

How is the diagnosis made?	History, digital rectal exam, elevated postvoid residual (PVR), urinalysis, cystoscopy, U/S
What lab tests should be performed?	Urinalysis, PSA, BUN, CR
What is the differential diagnosis?	**Prostate cancer** (e.g., nodular)—biopsy Neurogenic bladder—history of neurologic disease Acute prostatitis—hot, tender gland Urethral stricture—RUG, history of STD Stone UTI
What are the treatment options?	Pharmacologic—α-1 blockade Hormonal—antiandrogens Surgical—TURP, TUIP, open prostate resection Transurethral balloon dilation
What is Proscar?	Finasteride: 5-α-reductase inhibitor; blocks transformation of testosterone to dihydrotestosterone; may shrink BPH and slow progression of BPH
What is Hytrin?	Terazosin: α-blocker; may increase urine outflow by relaxing prostatic smooth muscles
What are the indications for surgery?	Due to obstruction: Urinary retention Hydronephrosis UTIs Severe symptoms
What is "TURP"?	**T**rans**U**rethral **R**esection of **P**rostate: resection of prostate tissue via a scope
What is "TUIP"?	**T**rans**U**rethral **I**ncision of **P**rostate
What percentage of tissue removed for BPH will have malignant tissue on histology?	Up to 10%!

What is the most likely outcome with TURP?

More than two-thirds of patients have improvement in urinary symptoms

What are the possible complications of TURP?

Immediate:
- Failure to void
- Bleeding
- Clot retention
- UTI
- Incontinence

TESTICULAR CANCER

What is the incidence?

Rare; 2 to 3 new cases per 100,000 men per year in the United States

What is its claim to fame?

Most common solid tumor of young adult men (20–40 years)

What are the risk factors?

Cryptorchidism (6% of testicular tumors develop in patients with a history of cryptorchidism)

What is cryptorchidism?

Failure of the testicle to descend into the scrotum

What is the relative risk of malignancy in a cryptorchid testicle?

Intraabdominal testis: 1 in 20
Inguinal testis: 1 in 80

Does orchiopexy as an adult remove the risk of testicular cancer?

NO; orchiopexy (placement of cryptorchid testis in scrotum) does not alter malignant potential

What are the symptoms?

Most patients present with a painless lump, swelling, or firmness of the testicle; often noticed after incidental trauma to the groin

What percentage present with symptoms of metastatic disease (back pain, anorexia)?

Approximately 10%

What are the classifications?

Germ cell tumors (95%):
- Seminomatous (35%)
- Nonseminomatous (65%)
- Embryonal cell carcinoma
- Teratoma
- Mixed cell
- Choriocarcinoma

Nongerminal (5%)
- Leydig cell
- Sertoli cell
- Gonadoblastoma

What is the major classification based on therapy?

Seminomas and nonseminoma tumors

What are the tumor markers for testicular tumors?

1. Human chorionic gonadotropin (HCG)
2. Alpha-fetoprotein (AFP)

What are the tumor markers by tumor type?

HCG—increased in choriocarcinoma (100%), embryonal carcinoma (50%), and rarely in pure seminomas (10%); (half of nonseminomatous tumors)

AFP—increased in embryonal carcinoma and yolk sac tumors (half of nonseminomatous tumors)

Which tumors almost never have an elevated AFP?

Choriocarcinoma and seminoma

In which tumor is HCG almost always found elevated?

Choriocarcinoma

How often is HCG elevated in patients with pure seminoma?

Only about 10% of the time!

What other tumor markers may be elevated and useful for recurrence surveillance?

LDH, CEA, human chorionic somatomammotropic (HCS), gamma-glutamyl transpeptidase (GGT), placental alkaline phosphate (PLAP)

What are the steps in workup?

PE, scrotal U/S, check tumor markers, CXR, CT (chest/pelvis/abd)

Define the stages (Boden and Gibb):	
A	Confined to testis/cord
B	Regional lymph node spread
C	Distant metastasis, spread beyond retroperitoneal nodes
Define the stages according to TMN staging (simplified):	
Stage I	Confined to testis/cord
Stage IIA	Microscopic regional retroperitoneal nodes
Stage IIB	Gross retroperitoneal nodes less than 5 cc
Stage IIC	"Bulky" retroperitoneal nodes (> 5 cc)
Stage III	Distant metastasis, positive nodes further than retroperitoneal basin, elevated tumor markers after retroperitoneal dissection
What is the treatment of seminoma at the various stages:	
Stage I?	Inguinal orchiectomy and radiation
Stages IIA and IIB?	Inguinal orchiectomy and radiation
Stages IIC and III?	Orchiectomy and chemotherapy
What is the treatment of nonseminomatous disease at the various stages:	
Stage I?	Orchiectomy and retroperitoneal lymph node dissection versus close follow-up for retroperitoneal nodal involvement
Stages IIA and IIB?	Orchiectomy, retroperitoneal node dissection; ± chemotherapy

Stage IIC and III?

Orchiectomy and chemotherapy, followed by retroperitoneal node dissection to evaluate the need for more chemotherapy

What percentage of stage I seminomas are cured after treatment?

Ninety-five percent

Which type is most radiosensitive?

Seminoma (think **s**eminoma = **s**ensitive to radiation)

Why not remove testis with cancer through a scrotal incision?

It could result in tumor seeding of the scrotum.

What is the major side effect of retroperitoneal lymph node dissection?

Impotence

TESTICULAR TORSION

What is it?

Torsion (twist) of the spermatic cord, resulting in venous outflow obstruction, and subsequent arterial occlusion→infarction of the testicle

What is the classic history?

Acute onset of scrotal pain usually after vigorous activity or minor trauma

What is a "bell clapper" deformity?

Bilateral nonattachment of the testicles by the gubernaculum to the scrotum (free like the clappers of a bell)

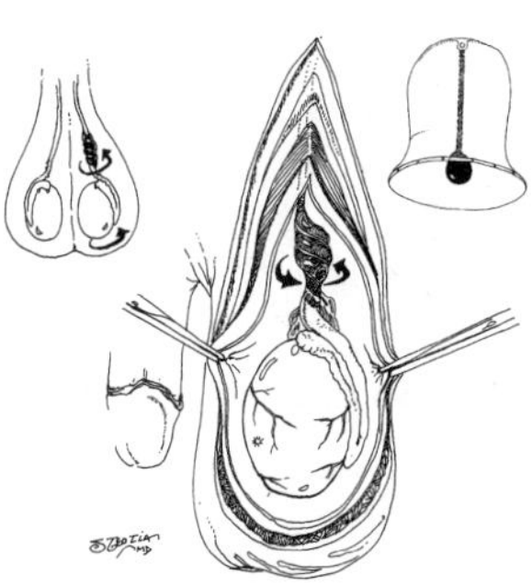

What are the symptoms?

Pain in the scrotum, suprapubic pain

What are the signs? Very tender, swollen, elevated testicle; nonillumination

What is the differential diagnosis? Testicular trauma, inguinal hernia, epididymitis, appendage torsion

How is the diagnosis made? Surgical exploration, U/S (solid mass) and Doppler flow study, cold Tc-99m scan

What is the treatment? Surgical detorsion and bilateral orchiopexy to the scrotum

How much time is available from the onset of symptoms to detorse the testicle? Less than 6 hours will bring about the best results

EPIDIDYMITIS

What is it? Infection of the epididymis

What are the signs/ symptoms? Swollen, tender testicle; dysuria; scrotal ache/pain; fever; chills; scrotal mass

What is the cause? Bacteria from the urethra

What are the common bugs in the following types of patients:

Elderly patients/ children? *E. coli*

Young men? STD bacteria: *Gonorrhea, Chlamydia*

What is the major differential diagnosis? Testicular torsion

What is the treatment? Rule out testicular torsion; administer antibiotics

IMPOTENCE

What is it? Inability to achieve an erection

What are the six major causes of impotence?

1. **Vascular:** decreased blood flow or leak of blood from the corpus cavernosus (most common cause)
2. **Endocrine:** low testosterone
3. **Anatomic:** structural abnormality of the erectile apparatus (e.g., Peyronie's disease)
4. **Neurologic:** damage to nerves (e.g., postoperative, IDDM)
5. **Medications** (e.g., clonidine, MAOIs)
6. **Psychologic** : performance anxiety, etc. (very rare)

What lab tests should be performed?

Fasting GLC (rule out diabetes and thus diabetic neuropathy)
Serum testosterone
Serum prolactin

What test evaluates for vascular causation of impotence?

Intracavernous vasoactive injection: injection of papaverine or PGE1 into the cavernous cavity of the penis and a full erection subsequently rules out a vascular cause of the impotence

What other diagnostic tests are often useful?

U/S with Doppler flow studies, cavernous pressures, arteriography (pudendal), penile monitoring for erection

What is the treatment?

Depends on the cause: vacuum pump, penile prosthesis, vasoactive injections (inject PGE1 , papaverine, phentolamine), psychologic therapy, testosterone injections

CALCULUS DISEASE

What is the incidence?

One in ten people will have stones

What are the risk factors?

Poor fluid intake, IBD, hypercalcemia ("CHIMPANZEES"), renal tubular acidosis, small bowel bypass

What are the types of stones?

1. Calcium oxalate/calcium PO_4 (75%)—secondary to hypercalciuria (increased intestinal absorption, decreased renal reabsorption, increased bone reabsorption)

2. Struvite (MgAmPh)(15%)—infection stones; E more than M; seen in UTI with urea-splitting bacteria (*Proteus*); may cause staghorn calculi; high urine pH
3. Uric acid (7%)—stones are radiolucent (think: **u**ric = **u**nseen); seen in gout, Lesch-Nyhan, chronic diarrhea, cancer; low urine pH
4. Cystine (1%)—genetic predisposition

What type of stones are not seen on AXR?

Uric acid (Think: **U**ric = **U**nseen)

What stone is associated with UTIs?

Struvite stones (Think: **S**truvite = **S**epsis)

What stones are seen in IBD/bowel bypass?

Calcium oxalate

What are the symptoms?

Severe pain; patient cannot sit still: renal colic (typically pain in the kidney/ureter that radiates to the testis or penis), hematuria (remember, patients with peritoneal signs are motionless)

What are the classic findings/symptoms?

Flank pain, stone on AXR, hematuria

What is the diagnosis?

KUB (90% radiopaque), IVP, urinalysis and culture, BUN/Cr, CBC

What is the significance of hematuria and pyuria?

Stone with concomitant infection

What is the treatment?

Narcotics for pain, vigorous hydration, observation
Further options: ESWL (lithotripsy), ureteroscopy, percutaneous litho., open surgery; metabolic workup for recurrence

What are the indications for intervention?

Urinary tract obstruction
Persistent infection
Impaired renal function

What are the contraindications of outpatient treatment?

Pregnancy, diabetes, obstruction, severe dehydration, severe pain, urosepsis/fever, pyelonephritis, previous urologic surgery/one functioning kidney

What are the three common sites of obstruction?

1. Ureteropelvic junction (UPJ)
2. Ureterovesicular junction (UVJ)
3. Intersection of the ureter and the iliac vessels

What are the preventive measures?

Increase urine volume
Ca—reduce Ca/oxalate load in diet, treat underlying disease
Struvite—treat underlying infection
Uric acid—decrease meat in diet, increase pH, allopurinol
Cystine—decrease meat, increase urine output, increase pH (D-penicillamine or α-mercaptopropionylglycine in refractory cases)

INCONTINENCE

What are the types of incontinence?

True incontinence, stress incontinence, overflow incontinence, urge incontinence, enuresis

Define the following terms:

True incontinence (TI)

Constant or periodic loss of urine without warning, caused by sphincter abnormality (e.g., exstrophy of bladder)

Stress incontinence (SI)

Loss of urine associated with coughing, lifting, exercise, etc.; seen most often in women, secondary to relaxation of pelvic floor following multiple deliveries

Overflow incontinence (OI)

Failure of the bladder to empty properly; may be caused by bladder outlet obstruction (BPH or stricture) or detrusor hypotonicity

Urge incontinence (UI)

Loss of urine secondary to detrusor instability in patients with stroke, dementia, Parkinson's disease, etc.

Enuresis — Bedwetting in children

How is the diagnosis made? — History (including meds), physical exam (including pelvic/rectal exam), urinalysis, postvoid residual (PR), urodynamics, cystoscopy/vesicocystourethrogram (VCUG) may be necessary

What is the treatment of the following disorders:

SI? — Bladder neck suspension, pessaries, estrogen therapy, α-adrenergic stimulation

UI? — Pharmacotherapy (anticholinergics, α-agonists) bladder denervation, and augmentation cystoplasty

OI? — Self-cath, surgical relief of obstruction; avoidance of indwelling catheters (UTIs)

TI? — Appropriate surgical intervention

UTI

What is it? — Urinary tract infection

What is the etiology? — Ascending infection, instrumentation, sex in females

What are the common organisms?

1. *E. coli* (≈90%)
2. *Proteus*
3. *Klebsiella, Pseudomonas*

What are the predisposing factors? — Stones, obstruction, reflux, diabetes mellitus, pregnancy, indwelling catheter/stent

What are the symptoms?

Lower UTI—frequency, urgency, dysuria, nocturia
Upper UTI—back/flank pain, fever, chills

How is the diagnosis made? — Symptoms, urinalysis (more than 10 WBCs/HPF, more than 10^5 CFU grown from clean-catch urine)

When should workup be performed?	After first infection in **male** patients (unless Foley is in place) After first pyelonephritis in prepubescent female patients
What is the treatment?	Lower: 1 to 4 days of oral antibiotics Upper: 3 to 7 days of IV antibiotics

WARD QUESTIONS

Does orchiopexy reduce the incidence of testicular neoplasms in undescended testis?	No
Why should orchiopexy be performed?	Decreases the susceptibility to blunt trauma Increases the ease of follow-up exams
In which area of the prostate does BPH arise?	Periurethral
In which area of the prostate does prostate cancer arise?	Periphery
What type of bony lesions are seen in metastatic prostate cancer?	Osteoblastic (radiopaque)
What percentage of renal cell carcinoma shows evidence of metastatic disease at presentation?	Approximately 33%
What is the most common site of distant metastasis in renal cell carcinoma?	Lung
What is the most common solid renal tumor of childhood?	Wilms' tumor
What type of renal stone is radiolucent?	Uric acid (Think: **U**ric = **U**nseen)

What are posterior urethral valves?	The most common obstructive urethral lesion in infants and newborns; occurs only in males; found at the distal prostatic urethra
What is the most common intraoperative bladder tumor?	A Foley catheter—don't fall victim!
What provides drainage of the left gonadal (e.g., testicular) vein?	Left renal vein
What provides drainage of the right gonadal vein?	IVC
What are the signs of urethral injury in the trauma patient?	"High-riding, ballottable" prostate, blood at the urethral meatus, severe pelvic fracture, ecchymosis of scrotum
What is the evaluation for urethral injury in the trauma patient?	RUG (**R**etrograde **U**rethro**g**ram)
What is the evaluation for a transected ureter introp?	IV indigo carmine and then look for leak of blue urine in the operative field
What aid is used to help identify the ureters in a previously radiated retroperitoneum?	Ureteral stents
How should a small traumatic preperitoneal bladder rupture be treated?	Foley catheter
How should a traumatic intraperitoneal bladder rupture be treated?	Operative repair

69

Ophthalmology

Define the following terms:

Esotropia	Eyes inward
Exotropia	Eyes outward
Hypertropia	Eyes upward
Hypotropia	Eyes downward
Diplopia	Double vision
Strabismus	Eye malalignment
Hyphema	Blood in anterior chamber of eye
Chemosis	Edema of the conjunctiva
Endophthalmitis	Intraocular infection
Ptosis	Eyelid droop
Anisocoria	Asymmetric pupil diameter
Nystagmus	Back and forth jerky movement of the eyes
Dacrocystitis	Lacrimal sac infection
Mydriasis	Pupil dilation (Think: my**D**riasis = **D**ilation)
Miosis	Pupil constriction
Myopia	Nearsightedness

OCULAR TRAUMA

What are the signs/ symptoms of corneal abrasions?	Pain! History of ocular trauma
How are corneal abrasions diagnosed?	Fluorescein test
With a laceration of the eyebrow, should the eyebrow be shaved prior to suturing closed?	NO; 20% of the time the eyebrow will not grow back!
What is a retinal detachment?	A **separation** of the neurosensory retina from the pigment epithelium and its supportive choroid, resulting in retinal infarction
What causes retinal detachment?	**Trauma,** ocular surgery, diabetes, spontaneous—small rent in retina allows fluid to insinuate itself in the subretinal space causing a retinal detachment
What are the signs/ symptoms of a retinal detachment?	Floaters, blind spots, flashing lights
What is the treatment for a retinal detachment?	Surgery—sclera buckling therapy
What is the major symptom of a lens detachment?	Blurred vision
What is the common ocular physical finding after a sinus fracture?	Conjunctivae emphysema
How are acid and alkali chemical eye burns treated?	Copious eye irrigation for both
What is sympathetic ophthalmia?	Autoimmune destruction of the contralateral **good eye** after penetrating injury causing blindness to ipsilateral eye; remove blind eye within 2 weeks following penetrating injury to avoid this condition

Should a penetrating eye object be removed?

NO! Call the ophthalmologist and do not remove.

GLAUCOMA

What is it?

An ocular disease complex primarily characterized by an **increased intraocular pressure**

What are the different types?

1. **Chronic open angle:** bilateral, insidious, slowly progressive; most common type (90%)
2. **Narrow angle:** acute obstruction of aqueous outflow; painful, **acute** visual loss, cloudy cornea
3. **Congenital:** genetically transmitted; often appearing in first year of life

What is the pathophysiology?

Increased ocular pressure related to increased intraocular aqueous humor production and/or decreased outflow of aqueous humor from the eye, leading to optic nerve degeneration

How is the diagnosis made?

1. Increased intraocular pressure
2. Retinoscopy (optic disc cupping)
3. Peripheral visual field testing

What is the treatment?

Decrease intraocular pressure through topical eyedrops and/or surgery

DIABETIC RETINOPATHY

What is it?

A progressive microangiopathy of retinal blood vessels in diabetic patients

What are the different types?

1. Preproliferative: retinoscopic hemorrhages *without* neovascularization (precursor of proliferative retinopathy)
2. Proliferative: advanced retinoscopic vascular changes *with* neovascularization

What are the symptoms?

Decreased visual acuity

How is the diagnosis made?

1. Retinoscopy
2. Fluorescein angiogram

What is the treatment?

1. **Preproliferative:** monitoring for signs and symptoms of proliferative retinopathy, blood sugar control
2. **Proliferative:** retinal photocoagulation with **argon laser** to peripheral retina

CORNEA

What is keratitis?

Inflammation of the **cornea** secondary to an infectious or mechanical etiology

What infectious agents are frequently involved?

Staphylococcus, Streptococcus, Pseudomonas, Herpes, Chlamydia

What predisposes the cornea to infection?

Exposure, trauma

What is the treatment of corneal opacities secondary to scarring?

Corneal transplant

THE RED EYE

What are the eight signs of serious ocular pathology in a red eye?

1. Visual loss
2. Pain
3. Opacities
4. Pupil irregularities
5. Perilimbal erythema
6. Increased pressure
7. History of eye disease
8. Refractory to treatment

Give the classic signs/ symptoms of the following conditions:

Bacterial conjunctivitis

Conjunctival redness with purulent discharge

Viral conjunctivitis

Conjunctival redness with serous discharge

Allergic conjunctivitis

Clear conjunctival discharge

Acute narrow angle glaucoma (congenital glaucoma)	Acute pain, cloudy cornea, perilimbal redness, blurred vision
Iritis	Perilimbal redness, irregular pupil, pain, decreased vision
Corneal ulcer	Epithelial defect with infiltrate, pain
Corneal abrasion	Epithelial defect, no infiltrate, pain
Orbital cellulitis?	Periocular swelling, erythematous ocular surface, decreased vision

OPHTHALMOLOGY QUESTIONS

What is a cataract?	Opacification of the lens (treated by surgical removal)
What is strabismus?	Misalignment of the eyes
Why is it important to correct strabismus?	To allow proper development of visual acuity and binocular vision
What is a pterygium?	A plaque-like extension of fibrovascular tissue onto the cornea
In what cases should a blind eye be removed?	Blind and painful, malignancy, blind traumatized eye, diagnostic purposes
What is Horner's syndrome?	Sympathetic nerve lesion of the neck resulting in: 1. Miotic pupil 2. Ptosis 3. Decreased facial diaphoresis

Index

Page numbers in *italics* represent figures; page numbers with *t* indicate tables.

Abbreviations, 11–18
Abdomen, 486
  acute, 184–185
    diagnosis, 185–187
Abdominal abscess, diagnosis, 189
Abdominal aortic aneurysms (AAA), 167, 455–460
  diagnosis, 189
  diagnostic tests, 458
  differential diagnosis, 457
  incidence, 456
  operative complications, 458
  repair, 460
  risk factors, 456
  risk of rupture, 456–457
  signs of rupture, 456
  symptoms, 456
  treatment, 457–458
Abdominal computer tomography, 214
Abdominal pain
  causes of diffuse, 187
  differential diagnosis
    scrotal, 187
    thoracic, 187
Abdominal Perineal Resection (APR), 279
Abdominal surgery, emergency, 34
Abdominal wall layers, 96, 193
Abdominal x-ray (AXR), 37, 167
Abdominoperineal resection (APR), 77
Abduction, 640
ABO crossmatching, 628
ABO typing, 633
Abrasion, 529
  corneal, 715
Abscess, 18, 156
  appendiceal, 265
  breast, 372
  pancreatic, 347
  perirectal, 293, 294
  peritoneal, 156–157
  peritonsillar, 557
Accelerated acute rejection, 628
ACE inhibitors, 468
Acetaminophen (Tylenol), 123
Achalasia, 592–593
Achilles tendon
  rupture, 655
  test for intact, 656
Achlorhydria, 18
Acholic stool, 18
Acid burns, 222
Acid secretion, 179
Acidosis
  metabolic, 100, 436
  respiratory, 100, 436
Acquired heart disease
  aortic insufficiency, 605–606
  aortic stenosis, 604–605
  artificial valve placement, 608
  cardiopulmonary bypass, 602–604
  coronary artery, 600–601
  coronary artery bypass graft, 601–602
  infectious endocarditis, 608–609
  mitral regurgitation, 607–608
  mitral stenosis, 606–607
  postpericardiotomy syndrome, 602
Acral lentiginous melanoma, 428
Acro-, 18
Acronyms, 18
Actinic keratosis, 426
Acute abdomen, 184–185
  diagnosis, 185–187
Acute acalculus cholecystitis, 333–334
Acute arterial occlusion, 453–455
Acute cholecystitis, 332–333
Acute compartment syndrome, 651–652
Acute gastritis, 229
Acute mesenteric ischemia, 461–462
Acute pancreatitis, 240
Acute rejection, 628, 629
Acute rhinitis, 552

Acute sinusitis, 553–554
Acute suppurative otitis media, 542–544
Addisonian crisis, 136–137
Adduction, 639
Adeno-, 18
Adenocarcinoma, 258, 696
  follicular, 396–397
  malignant mucoid, 266
  papillary, 395–396
Adenoma
  adrenal, 376
  hepatocellular, 311
  treatment, 381
  tubular, 281, 282
  tubulovillous, 281, 282
  villous, 282
Adhesions, 18, 34, 129
Admission orders, 10
Adnexa, 18
Adrenal adenoma, 376
Adrenal carcinoma, 376
Adrenal glands
  Conn's syndrome, 380–382
    signs/symptoms, 381
    treatment, 381–382
  Cushing's syndrome, 373–377
    cause of, 373
    diagnosis, 374–376
    medications, 376
    signs/symptoms, 374
  gluconoma, 383–384
  incidentaloma, 377
  insulinoma, 382
  multiple endocrine neoplasia, 387
    MEN type I, 387–388
    MEN type IIA, 388
    MEN type IIB, 388–389
  normal physiology, 373
  pheochromocytoma, 377–380
    diagnosis, 378
    rule of 10's, 379
    signs/symptoms, 378
    sites of, 379
  Whipple's triad, 382–383
  Zollinger-Ellison syndrome, 384–387
    complications, 385
    diagnosis, 385–386
    incidence, 384
    signs/symptoms, 384
    treatment, 386–387
Adrenal incidentaloma, 377
Adrenal tumor, 375, 376
Adrenocorticotropic hormone (ACTH), 373
  levels, 374
Adson maneuver, 573
Adson pickup, 44, *44*
Adult respiratory distress syndrome (ARDS), 32, 37
Adventitia, 18
Afferent, 18
Afferent loop syndrome, 32, 132, *132*
Aflatoxin as risk factor in hepatocellular carcinoma, 313
Afterload, 438, 600
Aganglionic megacolon, 499–502
A-gram, 449, 458, 464, 468
Air-fluid level, significance, 168
Airway, assessment, 204–205
Albumin, 122
Alcohol withdrawal, signs, 141
-algia, 18
Alkali burns, 222
Alkaline phosphatase, 309, 326
Alkaline reflux gastritis, 134
Alkalosis
  hypochloremic, 100
  metabolic, 100
  respiratory, 100, 436
Allen's test, 25, 137
Allergic rhinitis, 552–553
Allis clamp, 49, *49*
Allograft, 623
Allograft bone, 640
Amaurosis fugax, 18, 463
Amelanotic anal tumor, 292
American Joint Committee on Cancer (AJCC) stages, 430
Aminoglycosides, 118
Amphotericin, 119
Ampulla, 18
Amputations, lower extremity, 452–453
Amylase, 355
Anal basal cell carcinoma, 292
Anal bleeding, 291
Anal cancer, 291–292
Anal fissure, 294–295
Anal melanoma, 292, 432
Analgesic, 18
Anaphylactic shock, 151–152
Anaphylaxis, fatal, 316
Anaplastic carcinoma, 399–400
Anastomosis, 18
  hepatoenteric, 336

Anatomical snuff-box, 534
pain in, 656
Anchovy paste pus, 315
Anemia, microcytic, 112, 277
Anergy, 18
Anesthesia, 171–175
endotracheal, 171
epidural, 171
general, 171
local, 171
regional, 171
spinal, 171
Aneurysms, 455–460
abdominal aortic, 455–460
dissecting aortic, 619
false, 447
popliteal artery, 469
splenic artery, 469
treatment, 681
true, 447
Angio-, 19
Angiography, selective mesenteric, 230
Angiosarcoma, 419
Angulated fracture, 647
Anion gap, 434
acidosis, 434
Aniridia, 518
Anisocoria, 711
Ankle to Brachial Index (ABI), 449
Annular pancreas, 355, 517
Ano, fistula in, 271–273, *272*
Anomaly, 19
Anorectal fistulas, management, 272, 293
Anorectal malformations, 498
Anterior cord syndrome, 674
Anterior spinal syndrome, 459, 615
Antibiotics, 117–120
prophylactic, 159–160
Anticoagulation, 603
Antigen presenting cell (APC), 624
Antrectomy, 83, 236, 238, 240
with gastroduodenostomy, 75
with gastrojejunostomy, 75
Aorta, coarctation of, 417, 611–613
Aortic arterial branch occlusion, 618
Aortic dissection, 615–621, *616, 617, 618, 620*
surgery for, 619
Aortic graft infections, 459
Aortic insufficiency (AI), 605–606
Aortic stenosis (AS), 604–605
Aortoenteric fistula, treating, 460
Aortograms, thoracic, 214
Apley's law, 524
Apnea, 19
and bradycardia episodes, 525
Appendectomy, 79, *79*, 266, 269
laparoscopic, 264
Appendiceal abscess, 265
Appendiceal rupture, 38
Appendiceal tumors, 266
Appendicitis, 36, 186–187, 188, 258, 261–266, 507–508, 526
acute, 34, 37, 184, 189
causes, 261
complications, 265
diagnosis, 263–264
differential diagnosis, 263
radiographic signs, 167
symptoms, 261–263
treatment, 264–265
Appendix, 34, 96, 261–266
Appendix testis, 693
Aphthous ulcer, 176
Arachnoid cap cells, 677
Argon laser, 116
Army-Navy retractor, 52, *52*
Arterial anatomy, 447
Arterial bypass operation, 446
Arterial line complications, 137
Arterial oxygen content, 435
Arteriovenous malformations (AVM), 680
treatment, 681
Artery, layer of, 447
Artery of Adamkiewicz, 96, 459
Arthritis, 661–662
degenerative, 662
posttraumatic, 661, 662
rheumatoid, 662
septic, 658
Arthrodesis, 642
Arthroplasty, 642
Artificial heart valve, 40
Artificial valve placement, 608
Aspirated foreign body, 478–479
Aspiration pneumonia, 127–128, 598
Aspirin, 122, 450
Assist-control ventilation, 443
Astrocytomas, 676
cerebellar, 677–678
Atelectasis, 19, 35, 124
ATG/antithymocyte globulin, 626
Atherosclerosis
initiation, 446

risk factors, 446
ATLS history, 218
Atraumatic bowel clamp, 46, *46*
Atresia
biliary, 513–514
duodenal, 494–495
ileal, 495–496
jejunal, 495
Atrial fibrillation, *620*
Auscultation in abdominal physical exam, 185
Austin Flint murmur, 622
Autograft, 623
Autologous vein graft, 452
Avitene®, 116
Avulsion fracture, 647, *647*
AX FEM, 82, *82*
Axilla, boundaries, 357
Axillary node dissection, 357, 365–366
with cystosarcoma phyllodes tumor, 370
with ductal carcinoma in situ, 367
Azathioprine (AZA), 625–626
for inflammatory bowel disease, 306
Aztreonam (Azactam), 119

B cells, 624
Babcock clamp, 46, *46*
Balanitis, 692
Balanoposthitis, 692
Ballance's sign, 25
Banting, 41
Barany, 41
Bariatric, 19
Bariatric surgery, 250–251
Barium enema, 305
Barlow's maneuver, 663
Barnard, 40
Barotrauma, 444
Barrett's esophagus, 19, 247, 595
Basal cell carcinoma, 425
anal, 292
Basilar skull fracture, 210
signs of, 669
Bassini, Edoardo, 39
Bassini herniorrhaphy, 76
Batson's plexus, 697
Battle's sign, 25, 669
Beck's triad, 25, 207, 618
Beckwith-Wiedemann syndrome, 518
Bell clapper's deformity, 492, 690, 703
Bell's palsy, 546–547
Benign breast disease, 370–372
Benign prostatic hyperplasia (BPH), 692, 698–700, 709
Benign thyroid disease, 400–401
Bennett's fracture, 649
Benzodiazepines, 123
reverse, 175
Bergman's triad, 26, 139
Berry aneurysm, 680
Beta, 19
Betadine, 227
Bezold's abscess, 544
Bicuspid aortic valve, 605
Bier block, 175
Bifurcation, 19
Bilateral hyperplasia, 382
Bile, 326
main constituents, 182
Bile acids, absorption, 180
Bile duct obstruction, diagnosis, 189
Bile salts, 19
absorption, 144
Bili-, 19
Biliary atresia, 513–514
Biliary colic, 328, 331
Biliary tract, 325–340, 513
acute acalculus cholecystitis, 333–334
acute cholecystitis, 332–333
anatomy, 325–326
annular pancreas, 517
atresia, 513–514
carcinoma of gallbladder, 337–338
cholangiocarcinoma, 338–339
cholangitis, 334–335
cholelithiasis, 330–332, 516–517
diagnostic studies, 328–329
gallstone ileus, 336–337
obstructive jaundice, 329–330
pathophysiology, 327–328
physiology, 326–327
radiographic evaluation, 328
sclerosing cholangitis, 335–336
surgery, 329
Bilious vomiting, 523
Billroth, Theodor, 39
Billroth I (BI), 75, *75*, 235, *235*, 238
Billroth II (BII), 75, *75*, 235, *235*, 238
Biopsy
core, 420
excisional, 21, 420, 425, 430
incisional, 22, 420, 425
shave, 430

transrectal, 697
Bird's beak, 168, 289
Bites, human, 160
Black-pigmented stones, 330
Bladder cancer, 695–696
Bladder candidiasis, treatment, 153
Bladder fistulas, 273
Bladder pheochromocytoma, 380
Blanching erythema, 157
Blepharoplasty, 527
Blind eye, removal of, 715
Blind loop syndrome, 32, 130–131
Blood and blood products, 111–114
Bloody nipple discharge, 368
Blount's disease, 664
Blowout fracture, 569
Blue dot sign, 491
Blumer's shelf, 26, 248
Blunt trauma algorithm, 221
Boas' sign, 26, 331
Bochdalek's hernia, 192
Body fluid, 98
Boerhaave's syndrome, 32, 243
Boil, 19
Bolus, 103
Bone tumor, pediatric, 667
Bouchard's nodes, 662
Bovie, 19, 40, 115
Bowel obstruction, diagnosis of neonatal, in pediatric surgery, 486
Bowen's disease, 426
Boxer's fracture, 534, 649, *649*
Brachial plexus, nerves of, 653
Branchial cleft anomalies, 476–477
Breast, 357–360
abscess, 372
anatomy, 357–360
blood supply, 358–359
lymphatic drainage, 359
nerves, 357–358
cancer, 37
differential diagnosis, 361
incidence, 360–366
indications for biopsy, 362–363
male, 369–370
metastases, 364
preoperative staging workup, 363
risk factors, 360–361
screening recommendations for, 362
signs, 361
sites, 34
staging, 364
symptoms, 361
treatments, 364–366
types, 34, 361
ductal carcinoma in situ, 366–367
lobular carcinoma in situ, 368–369
reconstruction, 369
Breast milk
calories, 525
production, 360
Breathing, assessment, 205–207
Breslow classification, 430
Bronchial adenoma, 584–585
Bronchogenic carcinoma, 578–582
Brooke ileostomy, 76, 254, *254*
Brown-Séquard syndrome, 674
Budd-Chiari syndrome, 33, 321
Buerger's disease, 470
Bullous myringitis, 542
Bupivacaine (Marcaine), side effect of, 173
Burns, 222–228
acid, 222
alkali, 222
chemical eye, 712
dressing of major, 227
dressing of minor, 226
electrical, 222
first degree, 222
hospitalization criteria for, 224
rule of nines, 223, *223*
second degree, 222
signs of infection, 226
and smoke inhalation, 224–225
thermal, 222
third degree, 223
topical antibiotic agents, 227

Cachexia, 19
Calcaneus fracture, 653
Calcium absorption, 146, 181
Calcium oxalate stones, 706
Calculus, 19
Calculus disease, 705–707
Calor, 19
Calot's (Lund) node, 95, 325
Calot's triangle, 95, 325
Cancer, 188
adrenal, 376
anal, 291–292
basal cell, 425
bladder, 695–696
breast

differential diagnosis, 361
incidence of, 360–366
indications for biopsy, 362–363
preoperative staging workup, 363
risk factors, 360–361
screening recommendations for, 362
signs of, 361
sites of metastases, 364
staging, 364
symptoms, 361
treatments, 364–366
types, 361
in children, 524
colorectal, 275–280
epidermal, 292
epidermoid, 424
epithelial, 638
of gallbladder, 337–338
gastric, 247–249
hepatocellular, 310, 313–314
Hürthle cell thyroid, 398–399
medullary, 397–398
nasal cavity, 555
pancreatic, 352–355
location, 353
presentation, 353
prognosis, 355
risk factors, 352
treatment, 353–354
types, 353
parathyroid, 409–410
prostate, 696–698, 699, 709
renal cell, 693–694, 709
squamous cell, 424–425
testicular, 700–703
thyroid, 395
Candida albicans in burn wound infections, 226
Cannula, 19
Cantlie's line, 307
Captopril provocation test, 381, 468
Caput medusa, 320
Carbon dioxide retention, 440
Carbon monoxide inhalation overdose, treatment, 228
Carboxyhemoglobin level, 225
Carbuncle, 19, 161
Carcinoid, 258
Carcinoid syndrome, 32, 267–268
Carcinoid triad, 26
Carcinoid tumors, 266, 267–269, 584–585
Carcinoma. (*See* Cancer.)
Cardiac electrolytes, 600
Cardiac index, 434
Cardiac output, 433–434
increasing, 600, 622
Cardiac tamponade, 206–207, 618
Cardiac tumors, 614, 622
Cardiogenic shock, 150
Cardiopulmonary bypass (CPB), 602–604
Cardiovascular complications, 137
Cardiovascular surgery
abbreviations, 599
acquired heart disease
aortic insufficiency, 605–606
aortic stenosis, 604–605
artificial valve placement, 608
cardiopulmonary bypass, 602–604
coronary artery, 600–601
coronary artery bypass graft, 601–602
infectious endocarditis, 608–609
mitral regurgitation, 607–608
mitral stenosis, 606–607
postpericardiotomy syndrome, 602
aortic dissection, 615–621, *616, 617, 618, 620*
cardiac tumors, 614
coarctation of aorta, 611–613
congenital heart disease
patent ductus arteriosus, 610
ventricular septal defect, 609–610
cyanotic heart disease, 614
Ebstein's anomaly, 613
terminology in, 599–600
tetralogy of Fallot, 611
thoracic aortic aneurysm, 614–615
transposition of great vessels, 613
vascular rings, 613–614
Carotid artery stenosis, 464
Carotid endarterectomy (CEA), 40, 76, 278, 464
Carotid ultrasound/Doppler, 464
Carotid vascular disease, 463–465
Carrel, 40, 41
Caseation, 19
Cataract, 715
Catgut sutures, 54
Catheter
Coudé's, 690
femoral vein, 208
Foley, 690, 710
suprapubic, 691
Cauda equina syndrome, 683

Caudal, 20
Cauterization, 20
CCK, 182
Cecal volvulus, 289–290
  diagnosis, 290
  etiology, 290
  incidence, 290
  signs/symptoms, 290
  treatment, 290
Cecostomy tube, 86
Cecum, 96, 503
Cefazolin, 118
Cefoxitin, 118
Ceftazidime (Ceftaz), 118
Ceftriaxone (Rocephin), 118
Celiotomy, 20, 218
Cell-mediated immunity/rejection, 624
Cells
  antigen presenting, 624
  B, 624
  chief, 179
  plasma, 624
  Sternberg-Reed, 421
  T, 624
Cellulitis, 157
  orbital, 715
Central cord syndrome, 674
Central line, 92–93
  infections, 153–154
  placement, 170
Central nervous system (CNS) tumors, 524, 675
Central venous pressure, 434
Cephal-, 20
Cephalosporins, 117
Cerebellar astrocytomas, 677–678
Cerebral contusion, 672
Cerebral perfusion pressure, 669
Cerebrovascular accident, 463
Cervical disc disease, 683–684
Cervical spine injury, 213
Chance fracture, 674
Charcot's joint, 657, 662
Charcot's triad, 26, 334
Chemical eye burns, 712
Chemosis, 711
Chemotherapy
  for breast cancer, 366
  for colon cancer, 279
Chest, flail, 206
Chest tubes, 86, 87–91
  insertion, 87, *87*
    goals, 87
  positioning, 87
  removal, 91
Chest wall tumors, 573–574
Chest x-ray (CXR), 35
Chief cells, 179
Chiladidee's sign, 169
Child abuse, 667
  signs, 523
  treatment, 523
Child's classification, 309*t,* 309–310
Chin lift, 205
Cholangiocarcinoma, 328, 338–339
Cholangitis, 328, 334–335
  causes, 34
  management, 335
  sclerosing, 335–336
  suppurative, 335
Chole-, 20
Cholecyst-, 20
Cholecystectomy, 79, *79,* 326
  indications, 332
Cholecystenteric fistula, 271
Cholecystitis, 188, 328
  acute, 332–333
  diagnosis, 333
Cholecystokinin, 180
  release, 327
  sources, 327
Cholecystostomy tube, 85
Choledochal cyst, 514–516
Choledocho-, 20
Choledochojejunostomy, 79, *79*
Choledocholithiasis (gallstones), 328, 329–330, 334
  diagnosis, 331
  management, 332
Cholelithiasis, 36, 189, 328, 330–332, 516–517
  diagnosis, 188, 331
  treatment, 331, 333
Cholesteatoma, 541–542
Cholesterol gallstones, 330
  dissolving, 332
  pathogenesis, 330
Chondroblastoma, 659
Chondrosarcoma, 659, 661
Choriocarcinoma, 701
Christmas disease, 113
Chromium deficiency, 145
Chronic mediastinitis, 589
Chronic mesenteric ischemia, 461

Chronic pancreatitis, 347–349
Chronic rejection, 628, 629
Chronic sinusitis, 554
Chvostek's sign, 26, 107
Chyme, 20
Cicatrix, 20
Cilastatin, 118
Cimetidine (Tagamet), 122
Ciprofloxacin, 118
Ciprofloxicin, 119
Ciprofloxin, 117
Circulation, assessing, 207–209
Circumcision, contraindications to, 523
Cirrhosis
  and portal hypertension, 319–320
  as risk factor in hepatocellular carcinoma, 313
Cisapride (Propulsid), 123
Clark's classification, 429, *429*
Class I antigens, 623
Class II antigens, 623
Classic intraoperative inguinal hernia, 195–197, *196*, *197*
Claudication
  risk of limb loss with, 450
  treatment, 449
Clavicle fracture, 652
Clay shoveler's fracture, 649, 674
Clean wound, 154–155
Cleido-, 20
Clindamycin, 117, 118
Clinic note, 11
Clips, 116
Closed reduction, 640
Clostridial myositis, 158
Clostridium perfringens in clostridial myositis, 158
Clostridium tetani, 161
COAG mode on Bovie, 115
Coarctation of aorta, 417, 611–613
Cobblestoning, 305
Colic, 20
  biliary, 331
Colitis
  pseudomembranous, 158–159
  ulcerative, 414
Colles' fracture, 648, *648*
Colloid, 20
Colloid fluid, 110
Colon
  anatomic differences between small bowel and, 275
  arterial blood supply to, 274, *274*
  polyps, 280–282
  purpose of, 181, 275
  treatment of penetrating injury to, 220
Colon cancer, surgical margins, 279
Colon tumor/mass, differential diagnosis, 277
Colonic fistulas, 271
Colonic ischemia, 459
Colonic obstruction, 280
Colonic transition zone, 500
Colonic villous adenomas, 38
Colonic volvulus, 287
  types, 35
Colonoscopy, 20
Colon/rectal resection, preoperative preparation for, 279
Colorectal cancer, 275–280
  guaiac-positive stool test, 276
  incidence, 275
  left-sided lesions, 277
  male to female ratio, 275
  preoperative workup for, 278
  right-sided lesions, 276
  risk factors, 276
  screening, 276
Colostomy, 20, 252
  leveling, 500
Colovesical fistula, 271
Comminuted fracture, 644, *644*
Common bile duct obstruction, cause of, 34
Communicating hydrocele, 489, 691
Compartment syndrome, 33, 212, 454–455, 651–652, 667
  treatment, 455
Complete, 191
Complete blood count (CBC) differential, left shift on, 185
Compliance, 438, 600
Computer tomography (CT) scanning, 214
Congenital diaphragmatic hernia, 484–485
Congenital heart disease (CHD)
  patent ductus arteriosus, 610
  ventricular septal defect, 609–610
Congenital hip dislocation, 663
Congenital pyloric stenosis, 493–494
Conjoint tendon, 197
Conjunctivae emphysema, 712

Conn's syndrome, 380–382
signs/symptoms, 381
treatment, 381–382
Constipation, 20, 129
differential diagnosis of infant, in pediatric surgery, 486
Contaminated wound, 155
Continuous Positive Airway Pressure (CPAP), 443
Contractility, 438
Contrecoup injury, 672
Contusion, 529
cerebral, 672
Conventional cutting needle, 56, *56*
Cooper's hernia, 192
Cooper's ligaments, 359
tumor involvement, 361
Cor pulmonale, 20
Cord lipoma, 196, 490
Core biopsy, 420
Cornea, 714
Corneal abrasion, 715
Corneal ulcer, 715
Coronary arteries, major, 600
Coronary artery bypass graft (CABG), 40, 82, *82,* 601–602
indications, 622
Coronary artery disease (CAD), 600–601
Coronary blood flow, 600
Coronary ligament, 307
Coronary vein, 96
Corticosteroids
azathioprine, 625–626
cyclosporine, 626
Corticotropin-releasing hormone (CRH), 373
stimulation test, 375
Coudé's catheter, 92, 690
Courvoisier's gallbladder, 340
Courvoisier's law, 26
Courvoisier's sign, 353
Craniosynostosis, 688–689
Cricoid pressure, 171
Cricothyroidotomy, 205, 218, 570
Crohn's disease, 297, 301
comparison of, and ulcerative colitis, 302–306
and small bowel obstruction, 257
surgical indications, 34
Cronkite-Canada syndrome, 284
Croup (laryngotracheobronchitis), 560–561
Cryoprecipitate (cryo), 111
Cryptorchid testicle, 523, 700
Cryptorchidism, 488, 692, 700
CSF rhinorrhea/otorrhea, 669
Cullen's sign, 26, 346
Curettage, 20
Curling's ulcer, 176, 228, 239
Cushing, Harvey, 39, 41
Cushing's disease, 373, 375
Cushing's response, 418
Cushing's syndrome, 32, 373–377, 418
causes, 373
diagnosis, 374–376
medications, 376
signs/symptoms, 374
Cushing's triad, 26, 670
Cushing's ulcer, 176, 239
CUT mode on Bovie, 115
Cut-off sign, 168
Cyanotic heart disease, 614
Cyclosporine (CSA), 626
Cyproheptadine, 269
Cystic fibrosis, 497
Cystic hygroma, 478
Cystoduodenostomy, 352
Cystogastrostomy, 351
Cystogram, 690
Cystosarcoma phyllodes, 370
Cystoscope, 690
Cysts, 21
choledochal, 514–516
epidermal inclusion, 425
hydatid, 316
liver, 316
sebaceous, 426
thyroglossal duct, 476
unicameral bone, 659, 661
Cytomegalovirus (CMV) infection, 637
Cytoprotection, decreased, 237

D5W, 102
Dacryocystitis, 711
Daily note, progress, 10–11
Dakin solution, 84
Dance's sign, 27, 524
Dantrolene (Dantrium), 119
Dead space, 439
Deaver retractor, 51, *51*
Debakey, Michael, 40
Debakey classifications, *616,* 616–617, *617*
Debakey pickup, 43, *43*

Decompression
  Foley catheter bladder, 208
  gastric, 208, 209
Decortication, 575
Decreased cytoprotection, 237
Decubitus ulcer, 176
Degenerative arthritis, 662
Delayed primary closure, 84
Delayed splenic rupture, 411
DeQuervain's thyroiditis, 402
Dermatitis, 356
Desmoid tumors, 283
Dexamethasone suppression test
  high-dose, 374–375
  low-dose, 374
Diabetes, 356
Diabetes insipidus (DI), 136
Diabetic ketoacidosis (DKA), 135
Diabetic retinopathy, 713–714
Diaphragm, 97, 220
Diaphragmatic injuries, 214–217, *215*
Diaphragmatic irritation, 188
Diaphysis, 642, *643*
Diarrhea, postvagotomy, 133
Diastolic hypertension, 417
Dieulafoy's ulcer, 176, 239
Diffuse axonal injury, 672
Diffuse esophageal spasm, 593
  carcinoma, 596–598
  nutcracker esophagus, 593–594
  reflux, 594–595
  strictures, 595–596
Digastric muscle, 465
Digitalis, 462
Diphenhydramine hydrochloride (Benadryl), 122
Diplopia, 711
Direct bilirubin, 21
Direct inguinal hernia, 193–194
Dirty wound, 155
Disability, assessing, 209–210
Dislocations, 641
  elbow, 653, 654
  hip, 216, 653, 654
    congenital, 663
  knee, 654–655
    drawer test, 655
    ligaments, 655
    meniscus, 655
  shoulder, 653, 654
  unstable, 640
Dissecting aortic aneurysm, 619
Disseminated intravascular coagulation, 139, 140
Distal gastrectomy, 238
Diverticular abscess, treatment, 287
Diverticulitis, 189, 271, 286–287
  associated lab findings, 286
  barium enema findings, 286
  colonoscopic findings, 286
  complications, 286
  diagnosis, 189
  radiographic findings, 286
  signs/symptoms, 286
  therapy, 286–287
Diverticulosis, 284–285
  diagnostic approach, 285
  incidence, 285
  pathophysiology, 285
  risk, 285
  symptoms/complications, 285
  treatment, 285
Dobutamine, 437
Dolor, 21
Dopamine, 436–437
Double bubble sign on AXR, 525
Double-barrel colostomy, 252
Drains, purpose of, 85
Dressler's syndrome, 602
Dry gangrene, 452
Dubost, 41
Ductal carcinoma in situ (DCIS), 366–367
Ductus arteriosus, 475
Ductus venosus, 474, 475
Duhamel procedure, 501, *501*
Dukes' Astler-Coller modified staging system, 278–279
Dukes' classification, 280
Dumping syndrome, 32, 134–135
Duodenal atresia, 494–495
Duodenal perforation, treatment, 236
Duodenal ulcer, 34, 176, 231–233
  correction of bleeding, 236
  intractability, 236
Duodenostomy tube, 85
Duodenum, 255
Dupuytren's contracture, 534, 657
-dynia, 21
Dys-, 21
Dyspareunia, 21
Dysphagia, 21, 564
Dysuria, 691

Eagle-Barrett syndrome, 524
Ear
acute suppurative otitis media, 542–544
Bell's palsy, 546–547
bullous myringitis, 542
cholesteatoma, 541–542
facial nerve paralysis, 546
glomus tumors, 550
malignant otitis externa, 539–540
Meniere's disease, 549
mucoid otitis media, 544–545
otitis externa, 539
otosclerosis, 545
posterior fossa tumors, 551
sensorineural hearing loss, 547–548
serous otitis media, 544
tumors of external, 540
tympanic membrane (TM) perforation, 541
vertigo, 548–549
vestibular neuritis, 549–550
Ebstein's anomaly, 613
Ecchymosis, 21
-ectomy, 21
Ectopic adrenocorticotropic hormone (ACTH) source, 373
Ectopic adrenocorticotropic hormone (ACTH)-producing tumor, 375, 376
Edrophonium, 174
Edwards' procedure, 619
Efferent, 21
Efferent loop syndrome, 132–133
Eisenmenger's syndrome, 610
Ejection fraction, 600
Elbow dislocation, 653, 654
Elective lymph node dissection, 431
Electrical burns, 222
Electrical shock, 653
Electrocautery, 69
Electrolyte-mediated ileus, 110
Electrolytes
in colon, 182
imbalances, 104–110
Elemental tube feed, 146
Emphysema, 575
conjunctivae, 712
Encephalopathy, 324
stage III, 633
stage IV, 633
Enchondroma, 659
End colostomy, 252
Endarterectomy, 21
carotid, 464
Endocarditis, infectious, 608–609
Endocrine function of pancreas, 342
Endocrine glands. (*See* Adrenal glands; Parathyroid glands; Thyroid glands.)
Endophthalmitis, 711
Endoscopic cystogastrostomy, 352
Endoscopic retrograde cholangiopancreatography, 328
Endotracheal intubation, 205
End-to-side portacaval shunt, 324
Enema
barium, 305
Gastrografin, 289
Entamoeba histolytica, 315
Enteral feeding, advantages of, 145
Enteritis, 21
regional, 301
Enterococcus
in urinary tract infection (UTI), 153
in wound infections, 154
Enterocolitis, necrotizing, 511–512
Enterohepatic circulation, 180, 327
Enterolysis, 21, 79, 79
Entrapment, 569
Enuresis, 692, 708
Ependymomas, 676
Epidermal cancers, 292
Epidermal inclusion cyst, 425
Epidermoid carcinoma, 424
Epididymitis, 691, 704
Epidural analgesia, 173
Epidural anesthesia, 171
Epidural hematoma, 670–671
causes, 35
subdural, 212
Epidural hemorrhage, 689
Epigastric hernia, 192
Epigastric pain, 238
Epiglottitis, 561–562
Epilepsy surgery, 682
Epinephrine, 172, 437
Epispadias, 692
Epistaxis, 551–552
Epithelial cancers, 638
Epithelialization, 254, 527, 528
Eschar, 21
Escharotomy, 228
Escherichia coli
in urinary tract infection (UTI), 153
in wound infections, 154

Esophageal atresia
with tracheoesophageal fistula, *481,* 481–484, *482, 483*
without tracheoesophageal fistula, 480–481
Esophageal carcinoma, 596–598
Esophageal hiatal hernia, 198–200
Esophageal manometry, 593, 594
Esophageal reflux, 594–595
Esophageal strictures, 595–596
Esophageal varices, 320, 321
bleeding from, 242–243, 321
Esophagus, 275
diseases
achalasia, 592–593
anatomic considerations, 591
oropharyngeal dysphagia, 591–592
Esotropia, 711
Esthesioneuroblastoma, 571
Ethmoid sinus, 538
Eversion, 640
Ewing's sarcoma, 659, 660, 661
Excisional biopsy, 21, 420, 425, 430
Exocrine function of pancreas, 342
Exotropia, 711
Exploratory laparotomy, 81, *81*
Exposure, 210–212
Extended lymph node dissection, 249
External oblique muscle, 195
External pancreatic fistula, 273
Extra-anatomic bypass graft, 460
Extracellular fluid, subcompartments of, 98
Extracorporeal membrane oxygenation, 475
Extraperitoneal minor bladder rupture, treatment, 219
Extrathoracic metastases, 579
Exudate, properties of, 574
Eyeball orbit, bones, 538

Facelift, 527
Facial fractures
mandible, 566–567
midface, *567,* 567–568, *568*
Facial nerve paralysis, 546
Falciform ligament, 307
Fallopian tube, 490
False aneurysm, 447
Familial hypocalciuric hypercalcemia, 407
Familial polyposis, 282–283
Famotidine (Pepcid), 122
Fascia, 21
Fat emboli syndrome, 139
Fat necrosis, 370
Fatal anaphylaxis, 316
Fat-soluble vitamins, absorption, 144
Fatty acid deficiency, 145
Felon, 533
Femoral artery to popliteral artery distal bypass, 81, *81, 451*
Femoral fractures, 656
Femoral hernia, 198
definition, 192
Femoral vein catheter, 208
Femoral vessels, 95
Fentanyl, 175
Fetal circulation, 474–475
Fever, 163–164
in Intensive Care Unit (ICU), 433
postoperative, 163–164
Fibrin glue, 116
Fibroadenoma, 369, 371
Fibrocystic disease, 361, 370, 371
Fibroplasia, 528
Fibrosarcoma, 419, 420
Fibrous dysplasia, 659, 660
Fibrous histiocytoma, 420
Fibroxanthoma, 659
Figure of eight suture, 116, *116*
Fine needle aspiration, 395
First degree A-V block, 621
First degree burns, 222
treatment, 224
Fissure, anal, 294–295
Fistulas, 21, 270–273
in ano, 271–273, *273,* 293
bladder, 273
cholecystenteric, 271
colonic, 271
colovesical, 271
definition, 270
enterocutaneous, 270–271
external pancreatic, 273
gastrocolic, 271
pancreatic, 355
pancreatic enteric, 273
predisposing factors and conditions of, 270
refractory pancreatic, 273
vesicoenteric, 273
vesicovaginal, 273
Fitz-Hugh–Curtis syndrome, 31, 162
Fixation, 640

Flail chest, 206
Flexor digitorum profundus, 533
Flexor digitorum superficialis, 533
Fluconazole (Diflucan), 120
Fluids and electrolytes, 98–110
Flumazenil, 175
Focal nodular hyperplasia, 311–312
Fog reduction elimination device (FRED®), 203
Fogarty balloon catheter, 454
Folate deficiency, 144
Foley catheter, 22, 92, 175, 690, 710
  bladder decompression, 208
  contraindications to placement of, 209
Folic acid, 688
Follicular adenocarcinoma, 396–397
Foot dorsiflexion, 639
Foramen of Winslow, 245
Foramen ovale, 474
Forceps, 42, *42*, 43, *43*
Foregut, 95
Foreign body, aspirated, 478–479
Foreskin, disadvantages, 491
Forssman, 41
Fossa of Geraldi, 489
Fothergill's sign, 27
4/2/1 rule, 102
Four-compartment fasciotomy, 212
Fournier's gangrene, 160, 690
Fox's sign, 27, 346
Fractional excretion of sodium, 435–436
Fractures, 643–650
  angulated, 647
  avulsion, 647, *647*
  basilar skull, 210, 669
  Bennett's, 649
  blowout, 569
  boxer's, 534, 649, *649*
  calcaneus, 653
  chance, 674
  clavicle, 652
  clay shoveler's, 649, 674
  Colles', 648, *648*
  comminuted, 644, *644*
  displaced, 647, *647*
  Galeazzi, 650
  greenstick, 646, *646*, 663
  hangman's, 649, 674
  humeral shaft, 655
  humerus, 653
  impaction, 645
  intra-articular, 648
  Jefferson's, 674
  knee, 655–656
    drawer test of, 655
    ligaments of, 655
    meniscus of, 655
  laryngeal, 219
  Le Fort, *567*, 567–568, *568*
  longitudinal, 645
  mandible, 566–567
  mandibular, 211
  maxillofacial, 209
  midface, *567*, 567–568, *568*
  Monteggia's, 649
  oblique, 645, *645*
  odontoid, 674, 675, *675*
  open, 643, 651
  pathologic, 646, *646*
  pediatric, 667
  pelvic, 212, 216, 219, 650
  periarticular, 648
  Pott's, 650
  rotated, 647
  simple, 643
  skull, 673
  Smith's, 649
  spiral, 645, *645*
  stress, 646
  tibial, 649, 656
  torus, 646, 663
  transcervical, 649
  transverse, 644, *644*
  tripod, *568*, 568–569
  unstable, 640
Frank-Starling curve, 438
Free flap, 530
Frequency, 22, 691
Fresh frozen plasma (FFP), 111
Frey's syndrome, 570
5-FU for colon cancer, 279
Full-thickness injury, 228
Functional endoscopic sinus surgery (FESS), 554
Fundus of gallbladder, 326
Furosemide (Lasix), 122
Furuncle, 22, 161

G cells, 179
G6PD deficiency, 413
Galeazzi fracture, 650
Gallbladder
  carcinoma, 337–338
  emptying, 327

fundus of, 326
infundibulum, 326
porcelain, 339
valves, 326
Gallbladder emptying
inhibitors of, 180
stimulators, 180
Gallicurci, 393
Gallstone ileus, 336–337
Gallstone pancreatitis, 345–346
Gallstones, 182, 251
complications of, 331
radiopaque, 167
Gamekeeper's thumb, 535
Ganciclovir, complications of, 637
Gangrene
dry, 452
Fournier's, 160, 690
wet, 452
Gardner's syndrome, 31, 283
Gastrectomy, distal, 238
Gastric acid production, 237
Gastric bypass, 250, 251
Gastric cancer, 247–249
Gastric decompression, 208, 209
Gastric dilation, 128
Gastric distention, 524
Gastric outlet obstruction, 236
Gastric physiology, 245–246
Gastric ulcers, 176, 229, 237–239
Gastrin, 181, 246
Gastrinoma, 388
Gastrinoma triangle, 95, 386
Gastritis
acute, 229
stress, 241
Gastrocolic fistula, 271
Gastrocolic reflex, 183
Gastroduodenal artery, 94
Gastroduodenostomy, antrectomy with, 75
Gastroenteritis, 188
Gastroesophageal reflux disease (GERD), 246–247, 492–493
Gastrografin enema, 289
Gastrointestinal anastomosis (GIA) device, 60
Gastrointestinal (GI) bleeding
in pediatric surgery, 486
postoperative, 165
Gastrointestinal (GI) carcinoids, 34
Gastrointestinal (GI) complications, 128–135
Gastrointestinal (GI) hormones and physiology, 179–183
Gastrointestinal (GI) lymphoma, 423
Gastrojejunostomy, antrectomy with, 75
Gastropexy, 22
Gastroschisis, 504, 505–506
differences between omphalocele and, 506
Gastrostomy, 252
Gastrostomy tube, 85
General anesthesia, 171
General endotracheal anesthesia, 171
Gentamicin, 117, 118
Gerota's fascia, 94
GIA stapler, 48, *48*
Giant cell tumor, 659
Gibbon, John, 40
Gilbert's syndrome, 340
Glasgow Coma Scale (GCS), 209, 668–669
scoring system, 209–210
Glaucoma, 713
Gleason histologic grading system, 697–698
Gliomas, 676–677
Glisson's capsule, 307
Globus, 564
Glomus tumors, 550
Glottic lesions, 563–564
Glucagonoma, stimulation test used for, 384
Gluconoma, 383–384
Glutamine, 181
Goiter, toxic multinodular, 401
Gomco clamp, 690
Goodsall's rule, 27, 272, 293
Gout, 662
Grafts
skin, 529–530
treating infection, 460
Graham patch, 79, *79*, 233, *233*, 239, 240
Granulation tissue, 528
Graves' disease, 400–401
Greenfield filter, 127, *127*
Greenstick fracture, 646, *646*, 663
Grey Turner's sign, 27, 346
Grynfeltt-Lesshaft's triangle, boundaries of, 193
Grynfeltt's hernia, 191

Guarding
involuntary, 184
voluntary, 184
Gubernaculum, 94, 195, 490
Gunshot wound, treatment, 218
Gynecologic pain, differential diagnosis, 187
Gynecomastia, male, 372

Halsted, William, 39, 41
Hamburger sign, 264, 508
Hamman's sign/crunch, 27, 243
Hammerhead, 6
Hangman's fracture, 649, 674
Hardy, 41
Hartmann's pouch, 82, *82*, 252, 326
Hartmann's procedure, 77
Hashimoto's thyroiditis, 402–403
Hasson technique, 202
Head trauma, 668–670
Heart transplant, 40, 635
Heart-lung transplant, 41
Heberden's nodes, 662
Heel spur, 657
Heineke-Mikulicz pyloroplasty, 80, *80*
Helicobacter pylori in peptic ulcer disease, 231
Hemangioma, 22, 35, 310, 524
hepatic, 312–313
treatment, 524
Hematemesis, 22
Hematochezia, 229, 277, 298
Hematoma, 22
epidural, 670–671
subdural, 671–672
Hematuria, 692, 695, 706
Hemicolectomy, 82, *82*, 269
right, 266
Hemobilia, 317
Hemodynamic monitoring, 440–442
Hemophilia A, 113, 114
Hemophilia B, 113, 114
Hemoptysis, 22, 575–576, 576
Hemorrhage
epidural, 689
intracerebral, 681–682, 689
subarachnoid, 680–681, 689
traumatic subarachnoid, 672
Hemorrhagic pancreatitis, 346
Hemorrhoid quadrants, 296
Hemorrhoidectomy
complications, 296
contraindications, 297
Hemorrhoids, 295–297, 320
causes, 296
classification by degrees, 296
external, 296
internal, 296
signs/symptoms, 295
Hemothorax, 22
massive, 207, 219
Hemotympanum, 669
Henoch-Schönlein syndrome, 524
Heparin, 120–121
Heparin rebound, 604
Heparin-induced thrombocytopenic thrombosis (Hitt) syndrome, 33
Hepatic hemangioma, 312–313
Hepatic veins, thrombosis of, 321
Hepatic venous drainage, 308
Hepatitis B virus as risk factor in hepatocellular carcinoma, 313
Hepato-, 22
Hepatoblastoma, 522, 526
Hepatocellular adenoma, 311
Hepatocellular carcinoma, 310, 313–314
Hepatocytes, 309
Hepatoenteric anastomosis, 336
Hepatoma, 311
Hepatorenal syndrome, 317
Hernia sac, 195
Hernias, 34, 190–200
Bochdalek's, 192
classic intraoperative inguinal, 195–197, *196, 197*
congenital diaphragmatic, 484–485
Cooper's, 192
danger, 190
definition, 190
direct inguinal, 193–194
epigastric, 192
esophageal hiatal, 198–200
femoral, 192, 198
Grynfeltt's, 191
Hesselbach's, 192
hiatal, 193
incidence, 190
incisional, 191
indirect inguinal, 193, 194–195, 200
inguinal, 193, 486–491
internal, 191
intraparietal, 192
Littre's, 191, 260
lumbar, 191

Morgagni's, 192
obturator, 191
pantaloon, 191
paraesophageal hiatal, 198–199
Petit's, 191
precipitating factors, 190
properitoneal, 192
repair, 190
Richter's, 192
sliding, 191
sliding esophageal hiatal, 199–200, 200
spigelian, 191
umbilical, 192, 523
ventral, 191
Herniorrhaphy, 22
Herpes simplex virus (HSV), signs/symptoms of, 637
Hesitancy, 22, 691
Hess, 41
Hesselbach's hernia, 192
Hesselbach's triangle, 95, *196*, 196–197, 487
boundaries, 193
Heterotopic, 623
Heterotopic pancreatic tissue, 355
Hiatal hernia, 193
esophageal, 198–200
sliding, 199–200, 200
paraesophageal, 198–199
Hiatus, 22
Hickman® catheter, 93
Hickman-type catheter, 93
Hidradenitis, 22
High-dose dexamethasone suppression test, 374
Highly selective vagotomy, 78, *78*
Hindgut, 95
Hip dislocation, 216, 653, 654
congenital, 663
Hirschsprung's disease, 498, 499–502
surgery, 502
Histocompatibility antigens, 623
History and physical exam report, 8
HLA crossmatching, 628
Hodgkin's disease
histopathologic types of, 421
stages, 422
staging laparotomy, 421
Hodgkin's lymphoma, staging laparotomy, 422
Homans' sign, 27
Horizontal mattress stitch, 57, *57*
Horner's syndrome, 579, 689, 715
Howship-Romberg sign, 27, 200
5-HT, 268
Huggins, 41
Human bites, 160
Human chorionic gonadotropin (β-hCG), 186, 409
Human leukocyte antigen, 624
Humeral shaft fractures, 655
Humerus fracture, 653
Humoral immunity, 624
Hungry bone syndrome, 410
Hürthle cell adenoma, 399
Hürthle cell carcinoma, 399
Hürthle cell thyroid cancer, 398–399
Hutchinson's freckle, 429
Hydatid liver cysts, 316
Hydrocele, 489, 691
Hydrocephalus, 686–687
communicating versus noncommunicating, 686
Hydrocephalus ex vacuo, 687
Hydrops of gallbladder, 340
5-Hydroxyindoleacetic acid (5-HIAA), 268
Hyperacute rejection, 628
Hyperaldosteronism, 380, 418
secondary, 381
Hyperbilirubinemia, 513
Hypercalcemia, 106–107, 418
differential diagnosis, 407
Hyperchloremic acidosis, 498
Hyperglycemia, 108
Hyperkalemia, 104–105
Hypermagnesemia, 108
Hypernatremia, 105
Hyperparathyroidism, 405–406, 417–418
primary, 406–409
secondary, 408
tertiary, 408
Hyperplasia, 389
benign prostatic, 698–700
bilateral, 382
focal nodular, 311–312
parathyroid, 387
refractory, 405
unilateral, 382
Hypersplenism, 414
Hypertension
in cancer, 418
in coarctation, 417
in Conn's syndrome, 418

in Cushing's syndrome, 418
diastolic, 417
in hyperparathyroidism, 418
in increased intracranial pressure, 418
in neuroblastoma, 416
in pheochromocytoma, 417
portal, 318–324, 415
in renal artery stenosis, 417
in renal parenchymal disease, 418
surgically correctable, 416–418
Hyperthermia, malignant, 173–175
Hypertrophic pulmonary osteoarthropathy, 582
Hypertropia, 711
Hypervolemia, 100, 418
Hyphema, 711
Hypocalcemia, 107–108
Hypochloremic alkalosis, 100
Hypogastric artery, 96
Hypoglossal nerve, 465, 538
Hypoglycemia, 109
Hypokalemia, 105, 418
Hypomagnesemia, 108
Hyponatremia, 106
Hypospadiasis, 693
Hyposplenism, 414
Hypotension, 141
Hypothyroidism, 401
Hypotropia, 711
Hypoventilation, 440
Hypovolemia, 100
physiologic response, 99
Hypovolemic shock, 147–148, 208
Hypoxia, 141
Hytrin, 699

^{131}I uptake, 396
Icterus, 22
Idiopathic hypertrophic subaortic stenosis, 611
Ileal atresia, 495–496
Ileal conduit, 253
Ileoanal pull-through, 82, *82*
Ileostomy, 22
Ileum, 97, 255
Ileus, 22
meconium, 496–497
Ilioinguinal nerve, 195, 196
IMA artery, 392
^{131}I-MIBG scan, 379
Imipenem (Primaxin), 117, 118
Immunology, 623–624
Immunosuppression, 625, 631
Impaction fracture, 645
Imperforate anus, 498–499
Impotence, 693, 704–705
In situ vein graft, 452
Incarcerated, 190
Incision and drainage, 80, *80*
Incisional biopsy, 22, 420, 425
Incisional hernia, 191
Incisions, *69*, 69–74, *70, 71, 72, 73, 74*
Incomplete, 191
Incontinence, 692, 707–708
Increased intracranial pressure, 418
Indirect inguinal hernia, 193, 194–195, 200
Induration, 23
Infarction, *620*
Infections
aortic graft, 459
central line, 153–154
in transplant surgery, 637
urinary tract, 153
Infectious endocarditis, 608–609
Inflammation, 527
Inflammatory bowel disease (IBD), 301–302
Infundibulum of gallbladder, 326
Inguinal anatomy, 197, *197*
Inguinal hernia, 193, 486–491
classic intraoperative, 195–197, *196, 197*
direct, 193–194
indirect, 193, 194–195, 200
Inguinal herniorrhaphy, 196
Inhalational (volatile) anesthesia, side effects, 173
Inspection in abdominal physical exam, 185
Instrument knot, 63, *64,* 65
Insulinoma, 356, 382
Intensive care note, 11
Intensive Care Unit (ICU), 433
causes of fever in, 433
pneumonia in, 433
Intermittent claudication, 448
Intermittent mandatory ventilation (IMV), 443
Internal hernia, 191
Internal oblique muscle, 195
Interrupted stitch, 57, *57*
Interstitial fluid, 98
Intestinal metastasis, treatment, 431

Intra-abdominal injury, 212, 214
  seat-belt use, 219
Intra-aortic balloon pump (IABP), 621
Intra-articular fracture, 648
Intracavernous vasoactive injection, 705
Intracellular fluid, 98
Intracerebral hemorrhage, 681–682, 689
Intracranial pressure (ICP), 669
  decreasing, 670
Intraductal papilloma, 368, 370
Intramedullary rod placement, 656
Intraoperative cholangiogram, 328
  indications, 332
Intraparietal hernia, 192
Intraperitoneal bladder rupture, 710
Intravascular fluid, 98
Intravenous access, sites, 208
Intravenous pyelogram (IVP), 692
Intravenous pyelography, 468
Intrinsic factor, 179, 246
Intussusception, 23, 508–510, 526
Intussusceptum, 509, *509*
Inversion, 640
Involuntary guarding, 184
Ipsilateral decubitus CXR, 169
Irish's node, 248
Iritis, 715
Iron absorption, 144, 182
Ischemia, *620*
  acute mesenteric, 461–462
  chronic mesenteric, 461
  colonic, 459
Islet cell tumor, 356
Isoflurane, 689
Isograft, 623
Isolated adrenal metastasis, 432
Isolated lung metastasis, 432
Isoproterenol, 437
Isthmectomy, 399
-itis, 23
ITP, 414–415

J tube, 129
Jackson-Pratt (JP) drain, 85
Jaundice
  obstructive, 327, 329–330
  physiologic, 513
Jaw thrust, 205
Jefferson's fracture, 674
Jejunal atresia, 495
Jejunojejunostomy, 76
Jejunostomy, 252
Jejunostomy tube, 85
Jejunum, 97, 255
Jewett/Marshall system, 695
Juvenile nasopharyngeal angiofibroma, 555–556
Juvenile polyps, 284

Kanavel's sign, 533
Kaposi's sarcoma, 419
Kasai, 514
Kehr's sign, 27
Kelly clamp, 45, *45*
Kelly's sign, 27
Keloid, 529
Ketamine, 689
Kidney, ureters, and bladder (KUB), 167
Kidney stones, 37, 170
  patient position, 185
  radiopaque, 167
Kidney transplant, 72, *72*
  history, 630
  immunosuppression, 631
  rejection, 632
  statistics, 630–631
Kissing ulcers, 237, 240
Kjellberg, 670
Klatskin's tumor, 328, 339
Klebsiella in urinary tract infection (UTI), 153
Knee
  dislocation, 653, 654–655
  drawer test, 655
  ligaments, 655
  meniscus, 655
  pain, 653
Kocher, Theodor, 39, 41
Kocher clamp, 49, *49*
Kocher maneuver, 77, 342
Kocher's incision, 69, *69*
Kock pouch, 252
Krukenberg tumor, 27, 248

Laceration, 529
Lactated Ringer's (LR) solution, 101, 208
Lactic acidosis, 434
Lactulose for hepatic encephalopathy, 324
Ladd's bands, 503
Ladd's procedure, 503
Langer's lines, 527
Lap appy, 23, 79, *79*
Lap chole, 23, 79, *79*, 332

Laparoscopic appendectomy, 202, 264
Laparoscopic cholecystectomy, 201–202
Laparoscopic hernia, 202
Laparoscopic inguinal hernia repair, indications, 202
Laparoscopic-assisted procedure, 203
Laparoscopy, 23, 201–203
camera use during, 7
driving camera during, 203
Laparotomy, 23
Laplace's law, 28
Large bowel obstruction, 35
Laryngeal fracture, 219
Laryngomalacia, 477
Laryngotracheobronchitis, 560–561
Larynx
anatomy, 560
croup (laryngotracheobronchitis), 560–561
epiglottitis, 561–562
glottic lesions, 563–564
malignant lesions, 562
modified neck dissection, 565
radical neck dissection, 565
supraglottic lesions, 563
Le Fort fractures, *567*, 567–568, *568*
Left bundle branch block (LBBB), 621
Left hepatic lobectomy, 310
Left testicular vein, drainage, 94
Legg-Calvé-Perthes disease, 664
Leiomyoma, 23, 258
Leiomyosarcoma, 23, 419, 420
Lembert stitch, 60, *60*
Lens detachment, 712
Lentigo maligna melanoma, 428, 429
Leriche's syndrome, 31, 450
Levamisole chemotherapy for colon cancer, 279
Leveling colostomy, 500
Lichtenstein herniorrhaphy, 76
Lidocaine, 172
signs of toxicity, 174
Ligament of Berry, 392
Ligamentous C-spine injury, 169
Lipase, 355
Lipoid pneumonia, 479
Lipoma, cord, 196
Liposarcoma, 419, 420
Lister, Joseph, 39
Littre's hernia, 191, 260
Littre's inguinal hernia, 490
Liver
anatomy, *307*, 307–310, *308*
blood supply, 183
Child's classification, 309*t*, 309–310
malignancy, 35
tumors, 310–314
Liver abscesses, 314–316
amoebic, 315–316
bacterial, 314–315
hemobilia, 317
hydatid cysts, 316
Liver disease, signs/symptoms, 309
Liver failure, 633
Liver metastases, treatment, 280
Liver transplant, 40, 72, *72*, 632–634
rejection, 633–634
Lobectomy, 399
left hepatic, 310
right hepatic, 310
Lobectomy/isthmectomy, 397
Lobular carcinoma in situ, 368–369
Local anesthesia, 171
Longitudinal fracture, 645
Loop colostomy, 253, *253*
Low anterior resection (LAR), 77, 279
Low-dose dexamethasone suppression test, 374
Lower extremity amputations, 452–453
Lower extremity arterial insufficiency ulcer, 176
Lower gastrointestinal (GI) bleeding, 298–300
causes, 298
diagnostic tests, 298–300, *299*
signs, 298
symptoms, 298
treatment, 298, 300
Lucid interval, 689
Lumbar disc herniation, 682–683
Lumbar hernia, obturator, 191
Lumpectomy and radiation, 80, *80*, 365
Lung abscess, 575
hemoptysis, 575–576
mesothelioma, 576–578
spontaneous pneumothorax, 576
Lung transplant, 41, 636
Lungs
diseases
bronchogenic carcinoma, 578–582
carcinoid tumors, 584–585
pulmonary sequestration, 585
solitary pulmonary nodules, 582–583

Luschka, ducts of, 325
Lymph node metastasis, 367
Lymphangiosarcoma, 419
Lymphocytotoxic crossmatching, 628
Lymphoma, 258, 421–422, 571, 588
  gastrointestinal (GI), 423
  post-transplant, 638

Macrophage, 624
Mafenide, 227
Maintenance fluids, calculation, 102–104
Male breast cancer, 369–370
Male gynecomastia, 372
Malignancy in transplant surgery, 637–638
Malignant fibrous histiocytoma, 419, 420
Malignant hyperthermia, 173–175
Malignant melanoma, 659
Malignant mucoid adenocarcinoma, 266
Malignant neurilemmoma or schwannoma, 419
Malignant otitis externa (MOE), 539–540
Mallory-Weiss syndrome, 241–242
Malrotation, 526
  and midgut volvulus, 502–504
Mammary "milk line," 359
Mammogram, 363
Mammoplasty, 527
Mandible fractures, 566–567
Mandibular fracture, 211
Marginal ulcer, 176, 239
Marjolin's ulcer, 176, 425
Massive hemothorax, 207, 219
Mastectomy
  modified radical, 365
  simple, 79, *79*, 367
Mastitis, 372
Maxillofacial fracture, 209
McBurney, Charles, 39
McBurney's point, 28, 70, *70*, 96, 263
McBurney's sign, 28
McVay herniorrhaphy, 76
Mean arterial pressure, 435, 600
Mebendazole for hydatid liver cysts, 316
Mechanical ventilation, 442–445
Meckel's diverticulectomy, 259
Meckel's diverticulum, 37, 258–260, 510–511
  rule of 2s, 28
Meckel's scan, 260, 511
Meconium ileus, 496–497
Meconium peritonitis, 497
Meconium plug syndrome, 497–498
Median arcuate ligament syndrome, 462
Mediastinal anatomy, 585–586
Mediastinitis, 589
Mediastinum
  diseases
    chronic mediastinitis, 589
    lymphoma, 588
    mediastinal anatomy, 585–586
    mediastinitis, 589
    primary mediastinal tumors, 586–588
    superior vena cava syndrome, 589–591
Medullary carcinoma, 397–398
Medulloblastoma, 676, 678
Melanoma, 424, 427–432
  A, B, C, Ds, 25, 427
  acral lentiginous, 428
  anal, 292, 432
  definition, 427
  lentigo maligna, 428, 429
  in men, 428
  nodular, 428
  risk factors, 427
  sites, 427
  staging, 429–432
  superficial spreading, 428
  types, 34
  in women, 428
Melena, 23
Mendelson's syndrome, 33
MEN-I syndrome, 384
Meniere's disease, 549
  classic triad, 570–571
Meningeal carcinomatosis, 679
Meningiomas, 677
Meningitis, postneurosurgery, 689
Mental status change, 141
Meperidine (Demerol), 119
  side effects, 173
6-Mercaptopurine (6-MP) for inflammatory bowel disease, 306
Mesalamine for inflammatory bowel disease, 306
Mesenteric adenitis, 266
Mesenteric embolus, treatment, 462
Mesenteric ischemia, diagnosis, 189
Mesenteric lymphadenitis, 507
Mesoappendix, 261
Mesothelioma, 576–578
Metabolic acidosis, 100, 436
Metabolic alkalosis, 100

Metallic skin staples, 59, *59*
Metaphysis, 642, *643*
Metastatic tumors, 659, 678–679
Methimazole for Graves' disease, 401
Metoclopramide (Reglan), 122
Metronidazole (Flagyl), 117, 118, 119
Metzenbaum scissors, 47, *47*
Mezlocillin (Mezlo), 119
Microcytic anemia, 112, 277
Midface fractures, *567*, 567–568, *568*
Midgut, 95
Midline laparotomy, 70, *70*
Mikulicz's syndrome, 570
Milk leg, 469
Millard-Gubler syndrome, 689
Minute ventilation, 442
Miosis, 711
Mirizzi's syndrome, 33, 340
Mitotane, 376
Mitral regurgitation (MR), 607–608
Mitral stenosis (MS), 606–607
Mittelschmerz, 28
Modified radical mastectomy, 80, *80*, 365
Mohs' surgery, 426
Mondor's disease, 621
Monro-Kellie hypothesis, 669
Monteggia fracture, 649
Morbid obesity, 250
Morgagni's hernia, 192
Morphine, side effects, 173
Morison's pouch, 94
Motion pain, 184
Mucoepidermoid carcinoma, 571
Mucoid otitis media, 544–545
Mucous neck cells, 179
Mucus fistula, 77, 252
Multiple endocrine neoplasia, 387
  MEN type I, 387–388
  MEN type IIA, 388
  MEN type IIB, 388–389
Multiple myeloma, 659
Multiple organ failure (MOF), 436
Munchausen syndrome, 32
Murphy's sign, 28, 333
Murray, 40, 41
Myasthenia gravis, 587
Mydriasis, 711
Myelomeningocele, 687–688
Myocardial infarction, 138, 458
Myofibroblasts, 528
Myoglobinuria, 222
Myopia, 711
Myxoma, 614

Nafcillin, 119
Najarian, 41
Naloxone (Narcan), 175
Narcotics, reversing, 175
Nasal cavity cancer, 555
Nasal septal hematoma, 211
Nasogastric decompression, 226
Nasogastric tubes (NGT), 91–92
Nasotracheal intubation, 205
Neck, anatomy, 217, *217*
Necrosis, pancreatic, 347
Necrotic, 23
Necrotic sigmoid colon, 459
Necrotizing enterocolitis, 511–512
Necrotizing fasciitis, 157
Needle thoracostomy, 206
Needle-driver, 44, *44*
Needle-gauge size, 93
Negative feedback loop, 393
Nelson's syndrome, 377
Neoplastic polyps, subtypes, 281
Neostigmine, 174
Nephrolithiasis, 188
Nephrostomy, perc, 690
Neuhauser's sign, 496
Neural tube defects, 687–688
Neurilemmoma, 419
Neuroblastoma, 416, 519–521, 524, 526
Neurogenic shock, 150–151
Neurogenic tumors, 588
Neurosurgery, 668–689
  cerebral contusion, 672
  epidural hematoma, 670–671
  head trauma, 668–670
  pediatric
    craniosynostosis, 688–689
    hydrocephalus, 686–687
    spinal dysraphism/neural tube defects, 687–688
  skull fracture, 673
  spinal cord trauma, 673–674
  spine
    cervical disc disease, 683–684
    lumbar disc herniation, 682–683
    spinal epidural abscess, 684–685
    syringomyelia, 685
  subdural hematoma, 671–672
  traumatic subarachnoid hemorrhage, 672

tumors
cerebellar astrocytomas, 677–678
general, 675–676
gliomas, 676–677
medulloblastoma, 678
meningiomas, 677
metastatic, 678–679
vascular
epilepsy, 682
intracerebral hemorrhage, 681–682
occlusive cerebrovascular disease, 679
subarachnoid hemorrhage, 680–681
Nipple discharge, bloody, 368
Nissen, 79, *79*
Nitroglycerin (NTG), 437–438
Nitrous oxide, contraindications, 172
No man's land, 531
Nocturia, 691
Nodal metastasis, treatment, 431
Nodular melanoma, 428
Noncommunicating hydrocele, 489, 691
Nonpolarizing neuromuscular blocker pancuronium, side effect, 172
Nonseminomatous disease, 702
Non-union, 642
Norepinephrine, 437
Normal saline, 101
Nose and paranasal sinuses
acute, 553–554
acute rhinitis, 552
allergic rhinitis, 552–553
cancer of nasal cavity, 555
chronic, 554
epistaxis, 551–552
juvenile nasopharyngeal angiofibroma, 555–556
Nutcracker esophagus, 593–594
Nutrition
pediatric needs, 473–474
surgical, 143–146
Nylon, 55
Nystagmus, 711
Nystatin, 120

Obesity, morbid, 250
Oblique fracture, 645, *645*
Oblique muscle
external, 195
internal, 195
Obstipation, 23
Obstructive jaundice, 327, 329–330
Obturator hernia, 191
Obturator sign, 28, 262
Occlusive cerebrovascular disease, 679
Octreotide, 269, 273
Ocular trauma, 711–713
Odontoid fracture, 674, 675, *675*
Odynophagia, 23, 564
Ogilvie's syndrome, 31
OKT3, 627, *627*
Omeprazole (Prilosec), 122
Omohyoid muscle, 465
Omphalocele, 504–505
differences between gastroschisis and, 506
100/50/20 rule, 102
Op note, 9
Open fractures, 643
classification of, 651
risks in, 651
treatment, 651
Open reduction, 640
indications, 650
Operating room, 6–7
Operative wound classification, 154–157
Ophthalmology, 711–715
cornea, 714
diabetic retinopathy, 713–714
glaucoma, 713
ocular trauma, 712–713
red eye, 714–715
terminology in, 711
Opsonins, 414
Orbital cellulitis, 715
Orchidopexy, 523
Orchiectomy, 702
Orchiopexy, 709
Orchitis, 691
Organ preservation, 629–630
Organs of Zuckerkandl, 380
Oropharyngeal dysphagia, 591–592
-orraphy, 23
Ortho bowel routine (OBR), 129
Orthopaedic emergencies, 650–651
Orthopaedic infections
osteomyelitis, 657–658
septic arthritis, 658
Orthopaedic surgery
abbreviations, 639
arthritis, 661–662
dislocations
elbow, 654
hip, 654

knee, 654–655
shoulder, 654
fractures, 643–650
general principles, 642–643
infections
osteomyelitis, 657–658
septic arthritis, 658
knee dislocations, 655–656
drawer test of, 655
ligaments of, 655
meniscus of, 655
knee fractures, 655–656
drawer test of, 655
ligaments of, 655
meniscus of, 655
pediatric, 663–667
congenital hip dislocation, 663
Salter classification, 664–667, *666*, *667*
scoliosis, 663–664
rotator cuff, 656–657
terminology in, 639–642
trauma, 650–653
tumors, 658–660
Ewing's sarcoma, 661
osteosarcoma, 660–661
Orthopaedics, pediatric, 663–667
Orthotopic, 623
Ortolani's sign, 663
Osgood-Schlatter's disease, 664
Osteoarthritis, 661, 662
Osteochondroma, 659, 661, 667
Osteoid osteoma, 659
Osteomyelitis, 657–658
Osteosarcoma, 659, 660–661
Osteotomy, 642
Ostomies, 23, 252–254
Otitis externa (swimmer's ear), 539, 569
Otitis media, 569
Otolaryngology
anatomy, 536–539
ear
acute suppurative otitis media, 542–544
Bell's palsy, 546–547
bullous myringitis, 542
cholesteatoma, 541–542
facial nerve paralysis, 546
glomus tumors, 550
malignant otitis externa, 539–540
Meniere's disease, 549
mucoid otitis media, 544–545
otitis externa, 539
otosclerosis, 545
posterior fossa tumors, 551
sensorineural hearing loss, 547–548
serous otitis media, 544
tumors of external, 540
tympanic membrane (TM) perforation, 541
vertigo, 548–549
vestibular neuritis, 549–550
facial fractures
mandible, 566–567
midface, *567*, 567–568, *568*
larynx
anatomy, 560
croup (laryngotracheobronchitis), 560–561
epiglottitis, 561–562
glottic lesions, 563–564
malignant lesions, 562
modified neck dissection, 565
radical neck dissection, 565
supraglottic lesions, 563
nose and paranasal sinuses
acute, 553–554
acute rhinitis, 552
allergic rhinitis, 552–553
cancer of nasal cavity and, 555
chronic, 554
epistaxis, 551–552
juvenile nasopharyngeal angiofibroma, 555–556
oral cavity and pharynx
cancer of, 558
peritonsillar abscess, 557
pharyngotonsillitis, 556–557
salivary gland tumors, 559–560
-otomy, 23
Otosclerosis, 545
Ovarian torsion, position of patient with, 185
Ovary, 490
Overflow incontinence, 707, 708
Overwhelming postsplenectomy sepsis (OPSS), 413
Oxygen delivery, 435, 439
Oxygen saturation, 435, 440
Oxygenation, 442

Packed red blood cells (PRBCs), 111
Paget's disease of breast, 369
Paget-von Schroetter syndrome, 572

Pain
  abdominal, 184–189
  epigastric, 238
  motion, 184
  periumbilical, 261, 262
  referred, 187
Painless jaundice, 353
Palpable lymph node metastasis, treatment, 431
Palpation in abdominal physical exam, 185
Pancoast's tumor, 578
Pancreas, 341–342
  abscess, 347
  annular, 355, 517
  blood supply, 341
  ducts, 341
  endocrine function, 342
  exocrine function, 342
  regions, 341
  removal of head, 341
  transplant, 634–635
Pancreatic ascites/pleural effusion, 349–350
Pancreatic carcinoma, 352–355
  location, 353
  presentation, 353
  prognosis, 355
  risk factors, 352
  treatment, 353–354
  types, 353
Pancreatic divisum, 355
Pancreatic endocrine insufficiency, 348
Pancreatic enteric fistula, 273
Pancreatic exocrine insufficiency, 348
Pancreatic fistula, 355
Pancreatic injury, treatment, 220
Pancreatic necrosis, 347
Pancreatic pseudocyst, 350–352
Pancreatic somatostatinoma tumor, 356
Pancreatic transplant, 41
Pancreaticoduodenectomy, 353–354
Pancreaticojejunostomy, 273
Pancreatitis, 188
  acute, 240, 342–345
    complications, 343
    diagnosis, 343
    differential diagnosis, 342–343
    etiology of hypocalcemia, 345
    prognosis, 344
    Ranson's criteria, 344–345
    signs, 342, 343
    symptoms, 342
    treatment, 343
  causes, 34
  chronic, 347–349
  gallstone, 345–346
  hemorrhagic, 346
  pancreatic ascites/pleural effusion, 349–350
  pancreatic pseudocyst, 350–352
    complications, 351
    diagnostic, 350–351
    signs, 350
    symptoms, 350
    treatment, 351–352
  postoperative, 128
Pancuronium, 174
Pannus, 662
Pantaloon hernia, 191
Papillary adenocarcinoma, 395–396
Papilloma, intraductal, 370
Paradoxic alkalotic aciduria, 100
Paraesophageal hiatal hernia, 198–199
Paramedian, 71, *71*
Paranasal sinuses, cancer, 555
Paraneoplastic syndromes, 418, 579
Paraphimosis, 491, 692
Parasternal chest gunshot/stab wound, workup/treatment, 220
Parathyroid carcinoma, 409–410
Parathyroid glands
  anatomy, 404–405
  imaging, 405
  physiology, 405
    hyperparathyroidism, 405–406
    parathyroid carcinoma, 409–410
    primary hyperparathyroidism, 406–409
Parathyroid hyperplasia, 387
Paratopic, 623
Parkland formula, 225
Paronychia, 533
Parotitis, 160
Parrot's beak, 168
Patent ductus arteriosus (PDA), 610
Patent urachus, 525
Pathologic fracture, 646, *646*
Patient-controlled analgesia (PCA) pump, 175
PDS®, 55
Pectus carinatum, 480
Pectus deformity, 479
Pectus excavatum, 480

Pediatric bone tumor, 667
Pediatric fractures, 667
Pediatric neurosurgery
  craniosynostosis, 688–689
  hydrocephalus, 686–687
  spinal dysraphism/neural tube defects, 687–688
Pediatric orthopaedics, 663–667
Pediatric surgery
  abdomen, 486
  anorectal malformations, 498
  appendicitis, 507–508
  aspirated foreign body, 478–479
  biliary tract
    annular pancreas, 517
    atresia, 513–514
    choledochal cyst, 514–516
    cholelithiasis, 516–517
  chest, 479
  congenital diaphragmatic hernia, 484–485
  congenital pyloric stenosis, 493–494
  duodenal atresia, 494–495
  esophageal atresia
    with tracheoesophageal fistula, *481*, 481–484, *482, 483*
    without tracheoesophageal fistula, 480–481
  extracorporeal membrane oxygenation, 475
  fetal circulation, 474–475
  gastroesophageal reflux disease, 492–493
  gastroschisis, 505–506
  Hirschsprung's disease, 499–502
  ileal atresia, 495–496
  imperforate anus, 498–499
  inguinal hernia, 486–491
  intussusception, 508–510
  IV fluids and nutrition, 473–474
  jejunal atresia, 495
  malrotation and midgut volvulus, 502–504
  Meckel's diverticulum, 510–511
  meconium ileus, 496–497
  meconium peritonitis, 497
  meconium plug syndrome, 497–498
  neck, 476
    branchial cleft anomalies, 476–477
    cystic hygroma, 478
    stridor, 477–478
    thyroglossal duct cyst, 476
  necrotizing enterocolitis, 511–512
  omphalocele, 504–505
  pectus carinatum, 480
  pectus deformity, 479
  pectus excavatum, 480
  pulmonary sequestration, 485–486
  testicular torsion, 491–492
  tumors
    hepatoblastoma, 522
    neuroblastoma, 519–521
    rhabdomyosarcoma, 521–522
    Wilms', 517–518
Pelvic fractures, 212, 216, 650
  treatment, 219
Penetrating eye object, 713
Penicillin, 117
Penicillin G, 161
Penrose drain, 85
Pentalogy of Cantrell, 505, 525
Pepsin, 179, 246
Pepsinogen, 246
Peptic ulcer, 176
  perforated, 239–240
Peptic ulcer disease (PUD), 231
Perc nephrostomy, 690
Percentage of recurrence, 289
Percocet, 119
Percussion in abdominal physical exam, 185
Percutaneous, 23
Percutaneous endoscopic gastrostomy (PEG), 80, *80*
Percutaneous transhepatic cholangiogram, 328
Perforated peptic ulcer, 239–240
Perianal warts, 295
Periarticular fracture, 648
Pericarditis, 621
Peripheral nerve injury, 653
Peripheral vascular disease, 447–452
  definition, 447
  signs, 448
  surgical treatment, 449
  symptoms, 448
  ulcers, 448
Perirectal abscess, 293, 294
Peritoneal abscess, 156–157
Peritoneal lavage (DPL), 214–216, 523
Peritoneal signs, 184
Peritoneal tap, positive, 218
Peritonitis, position of patient with, 185
Peritonsillar abscess, 557

Periumbilical pain, 261, 262
Petit's hernia, 191
Petit's triangle, boundaries, 193
Peutz-Jeghers syndrome, 31, 284
-pexy, 24
Peyer patches, 183
Peyronie's disease, 692
Pfannenstiel's incision, 71, *71*
Pharyngotonsillitis, 556–557
Pharynx
  cancer, 558
  peritonsillar abscess, 557
  pharyngotonsillitis, 556–557
  salivary gland tumors, 559–560
Pheochromocytoma, 377–380, 416–417
  bladder, 380
  diagnosis, 378
  rule of 10s, 28, 379
  signs/symptoms, 28, 378
  sites, 379
Phimosis, 491, 692
Phleb-, 24
Phlebolith, 24
Phlegmon, 24
Photon scan, 405
Physiologic jaundice, 513
Physis, 642, *643*
Pigment stones, 330
Plantarflexion, 639
Plasma cells, 624
Plasmapheresis, 415
Plastic surgery, 527
  flaps, 530–531
  hands, 531
    sensory supply to, 532–535
  skin grafts, 529–530
  wound healing, 527–528
    contraction, 528–529
    epithelialization, 528
Platelets, 111
  normal life, 113
Platysma muscle, 465
Pleomorphic adenoma, 571
Pleural effusion, 574–575
Pleurovac® chambers, 88–90, *88–90*
Plica, 24
Plicae circulares, 24, 97
Plicae semilunares, 24
Plummer-Vinson syndrome, 31
Pneumatic equalization tube, 544
Pneumatosis intestinalis, 169
Pneumaturia, 24, 692
Pneumonia, 35
  aspiration, 127–128, 598
  lipoid, 479
Pneumothorax, 24, 206
PO metronidazole (Flagyl) for Crohn's disease, 306
Poland's syndrome, 525
Polydactyly, 527
Polyps
  colon, 280–282
  juvenile, 284
  neoplastic, 281
  rectum, 280–282
Polyuria, 691
Popcorn calcification, 582
Popliteal artery aneurysm, 469
Pop-off suture, 61, *61*
Porcelain gallbladder, 339
Portacath®, 93
Portal hypertension, 318–324, 415
  anatomy, 318
  blood drainage, 318–319
  causes, 319
  and cirrhosis, 319–320
  clinical findings, 320
  pathophysiology, 319
Portal pressure, measurement, 320
Portal vein, 308
Portal-systemic collateral circulation, 320
Positive End Expiration Pressure (PEEP), 444, 445
Positive pressure ventilation, 444
Posterior cord syndrome, 674
Posterior fossa tumors, 551
Posthitis, 491, 691
Postlaparoscopic shoulder pain, 203
Postneurosurgery meningitis, 689
Postoperative atrial fibrillation, 137
Postoperative fever, 163–164
Postoperative gastrointestinal (GI) bleeding, 165
Postoperative note, 9–10
Postoperative pancreatitis, 128
Postoperative renal failure, 139
Postoperative respiratory failure, 124–125
Postoperative SBO/ileus, 129–130
Postpericardiotomy syndrome, 602
Postsplenectomy, complications, 413
Post-transplant lymphoma, 638
Post-transplant lymphoproliferative disease, 638

Posttraumatic arthritis, 661, 662
Postvagotomy diarrhea, 133
Postvoid residual, 692
"POTTS" a vessel, 446
Pott's disease, 650
Pott's fracture, 650
Pott's scissors, 48, *48*
Pouch of Douglas, 96
Pouchitis, 131
Poupart's ligament, 195, 197, *197*
Prednisone, 625
Prehn's sign, 691
Preload, 438, 600
Preoperative note, 8–9
Preperitoneal fat stripe, 169
Presenting on rounds, 5
Pressure support, 444
Priapism, 674, 692
Primary hyperparathyroidism, 406–409
Primary intention, 55
Primary mediastinal tumors, 586–588
Primary survey, 204–212
  airway, 204–205
  breathing, 205–207
  circulation, 207–209
  disability, 209–210
  exposure, 210–212
Primary wound closure, 84
Pringle maneuver, 80, *80*, 317
Prolactin, 360
Prolene, 55
Promethazine (Phenergan), 122
Pronation, 639
Properitoneal hernia, 192
Prophylactic antibiotics, 159–160
Propylthiouracil for Graves' disease, 401
Proscar, 699
Prostate cancer, 696–698, 699, 709
Protamine, side effect of, 622
Proteus in urinary tract infection (UTI), 153
Proximal bile duct cholangiocarcinoma, management, 339
Proximal gastric vagotomy, 234, 236
Pruritus, 353
Pseudocapsule, 421
Pseudocyst, 24
Pseudogout, 662
Pseudohermaphroditism, 691
Pseudohyponatremia, 106
Pseudomembranous colitis, 158–159
Pseudomonas in burn wound infections, 226
Pseudopolyps, 305
Psoas shadow, loss of, 168
Psoas sign, 28, 262
Pterygium, 715
Ptosis, 711
Puestow procedure, 78, *78*, 355
Pulmonary capillary wedge pressure, 434, 441–442
Pulmonary embolism, 125–127
Pulmonary hypertrophic osteoarthropathy, 583
Pulmonary sequestration, 485–486, 585
Pulmonary vascular resistance, 435, 600
Pulse volume recordings, 449
Purse-string suture, 59, *59*
Pus, 24
Pyloric stenosis, 526
Pylorus-preserving Whipple, 354
Pyramidal lobe, 392
Pyridostigmine, 174
Pyuria, 692, 706

Raccoon eyes, 28, 669
Radiation therapy for colon cancer, 279
Radiopaque fecalith, 167
Ranitidine (Zantac), 122
Ranson's criteria, 344–345
Ranula, 570
Rapid-sequence anesthesia induction, 172
Rash, 356
Ray amputation, 453
Raynaud's phenomenon, 470
Rebound tenderness, 184
Reconstruction, breast, 369
Rectal cancer
  incidence, 277
  signs/symptoms, 277
  surgical margin, 279
Rectal disease, 188
Rectal exam, 212
Rectal pain, 188
Rectal penetrating injury, treatment, 219
Rectum
  blood supply, 275
  polyps, 280–282
  venous drainage, 275
Red blood cells (RBCs), normal life, 113
Red eye, 714–715
RED reaction syndrome, 31
Reducible, definition, 190

Reduction, 640
Refeeding syndrome, 33, 145
Referred pain, 187
Reflux, 199
Refractory hyperplasia, 405
Refractory pancreatic fistula, 273
Regional anesthesia, 171
Regional enteritis, 301
Reitz, 41
Rejection, 632, 633–634, 635–636
Relaxing incision, 197
Renal artery stenosis, 417, 467–468
Renal cell carcinoma, 693–694, 709
Renal failure, postoperative, 139
Renal parenchymal disease, 418
Renal stones, 709
Renal transplant, 40
Renal vein renin ratio, 468
Rendu-Osler-Weber (ROW) syndrome, 32
Replogle tube, 525
Respiratory acidosis, 100, 436
Respiratory alkalosis, 100, 436
Respiratory failure, postoperative, 124–125
Respiratory quotient, 143–144
Rest pain, 448
  risk of limb loss with, 450
Retinal detachment, 712
Retinopathy, diabetic, 713–714
Retractor
  Army-Navy, 52, *52*
  Deaver, 51, *51*
  Richardson, 53, *53*
  Sweetheart, 51, *51*
  Weitlander, 52, *52*
Retrograde pyelogram, 690
Retrograde urethrogram (RUG), 216, 690, 710
Retroperitoneal calcification, differential diagnosis, 168
Retroperitoneal injury, 214
Retroperitoneal node dissection, 702
Retroperitoneal varices, 320
Reversible ischemic neurologic deficit (RIND), 463
Reynold's pentad, 29, 334
Rhabdomyosarcoma, 419, 420, 521–522, 571
Rheumatoid arthritis, 662
Rhinitis
  acute, 552
  allergic, 552–553
Rhinoplasty, 527
Rhoades, 40
Rib, blood vessels, 95
Richardson retractor, 53, *53*
Richter's hernia, 192, 490
Riedel thyroiditis, 403
Right bundle branch block (RBBB), 621
Right hepatic lobectomy, 310
Right testicular vein, drainage of, 94
Right-angle clamp, 45, *45*
Ring-enhancing brain lesion, 675
Rotated fracture, 647
Rotator cuff, 656–657
Rotter's lymph nodes, 94
Rotter's nodes, 359
Rounds
  preparation, 4
  presenting, 5
Roux stasis syndrome, 133
Roux-en-Y cystojejunostomy, 352
Roux-en-Y limb, 76, *76*
Rovsing's sign, 29, 262
Rubor, 24
Rugae, 245
Rule of fives, 513
Rule of nines, 223, *223*
Rule of twos, 259, 511
Rule of two-thirds of portal hypertension, 321
Ruptured abdominal aortic aneurysm, 189

Sabiston, David, Jr., 40
Sacral sparing, 673
Saddle embolus, 126
Saint's triad, 29
Saline infusion, 381
Salivary gland tumors, 559–560
Salter classification, 665–667, *666, 667*
Santorini duct, 341
Sarcomas, 258
  soft tissue, 419–421
  types of malignant, 419
Scalpel blades, 50, *50,* 69
Schistosomiasis, 321
Schwannoma, 419
Schwartze's sign, 545
Sciatica, 683
Scissors/needle-driver/clamp, 42, *42*
Sclera buckling therapy, 712
Sclerosing cholangitis, 335–336

Sclerotherapy, 322
via endoscope, 242
Scoliosis, 663–664
Scrotum, attachment of testicle to, 195
Sebaceous cyst, 426
Seborrheic keratosis, 426
Second degree A-V block, 621
Second degree burns, 222
treatment, 224
Secondary hyperaldosteronism, 381
Secondary hyperparathyroidism, 408
Secondary intention, 55
Secondary wound closure, 84
Secretin, 180–181
Secretin stimulation test, 385
Sedative, pediatric, 523
Seizures, 653
Seldinger technique, 77
Selective mesenteric angiography, 230
Selenium deficiency, 145
Seminoma, 701, 702, 703
Sengstaken-Blakemore tamponade balloon, 242
Sensorineural hearing loss, 547–548
Sentinel loops, 168
Septic arthritis, 658
Septic shock, 149–150
Serous otitis media, 544
Serum cortisol, direct test, 374
Sestamibi scan, 405
Seton, 272
Shave biopsy, 430
Sheehan's syndrome, 686–687
Shin splints, 657
Shock
anaphylactic, 151–152
cardiogenic, 150
definition, 147
hypovolemic, 147–148, 208
neurogenic, 150–151
septic, 149–150
signs, 147
spinal, 151
Short bowel syndrome, 129
Short-chain fatty acids, 181
Shoulder dislocation, 653, 654
Shouldice herniorrhaphy, 77
Shunt
end-to-side portocaval, 324
side-to-side portocaval, 324
Shunt fraction, 439–440
Shunt series, 687
Sickle cell disease, 658
Side-to-side portocaval shunt, 324
Sigmoid volvulus, 35, 287, 288–289
diagnosis, 288–289
etiologic factors, 288
incidence, 288
signs/symptoms, 288
treatment, 289
Silastic silo, 506
Silk, 55
Silk glove sign, 29, 200
Silver nitrate, 227
Silver sulfadiazine (Silvadene), 227
Simple fracture, 643
Simple mastectomy, 367
Simple running (continuous) stitch, 58, *58*
Sinusitis
acute, 553–554
chronic, 554
Sipple's syndrome, 32, 388
Sister Mary Joseph's sign, 29, 40, 248
Sitz bath, 293
Skin grafts, 529–530
Skin lesions, 424–426
Skin sutures, removal, 62
Skull fracture, 673
Sliding esophageal hiatal hernia, 199–200, *200*
Sliding hernia, 191
Slipped capital femoral epiphysis, 664
Small bowel, 35, 188
anatomic differences between colon and, 275
anatomy, 255
injury treatment, 220
Meckel's diverticulum, 258–260
obstruction, 34, 35, 255–258, 525
tumors, 258
Smith's fracture, 649
Smoke inhalation
lab assessment, 225
signs, 224
Soave procedure, 502, *502*
Sodium nitroprusside (SNP), 438
Soft tissue sarcomas, 419–421
Solitary pulmonary nodules, 582–583
Somatostatin, 181
Somatostatinoma, 356
Space of Retzius, 96, 692
Spermatic cord, 195
contents, 193

Spigelian hernia, 191
Spina bifida occulta, 687
Spinal anesthesia, 171
  side effects, 173
Spinal cord trauma, 673–674
Spinal dysraphism, 687–688
Spinal epidural abscess, 684–685
Spinal immobilization, 204
Spinal shock, 151, 673
Spine
  cervical disc disease, 683–684
  lumbar disc herniation, 682–683
  spinal epidural abscess, 684–685
  syringomyelia, 685
Spiral fracture, 645, *645*
Spironolactone, 381
Spleen, 35, 341
  arterial supply, 411
  functions of, 411
  injuries, 411–412
  treatment of injuries, 412–415
  venous drainage, 411
Splenectomy, 249, 414
  immunizations to patients, 413
  indications, 412–413
  need for NG tube after, 413
Splenic artery aneurysm, 469
Splenic injuries, treatment, 523
Splenic vein thrombosis, 345, 414
Splenomegaly, 320, 414, 415
Splenorrhaphy, 412
Split thickness skin graft (STSG), 527
Split-thickness injury, 228
Spontaneous pneumothorax, 576
Spurling's sign, 684
Squamous cell carcinoma, 424–425
Stab wound to belly, treatment, 218
Staging laparotomy for Hodgkin's lymphoma, 422
Stamm gastrostomy, 78, *78*
Stanford classification, *617*, 617–618, *618*
Staphylococcus aureus
  in burn wound infections, 226
  in infectious endocarditis, 609
  in suppurative hidradenitis, 158
  in urinary tract infection (UTI), 153
  in wound infections, 154
Staphylococcus epidermidis, 161
  in infectious endocarditis, 609
Staphylococcus in parotitis, 160
Staple remover device, 59, *59*
Starr, 40
Starzl, 40
Steatorrhea, 24
Stenosis, 24
  renal artery, 417, 467–468
Stenson's duct, 537
Step off, 569
Sterile field, 24
Sterility, 693
Sternberg-Reed cells, 421
Sternotomy, 73, *73*
Steroids, 120
Stick tie, 61, *61*
Stitch abscess, 157
Stomach
  anatomy, *244*, 244–245
  blood supply, 245, *245*
  gastric cancer, 247–249
  gastric physiology, 245–246
  gastroesophageal reflux disease, 246–247
Strabismus, 711, 715
Strangulated, definition, 190
Strangulation, risk of, in inguinal hernia, 194
Streptococcus in burn wound infections, 226
Streptococcus viridans in infectious endocarditis, 609
Stress fracture, 646
Stress gastritis, 241
Stress incontinence, 707, 708
Stridor, 477–478
String sign, 168
Stroke, 464
Stroke volume, 434
Struvite stones, 706
Subarachnoid hemorrhage, 680–681, 689
  complications, 680–681
  signs/symptoms, 680
Subclavian steal syndrome, 466–467
Subcutaneous air, significance, 211
Subcutaneous emphysema, treatment, 219
Subcuticular stitch, 58, *59*
Subdural hematoma, 671–672
Subluxation, 642
Succinylcholine
  antidote to reverse, 174
  contraindications, 172
  duration of action, 174
Succus, 24
Sucralfate (Carafate), 122

Superficial spreading melanoma, 428
Superinfection, 153
Superior mesenteric artery, 462
Superior thyroidal artery, 465
Superior vena cava syndrome, 32, 589–591
Supination, 639
Suppurative cholangitis, 335
Suppurative hidradenitis, 158, 161
Supraglottic lesions, 563
Suprapubic catheter, 691
Suprapubic pain, causes, 187
Surgeon's knot, 61
Surgery (See *Cardiovascular surgery; Neurosurgery; Orthopaedic surgery; Pediatric surgery; Plastic surgery; Thoracic surgery.*)
Surgery clerkship, studying for, 3–4
Surgery signs, triads, 25–30
Surgical gloves, 41
Surgical hemostasis, *115*, 115–116, *116*
Surgical history, 39–41
Surgical infection, 153–162
Surgical instruments, 42–53
Surgical intensive care (SICU), 433–445
  basics, 433
  drugs, 436–438
  physiology, 438–440
Surgical knot, 61
  tying, 63–68, *64, 65, 66–68*
Surgical notes, 8
Surgical nutrition, 143–146
Surgical percentages, 36–38
Surgical prophylaxis, 165–166
Surgical radiology, 167–170
Surgical student
  appearance of, 4
  equipment carried by, 4
  perfect, 5–6
  preparation for rounds, 4
Surgical syndromes, 31–33
Surgical ulcers, 176
Surgicel®, 116
Sutures
  classification, 54
  definition, 54
  materials, 54–55
  size, 54
  techniques, 56–61
Swan-Ganz catheter, 440
Swan-Ganz waveforms, 441
Sweetheart retractor, 51, *51*
Swenson procedure, 501, *501*
Swimmer's ear, 539, 569
Sympathetic ophthalmia, 712
Synchronous IMV, 443
Syndactyly, 527
Syndrome of inappropriate antidiuretic hormone (SIADH), 31, 136
Synthetic mesocaval H-graft, 324
Synthetic portocaval H-graft, 324
Syringomyelia, 685
Systemic Inflammatory Response Syndrome (SIRS), 436
Systemic vascular resistance, 434, 600
Systemic vascular resistance index, 434–435

T cells, 624
Tachycardia, causes, 141
Tail of Spence, 360
Takayasu's arteritis, 470
Tamoxifen, 366
Taper-point needle, 56, *56*
Temperature, monitoring of, in burn patient, 226
Temporary monocular blindness, 463
Tenckhoff catheter, 93
Tenesmus, 24
Tennis elbow, 657
Tenosynovitis, 533
Tension pneumothorax, 206
Teratomas, 587–588
Tertiary hyperparathyroidism, 408
Tertiary intention, 56
Testicle
  attachment of, to scrotum, 195
  cryptorchid, 700
Testicular appendage, 196
Testicular cancer, 700–703
Testicular torsion, 491–492, 703–704
  position of patient with, 185
Tetanus
  causes, 161
  infection, 166
  prophylaxis, 228
  signs, 162
Tetralogy of Fallot (TOF), 611
Thermal burns, 222
Thermodilution, 442
Third-degree burns, 223
  treatment, 224
Third spacing, 99–101
Third-degree A-V block, 621

Third-nerve palsy, 689
33 to 1 rule, 406
35-40 rule of blood gas values, 445
Thoracentesis, 574
Thoracic aortic aneurysm, 614–615
Thoracic aortograms, 36, 214
Thoracic arch aortogram, 213
Thoracic great vessel injury, 211, 213
Thoracic outlet syndrome, 32, 572–573
Thoracic surgery
 chest wall tumors, 573–574
 diffuse esophageal spasm
  carcinoma, 596–598
  nutcracker esophagus, 593–594
  reflux, 594–595
  strictures, 595–596
 esophageal diseases
  achalasia, 592–593
  anatomic considerations, 591
  oropharyngeal dysphagia, 591–592
 lung abscess, 575
  hemoptysis, 575–576
  mesothelioma, 576–578
  spontaneous pneumothorax, 576
 lung diseases
  bronchogenic carcinoma, 578–582
  carcinoid tumors, 584–585
  pulmonary sequestration, 585
  solitary pulmonary nodules, 582–583
 malignant tumors, 574
 mediastinum diseases
  chronic mediastinitis, 589
  lymphoma, 588
  mediastinal anatomy, 585–586
  mediastinitis, 589
  primary mediastinal tumors, 586–588
  superior vena cava syndrome, 589–591
 outlet syndrome, 572–573
 pleura
  effusion, 574–575
Thoracostomy
 needle, 206
 tube, 86, 206, 207
Thoracotomy, 25, 74, *74*
"3-for-1" rule, 217
Thrombocytopenia, 112, 414
 causes, 112
Thrombophlebitis of superficial breast veins, 370
Thrombosis, splenic vein, 414
Thrombotic thrombocytopenic purpura treatment, 415
Throws, 62
Thumbprinting, 169
Thymoma, 587
Thymus gland, 404
Thyroglossal duct cyst, 476
Thyroid carcinoma, 395
Thyroid glands
 anatomy, 390–393
  arterial blood supply, 391
  venous drainage, 391
 physiology, 393
  anaplastic carcinoma, 399–400
  benign disease, 400–401
  carcinoma, 395
  follicular adenocarcinoma, 396–397
  Hürthle cell cancer, 398–399
  malignant nodules, 394–395
  medullary carcinoma, 397–398
  nodule, 393–394
  papillary adenocarcinoma, 395–396
  thyroiditis, 402–403
  toxic multinodular goiter, 401
Thyroid hormones, 393
Thyroid storm, 135–136
Thyroid suppression of thyroid nodule, 394
Thyroid surgery, 39
Thyroidectomy, 392–393, 396, 397
 total, 399
Thyroiditis, 402–403
 acute, 402
 chronic, 402
 DeQuervain's, 402
 Hashimoto's, 402–403
 Riedel, 403
 subacute, 402
Thyroid-stimulating hormone, 393
Thyrotropin-releasing hormone, 393
Tibial fractures, 656
Tibial plateau fracture, 649
Tidal volume, 442
Tie-over bolus dressing, 530
Tietze's syndrome, 31, 598
Tinel's test, 573
Tissue ischemia, lab test for, 439
^{201}TI(technetium)-thallium subtraction scan, 405
TMN staging, 702
Tonsil clamp, 47, *47*
TORCHES, 523

Torus fracture, 646, 663
Total body surface area (TBSA), 223, 224
Total parenteral nutrition (TPN), 40
  complications, 145
  indications, 145
Total thyroidectomy, 399
Toxic megacolon, 305
  incidence, 304
Toxic multinodular goiter, 401
Toxic shock syndrome, 31
Tracheobronchomalacia, 478
Tracheoesophageal fistula
  with esophageal atresia, *481*, 481–484, *482*, *483*
  esophageal atresia without, 480–481
Tracheostomy, indications for, 570
Transcervical fracture, 649
Transect, 25
Transfusion hemolysis, 112
Transient ischemic attack (TIA), 463
Transjugular intrahepatic portal caval shunt (TIPS), 322, 323, 324
Translocation, 162
Transplant surgery
  ATG/antithymocyte globulin, 626
  basic immunology, 623–624
  cells
    B, 624
    T, 624
  complications
    infection, 637
    malignancy, 637–638
  corticosteroids, 625
    azathioprine, 625–626
    cyclosporine, 626
  heart, rejection, 635–636
  heart-lung, 41
  immunosuppression, 625
  kidney, 72, *72*
    history, 630
    immunosuppression, 631
    rejection, 632
    statistics, 630–631
  liver, 72, *72*, 632–634
    rejection, 633–634
  lung, 41, 636
  macrophage, 624
  matching of donor and recipient, 628
  OKT3, 627, *627*
  organ preservation, 629–630
  pancreatic, 41, 634–635
  rejection, 628–629
  terminology, 623
Transposition of great vessels, 613
Transrectal biopsy, 697
Transudate, properties of, 574
Transurethral incision of prostate (TUIP), 699
Transurethral resection of bladder (TURB), 696
Transurethral resection of prostate (TURP), 81, *81*, 200, 692, 699, 700
Transverse abdominal, 73, *73*
Transverse fracture, 644, *644*
Transverse rectus abdominis myocutaneous (TRAM) flap, 369, 530
Trauma, 204–221
  orthopaedic, 650–653
Trauma studies, 213–214
Trauma, Whipple, 219
Traumatic aortic injury, 167
Traumatic hyphema, 211
Traumatic myositis ossificans, 657
Traumatic subarachnoid hemorrhage, 672
Trendelenburg, 25
Trental (pentoxifylline), 450
Triangle of Calot, 326
Triangular ligaments of liver, 307
Triple therapy, 625
Tripod fracture, *568*, 568–569
Trisegmentectomy, 310
Trisomy 21, 525
Trophic tube feeds, 146
Trousseau's sign, 29, 107
Trousseau's syndrome, 33
True aneurysm, 447
True incontinence, 707, 708
Truncal vagotomy, 82, *82*, 234, 238
T-tube, *85*, 85–86
Tube check, 254
Tube thoracostomy, 206, 207
Tubular adenoma, 281, 282
Tubulovillous adenoma, 281, 282
Tullio's phenomenon, 549
Tumors, 517
  appendiceal, 266
  carcinoid, 266, 267–269
  cerebellar astrocytomas, 677–678
  desmoid, 283
  general, 675–676
  gliomas, 676–677
  hepatoblastoma, 522
  Klatskin, 339
  liver, 310–314

medulloblastoma, 678
meningiomas, 677
metastatic, 678–679
neuroblastoma, 519–521
orthopaedic, 658–660
rhabdomyosarcoma, 521–522
small bowel, 258
Wilms', 517–518
Tunica vaginalis, 490
Turcot's syndrome, 284
Turf toe, 657
Two-hand tie, *65*, 65–66, *66–68*
Tympanic membrane (TM) perforation, 541
Type and cross, 112
Type and screen, 112

Ulcer disease, peptic, 231
Ulcerative colitis, 301, 414
comparison of Crohn's disease and, 302–306
Ulcers
aphthous, 176
corneal, 715
Curling's, 176, 228, 239
Cushing's, 176, 239
decubitus, 176
Dieulafoy's, 176, 239
duodenal, 176, 231–233
gastric, 176, 229, 237–239
LE arterial insufficiency, 176
marginal, 176
Marjolin's, 176, 425
peptic, 176
perforated peptic, 239–240
peripheral vascular disease, 448
venous stasis, 176, 448
Umbilical arteries, 474, 475
Umbilical hernia, 192, 523
Umbilical veins, 474, 475
Unhappy triad, 655
Unicameral bone cyst, 659, 661
Unilateral hyperplasia, 382
Universal donor, 111
Unresectable brain metastasis, treatment, 432
Unstable fracture or dislocation, 640
Upper gastrointestinal (GI) bleeding, 229–243
causes, 229
definition, 229
diagnostic tests, 230
signs/symptoms, 229
treatment, 230–231
Urachus, 475
Uremic platelet dysfunction, 112
Ureteral stents, 690, 710
Urethral injury, 710
Urge incontinence, 707, 708
Urgency, 25, 691
Uric acid stones, 706, 709
Urinary tract infection (UTI), 153, 692, 708–709
bacterial cause, 35
Urine analysis, positive, 153
Urine output
causes of decreased, 142
for children, 473
Urology, 690–710
benign prostatic hyperplasia, 698–700
bladder cancer, 695–696
calculus disease, 705–707
epididymitis, 704
impotence, 704–705
incontinence, 707–708
prostate cancer, 696–698
renal cell carcinoma, 693–694
terminology, 690–693
testicular cancer, 700–703
testicular torsion, 703–704
urinary tract infection, 708–709
urologic differential diagnosis, 693
ward questions, 709–710
Uterine pain, 188

Vagotomy, 236
and antrectomy, 234
and pyloroplasty, 234, *234*
truncal, 238
Vagus nerve, 94
Valgus, 641
Vancomycin, 117, 119
Variceal bleeding, treatment, 322
Varices
esophageal, 320
retroperitoneal, 320
Varicocele, 691
Varus, 641
Vascular anastomosis, 40
Vascular neurosurgery
epilepsy surgery, 682
intracerebral hemorrhage, 681–682
occlusive cerebrovascular disease, 679
subarachnoid hemorrhage, 680–681

Vascular rings, 613–614
  symptoms, 478
Vascular surgery, 446–470
Vecuronium, 174
Vein of Mayo, 96
Venous stasis ulcer, 176, 448
Ventilation, 442
Ventilator settings, typical initial, 444
Ventral hernia, 191
Ventricular aneurysm, *620*
Ventricular assist device (VAD), 621
Ventricular septal defect (VSD), 609–610
Veress needle, 202
Vertical mattress stitch, 57, *57*
Vertical-banded gastroplasty, 251
Vertigo, 548–549
Vesicoenteric fistula, 273
Vesicoureteral reflux, 693
Vesicovaginal fistula, 273
Vestibular neuritis, 549–550
Vicryl® suture, 55
Villous adenoma, 282
Virchow's node, 29, 248
Virchow's triad, 29
Vitamin A, 84
  deficiency, 144
Vitamin B_{12}
  absorption, 144, 182
  deficiency, 131, 144
Vitamin C deficiency, 144
Vitamin K deficiency, 145
Vitamin K-dependent clotting factors, 146
Volarflexion, 640
Volatile anesthetics, cardiovascular effects, 175
Volkmann's contracture, 656–657
Volume status, monitoring of, in burn patient, 226
Voluntary guarding, 184
Volvulus
  cecal, 289–290
  sigmoid, 287, 288–289
Vomiting, bilious, 523
von Willebrand's disease, 114

Ward emergencies, causes, 141–142
Warfarin (Coumadin), 121–123
Warren selective shunt, 322
Warren shunt, 242, 323
Warts
  perianal, 295
WDHA (water, diarrhea, hypokalemia, achlorhydria) syndrome, 355
Weitlander retractor, 52, *52*
Wenckebach phenomenon, 621
Werner's syndrome, 33
Westermark's sign, 29
Wet gangrene, 452
Wet-to-dry dressing, 25, 84
Wharton's duct, 537
Whipple procedure, 83, 353–354, 386
Whipple's triad, 30, 356, 382–383
White lines of Toldt, 96, 275
Whole blood, 111
  storage, 111
Wilms' tumor, 517–518, 526, 709
Wirsung duct, 341
Wisconsin, University of, solution, 629
Wolff-Parkinson-White syndrome, 621
Wound closure, general information, 55–56
Wound contraction, 528–529
Wound healing, 527–528
  contraction, 528–529
  epithelialization, 528
  inhibition, 84
  types, 55
Wound infection, 154–162
Wrist dorsiflexion, 640

Xenograft, 623

Yankauer suction, 50, *50*
Yersinia in mesenteric adenitis, 266

Zenker's diverticulum, 592
Zinc deficiency, 145
Zollinger-Ellison syndrome, 33, 356, 384–387, 389
  complications, 385
  diagnosis, 385–386
  incidence, 384
  signs/symptoms, 384
  treatment, 386–387
Z-plasty, 531

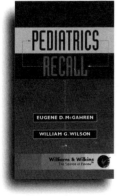